WOMEN'S HEALTH MADE EASY

WOMEN'S HEALTH MADE EASY

Carys Sonnenberg

MBChB, DCH, DRCOG, DFFP, MRCGP, British Menopause Society Registered Menopause Specialist, PgDip Obesity & weight management
GP in Hampshire; Founder of Rowena Health

Angela Wright

MBChB, MRCGP, DFSRH, Dip Pall Med, FECSM, DIPM, RegCOSRT, British Menopause Society Registered Menopause Specialist
GP with Special Interest in Menopause and Clinical Sexology in Hull and The Portland Hospital in London; Co-founder of Spiced Pear Health

Angela Sharma

BSc (Hons), MBCHB, DCH, DRCOG, DFFP, MRCGP, FECSM, British Menopause Society Registered Menopause Specialist
GP in London; Co-founder of Spiced Pear Health

Scion

First published 2026

A CIP catalogue record for this book is available from the British Library.

ISBN 9781914961649

Scion Publishing Limited
Long Hanborough, Oxfordshire, UK

www.scionpublishing.com

Important Note from the Publisher

The information contained within this book was obtained by Scion Publishing Ltd from sources believed by us to be reliable. However, while every effort has been made to ensure its accuracy, no responsibility for loss or injury whatsoever occasioned to any person acting or refraining from action as a result of information contained herein can be accepted by the authors or publishers.

Readers are reminded that medicine is a constantly evolving science and while the authors and publishers have ensured that all dosages, applications and practices are based on current indications, there may be specific practices which differ between communities. You should always follow the guidelines laid down by the manufacturers of specific products and the relevant authorities in the country in which you are practising.

Although every effort has been made to ensure that all owners of copyright material have been acknowledged in this publication, we would be pleased to acknowledge in subsequent reprints or editions any omissions brought to our attention.

Registered names, trademarks, etc. used in this book, even when not marked as such, are not to be considered unprotected by law.

Cover design by Andy Magee
Typeset by Dataworks in India
Printed in the UK

Last digit is the print number: 10 9 8 7 6 5 4 3 2

Contents

Detailed contents

Preface

Women's health is often described as "complex". It is probably more accurate to say it has been made so by decades of under-research, under-teaching, and historical bias within medicine.

For too long, women's symptoms have been minimised, normalised, or attributed to psychology. At the same time, clinicians have been expected to manage high-impact, intimate areas of care with limited formal training, patchy evidence and inconsistent guidance. This has created significant and systemic challenges in women's health: shown through delayed diagnoses, fragmented care and a growing sense of loss of trust in healthcare.

Women's Health Made Easy was written in response to these gaps. Invited to develop this text through the Primary Care Women's Health Society, we set out to create a practical, clinically useful resource that was grounded in real consultations. Drawing on our combined experience as GPs, menopause specialists and sexologists, we focus on areas historically underrepresented in training, including sexual health, vulval conditions, menstrual disorders, fertility and menopause, alongside communication, safeguarding, perinatal mental health and the interaction between hormonal and psychological wellbeing.

Improving women's healthcare requires better education, better support, and access to safe, pragmatic advice based on good evidence. This book is one contribution towards that change.

Note: throughout the text we use the words 'woman' and 'women', but the information and advice in these pages is intended to include all those assigned female at birth.

Carys Sonnenberg
Angela Wright
Angela Sharma

Acknowledgements

We are grateful for the mutual support we have given one another through the long hours of writing and proofreading, and want to extend our thanks to the Primary Care Women's Health Society for giving us the opportunity to write this book. We are also grateful to Scion Publishing Limited for their advice and guidance along the way. A huge thank you goes to our families for their patience, care and constant support throughout this process. We would also like to thank all the women we have met and cared for throughout our careers. You have shown us the value of listening and the impact that can be made when we get it right; and you have inspired us to do what we can to help to change and improve women's healthcare in the future.

Thanks are also due to Dr Anne Connelly, Professor Vikram Talaulikar, Dr Toni Hazell, Dr Sarah Gray, Dr Rachael Chrystal, Dr Alison Macbeth, Dr Zoe Hodson, Dr Sarah Ball, Dr Claire Phipps, Dr Alice Duffy, Dr Jill Crowfoot, Dr Clare Grove, Dr Kayo Oshiga, Dr Louise Payne, Dr Georgia Weeks, Melinda McDougall, Fiona Clark and Diane Danzebrink for their teaching, proofreading and support.

About the authors

Carys Sonnenberg

Dr Carys Sonnenberg is an experienced NHS GP and a British Menopause Society (BMS) Registered Menopause Specialist. She has practised as a GP since 2002 and leads women's health services within her NHS practice, including contraception, LARC provision and complex menopause management.

She is a member of the Royal College of General Practitioners (MRCGP) and holds the Diploma in Child Health (DCH), the Diploma of the Royal College of Obstetricians & Gynaecologists (DRCOG) and the Diploma of the Faculty of Sexual & Reproductive Health (DFFP). She was awarded the BMS Advanced Certificate in the Principles and Practice of Menopause Care after completing training at University College London Hospital, and is trained in cognitive behavioural therapy (CBT) for menopause.

She is a member of the wider board of the Primary Care Women's Health Society (PCWHS), contributing to speaking at national educational events, teaching sessions and written articles. Alongside her broader educational work, she regularly delivers talks to local women and provides menopause and women's health training for corporate organisations.

Her clinical interests extend to metabolic health and to extend her knowledge, she undertook nutrigenomics training and completed the Nutrigenomics Practitioner Programme with LifeCodeGx. In 2026 she completed a Postgraduate Diploma in Obesity and Weight Management (PgDip) at the University of South Wales.

She founded and is a director of Rowena Health, a private online menopause clinic, extending her care to women across the UK. She provides personalised, holistic care, equipping women with clear, evidence-based knowledge about their hormonal health and supporting long-term wellbeing.

Angela Sharma

Dr Angela Sharma is a GP Partner, a British Menopause Society (BMS) registered menopause specialist and a clinical sexologist, as well as the co-founder of Spiced Pear Health, an online menopause and sexology clinic.

She has been a GP in Notting Hill, London, for 23 years. She has set up and leads a menopause service in her own NHS practice, and is also the women's health lead as well as leading in antenatal and postnatal care. She is passionate about changing the lives and health of women for the better.

She has a BSc in Immunology & Oncology, and is a member of the Royal College of General Practitioners (MRCGP) and has Diplomas in Child Health (DCH), the Royal College of Obstetricians & Gynaecologists (DRCOG) and the Faculty of Sexual & Reproductive Health (DFFP). She undertook her training in Advanced Menopause Care at King's College Hospital in London, where she acquired experience in managing complex menopause cases, and is also trained in cognitive behavioural therapy for menopause. She has trained further in clinical sexology by attending the European Society of Sexual Medicine (ESSM) School of Sexual Medicine, and has become a Fellow of the European Committee of Sexual Medicine (FECSM). She is qualified in both the psychosexual therapeutic techniques and the medical aspects of sexual dysfunction. She also volunteers at Maggie's in west London, running menopause and intimacy after cancer workshops.

She is currently a member of the Medical Advisory Council for the BMS, and is also a trustee and medical advisory board member for the Menstrual Health Project, a charity that educates and empowers women on all menstrual health conditions. She speaks regularly to women, corporates and her peers about women's health issues, menopause and sexology.

Angela Wright

Dr Angela Wright is a GP, Menopause Specialist and Clinical Sexologist. She is also qualified in Palliative Medicine and worked in hospice medicine for over a decade. She is particularly interested in improving sexual function and menopausal symptoms in women who have undergone cancer treatment.

Angela completed her Advanced Menopause Care training in Hull. She now has a permanent NHS clinic there, seeing patients with complex menopause issues, female sexual dysfunction and premenstrual disorders. She also consults as a Clinical Sexologist for the Portland Hospital in London and the Wilmslow Hospital in Cheshire, and online at Spiced Pear Health. Her 2-year Clinical Sexology training was with the Contemporary Institute of Clinical Sexology (CICS), and she went on to attend the European Society of Sexual Medicine's Advanced School of Sexual Medicine. She then passed the examination to become a Fellow of the European Committee of Sexual Medicine (FECSM). She is a Diplomate of the Institute of Psychosexual Medicine. She is also trained in CBT for menopause, and in EMDR and Somatic Trauma Therapy.

Angela is passionate about women's health and sexology and is frequently asked to teach or talk about this subject. She is a registered trainer for the BMS & CoSRH, involved in training future menopause specialists and is also part of the Faculty for the sexology course she trained on, teaching the biomedical part of the course. She is an active committee member of the British Society of Sexual Medicine, the education committee of the Primary Care Women's Health Society, and a trustee for The Wellness Gateway, a charity providing trauma therapy to those who need it.

Abbreviations

ACE	angiotensin-converting enzyme
ADHD	attention deficit hyperactivity disorder
AIDS	acquired immune deficiency syndrome
AN	anorexia nervosa
ARB	angiotensin II receptor blocker
ART	antiretroviral therapy
ASD	autism spectrum disorder
BASHH	British Association for Sexual Health and HIV
BDD	body dysmorphic disorder
BMD	bone mineral density
BMI	body mass index
BMS	British Menopause Society
BP	blood pressure
BPS	bladder pain syndrome
BSO	bilateral salpingo-oophorectomy
BV	bacterial vaginosis
CAM	complementary and alternative medicine
CAP	complementary and alternative practices
CBT	cognitive behavioural therapy
CBTi	CBT for insomnia
ccHRT	continuous combined HRT
CEE	conjugated equine oestrogen
CHC	combined hormonal contraception
CHD	coronary heart disease
CIN	cervical intraepithelial neoplasia
COC	combined oral contraceptive
COCP	combined oral contraceptive pill
CoSRH	College of Sexual & Reproductive Healthcare
COSRT	College of Sexual and Relationship Therapists
CTP	contraceptive transdermal patch
Cu-IUD	copper IUD
CUV	cliterourethrovaginal
CVD	cardiovascular disease
CVR	contraceptive vaginal ring
DCIS	ductal carcinoma *in situ*
DES	diethylstilboestrol
DEXA	dual-energy X-ray absorptiometry
DHEA	dehydroepiandrosterone
DHT	dihydrotestosterone
DMPA	depot medroxyprogesterone acetate
DRSP	drospirenone
DSG	desogestrel
DSM	*Diagnostic and Statistical Manual of Mental Disorders*
DYG	dydrogesterone
EC	emergency contraception
ECG	electrocardiogram
ED	everyday
EE	ethinylestradiol
EPAU	Early Pregnancy Assessment Unit
EPO	evening primrose oil
FAI	free androgen index
FGM	female genital mutilation
FRAX	fracture risk assessment tool
FSH	follicle-stimulating hormone
GAG	glycosaminoglycan
GBMSM	gay and bisexual and men who have sex with men
GMC	General Medical Council
GnRH	gonadotrophin-releasing hormone
GPD	genito-pelvic dysthesia
GSM	genitourinary syndrome of the menopause
GUM	genitourinary medicine
HDL	high-density lipoprotein
HER2	human epidermal growth receptor 2
HFI	hormone-free interval
HIV	human immunodeficiency virus
HMB	heavy menstrual bleeding
HPO	hypothalamic–pituitary–ovarian
HPV	human papillomavirus
HRT	hormone replacement therapy
HSV	herpes simplex virus
HVS	high vaginal swab
IC	interstitial cystitis
ICD	*International Classification of Diseases*
IDVA	independent domestic violence advisor
IGF	insulin-like growth factor
IMB	intermenstrual bleeding
IMP	implant
IMS	International Menopause Society
IPM	Institute of Psychosexual Medicine
ISPMD	International Society for Premenstrual Disorders

IUD	intrauterine device
IV	intravenous
IVF	*in vitro* fertilisation
LARC	long-acting reversible contraceptive
LCIS	lobular carcinoma *in situ*
LFT	liver function test
LH	luteinising hormone
LMP	last menstrual period
LNG	levonorgestrel
LNG-EC	levonorgestrel emergency contraception
LNG-IUD	levonorgestrel intrauterine device
MARAC	multi-agency risk assessment conference
MC&S	microscopy, culture and sensitivities
Mgen	*Mycoplasma genitalium*
MHRA	Medicines and Healthcare products Regulatory Agency
MHT	menopause hormone therapy
MI	myocardial infarction
MP	micronised progesterone
MPA	medroxyprogesterone acetate
MRI	magnetic resonance imaging
MS	multiple sclerosis
MSM	men who have sex with men
MSU	mid-stream urine
NAPS	National Association for Premenstrual Syndromes
NET	norethisterone NFS non-fatal strangulation
NFS	non-fatal strangulation
NOGG	National Osteoporosis Guidelines Group
NSAID	non-steroidal anti-inflammatory drug
OAB	overactive bladder
OCD	obsessive–compulsive disorder
OGTT	oral glucose tolerance test
OSA	obstructive sleep apnoea
OSFED	other specified feeding or eating disorder
OTC	over the counter
PCB	postcoital bleeding
PCOS	polycystic ovary syndrome
PCR	polymerase chain reaction
PCWHS	Primary Care Women's Health Society
PEP	post-exposure prophylaxis
PFMT	pelvic floor muscle training
PGAD	persistent genital arousal disorder
PID	pelvic inflammatory disease
PMB	postmenopausal bleeding
PMD	premenstrual disorder
PMDD	premenstrual dysphoric disorder
PMS	premenstrual syndrome
PN	pudendal neuralgia
PND	postnatal depression
POI	premature ovarian insufficiency
POP	progestogen-only pill
POP-Q	pelvic organ prolapse quantification
POTS	postural orthostatic tachycardia syndrome
PrEP	pre-exposure prophylaxis
RCOG	Royal College of Obstetricians & Gynaecologists
RCT	randomised controlled trial
RED-S	relative energy deficiency in sport
SARC	Sexual Assault Referral Centre
SCC	squamous cell carcinoma
SHBG	sex hormone-binding globulin
sHRT	sequential combined HRT
SNRI	serotonin–noradrenaline reuptake inhibitor
SPC	Summary of Product Characteristics
SSRI	selective serotonin reuptake inhibitor
STI	sexually transmitted infection
T2DM	type 2 diabetes mellitus
TCA	tricyclic antidepressant
TENS	transcutaneous nerve stimulation
TOP	termination of pregnancy
TV	trichomonas vaginalis
U&Es	urea and electrolytes
UCP	urgent care pathway
UFED	unspecified feeding or eating disorder
UK NSC	UK National Screening Committee
UKMEC	UK Medical Eligibility Criteria for Contraceptive Use
UPA	ulipristal acetate
USC	urgent suspected cancer
UTI	urinary tract infection
UUI	urge urinary incontinence
VIN	vulval intraepithelial neoplasia
VMS	vasomotor symptom
VTE	venous thromboembolism
WHI	Women's Health Initiative
WHO	World Health Organization

Chapter 1
Female anatomy and physiology

1.1 Female anatomy

This chapter provides details of female anatomy, female hormones, the physiology of the ovary, the menstrual cycle, puberty and menopause, to support you to manage gynaecological issues which may be caused by structural or hormonal problems.

1.1.1 The pelvis

- The pelvis is the lower portion of the trunk, located between the abdomen and the thighs, formed by the bony pelvis and enclosing the pelvic cavity.
- The pelvic cavity is the space enclosed by the bony pelvis, below the abdominal cavity and above the pelvic floor.
  - This contains the urinary bladder, pelvic colon, the rectum, internal reproductive organs, and other internal structures including muscles, arteries, veins and nerves.
- The pelvic floor is the inferior muscular layer, which separates the pelvic cavity superiorly from the perineum inferiorly.
  - The pelvic floor supports the internal organs including the bladder, uterus and rectum.
  - Pelvic floor dysfunction occurs when the muscles and the supporting tissues of the muscle floor do not function properly, leading to a variety of symptoms.
    - The muscles can be either too tight (hypertonic) or too weak (hypotonic) or have difficulty coordinating properly.
    - Symptoms include pelvic pain, sexual problems (painful sex, decreased sensation and weaker orgasms), problems opening bowels (constipation, straining, incomplete evacuation), urinary incontinence (especially when laughing, coughing or sneezing); faecal incontinence (leaking stool or difficulty controlling bowel movements) and prolapse of the internal organs.
    - This condition can significantly affect quality of life. It is important to correctly diagnose and treat it. Treatment can vary, and may include pelvic floor training, medication, and in some cases surgery. Refer to *Chapter 9* for details about management.
- The perineum is the area of skin between the vagina and the anus.

1.1.2 The vulva

- The vulva (see *Fig. 1.1*) describes all the structures that make the external part of the female genitalia. Vulvas are unique and come in a variety of shapes and sizes.
- An examination of the vulva should include visualising the anus and the natal cleft.
- The vulva has a role in reproduction and urination.

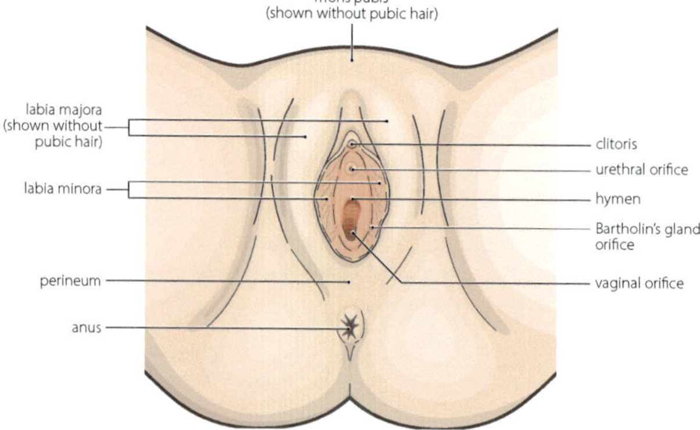

Figure 1.1: External female anatomy. Reproduced from *Anatomy and Physiology: an introduction for nursing and healthcare* (2020) with permission from Lantern Publishing Ltd.

Structures in the vulva

Mons pubis

- The mons pubis is a pad of fat anterior to the pubic symphysis which is covered by hair-bearing skin.
- Pubic hair has many benefits; it protects the vulva and vagina from dirt, infections and skin irritation.
- The mons pubis consists largely of fatty tissue which protects the pubic bone and provides cushioning during sexual intercourse. The sebaceous glands located within it secrete pheromones to induce sexual attraction.

Labia majora

- The outer skin folds, which after puberty are covered with hair.
- They can vary in size and be asymmetrical.
- They start at the mons pubis and extend down, lying outside the inner skin folds, joining together at the perineum.
- They consist mainly of fatty tissue but also contain a thin muscular layer, erectile tissue, sweat glands, sebaceous glands, nerve endings, hair follicles and blood vessels. They swell and become more sensitive during arousal.

Labia minora

- Two hairless folds of skin that sit between the labia majora. They extend down from the frenulum of the clitoral glans towards the back of the vulva and join there in a fold of skin called the fourchette.
- They protect the vestibule and vagina from irritation, friction and dirt.
- They contain nerve endings, blood vessels and erectile tissue, and when aroused, the increase in blood flow makes them become more sensitive and swollen, and they act as a cushion to make sex more comfortable.
- They can be asymmetrical and vary in size, shape, colour and texture.
- They are often longer and more prominent than the labia majora. They may be barely visible, or they can extend up to several centimetres long, protruding outside the labia majora. Their colour can vary between pink, red, brown and black.
- Some women may ask about labioplasty surgery (a surgical procedure which alters the appearance of the labia and/or clitoral hood). An increasing number of younger women are requesting this procedure, thinking that they do not have a 'normal' vulva. It is important to reassure them that every vulva is different. More information can be found at www.thevulvagallery.com.

Urethral opening

- An extension of the tube from the bladder, for excretion of urine.
- It opens within the vulval vestibule below the clitoral hood and above the vaginal entrance.

Vestibule

- The area enclosed by the labia minora containing the openings of the vagina (external vaginal orifice, vaginal introitus) and the urethra.

Bartholin's glands

- Also known as vulvovaginal glands, these are two pea-sized glands located either side of the vaginal opening at 5 and 7 o'clock.
- They play a role in lubricating the area around the vaginal opening.

Paraurethral glands

- Also known as Skene's glands, these are located inside around the urethra and play a role in both sexual and urinary health, producing fluid during orgasm and lubricating the urethral opening.

Clitoris

- The female sex organ, a sensory organ (see *Fig. 1.2*).
- It consists of a glans, a body, two crura and bulbs. Only the glands and part of the body can be seen externally; the rest is buried under the vulva and sits around the urethra and the vagina. The glans varies in size and may be only barely visible, or up to several centimetres long, or only become visible during arousal.
- The clitoral hood covers the glans and varies in size; it protects from dryness and chafing.
- The glans clitoris is innervated by about 8000 nerves and has a rich blood supply. It becomes erect and engorged during sexual stimulation and intercourse.
- It forms part of the cliterourethrovaginal (CUV) complex, informally known as the 'G-spot', an area of increased sensitivity and sexual significance about 2cm internally on the anterior wall of the vagina.
- The overall size of the clitoris is 9–11cm.

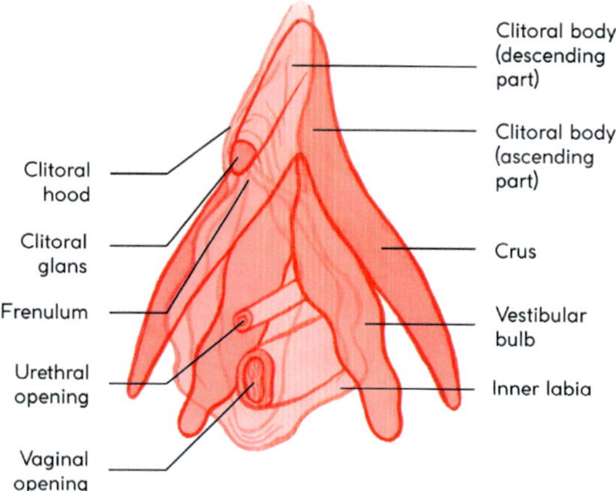

Figure 1.2: The clitoris in an erect state. Reproduced from www.thevulvagallery.com/anatomy.

Hymen

- The hymen is a small, flexible tissue that forms a ridge around the opening to the vagina. It may not be visible on examination.

1.1.3 The vagina

- The vagina is an elastic muscular tube which extends from the external vulval vestibule to the cervix. At the proximal end the vagina surrounds the cervix, creating an anterior and posterior fornix.
- It has several roles:
  - Sexual intercourse, receiving the penis during penis and vagina sex, and acting as a reservoir for semen.
  - Childbirth, when it expands to provide a channel for delivery of a newborn from the uterus.
  - Menstruation, as an outflow tract for menstrual blood.

Vaginal discharge

- Vaginal discharge is normal if it is odourless, clear or white, thick and sticky, slippery and wet.
- The amount of discharge can vary and can increase during pregnancy, with some forms of contraception or in women who are sexually active. For more information, refer to *Section 4.1*.
- There is no need to clean inside the vagina, and women should be advised not to douche.

Changes in the vagina and vulva

- In premenopausal women vaginal fluid is acidic, with a pH ranging from 3.8 to 4.5.
  - In a healthy vagina, acidity is maintained by the regular shedding of superficial epithelial cells, which release glycogen. Sugars derived from this glycogen are broken down by *Lactobacillus* spp., the normal vaginal bacteria, to produce lactic acid. This acidic environment helps prevent the overgrowth of organisms such as *E. coli* and other harmful bacteria.
- In postmenopausal women, vaginal pH is less acidic (>5).
  - Oestrogen deficiency causes thinning of the vaginal mucosa and a reduction in epithelial cells, leading to a reduction in glycogen.
  - *Lactobacillus* is no longer the predominant flora, and *E. coli* and other Gram-negative bacteria dominate.
  - Changes can be seen on inspection of the vulva, including decreased vaginal moisture, a loss of elasticity, shrinkage of the labia, loss of vaginal folds and thinning of the tissues of the vagina and vulva.
  - Women may experience vaginal dryness, soreness and discomfort during sex. Bladder symptoms can include urinary frequency and urgency. The change in vulval tissues can result in exposure of the urethra to infection. This condition is called genitourinary syndrome of the menopause. Treatment includes vulval skin care, use of good-quality non-hormonal moisturisers and lubricants during sex, and oestrogen (systemic and/or low-dose localised oestrogen) which can relieve these symptoms. Refer to *Section 6.7.*

1.1.4 The cervix

- The cervix (see *Fig. 1.3*) has two main functions:
  - It allows sperm to reach the body of the uterus, and it helps to maintain sterility of the upper female reproductive tract.
- The cervix is the lower part of the uterus; it connects the vagina with the main body of the uterus. It is approximately 4cm long and 3cm in diameter.
- It has two parts:
  - The ectocervix (the outer surface of the cervix that opens into the vagina)
  - The endocervix (the inside canal of the cervix).
- The endocervical canal is lined with a mucus-secreting columnar epithelium (often referred to as glandular epithelium). The internal os separates the top of the endocervical canal with the uterine cavity.

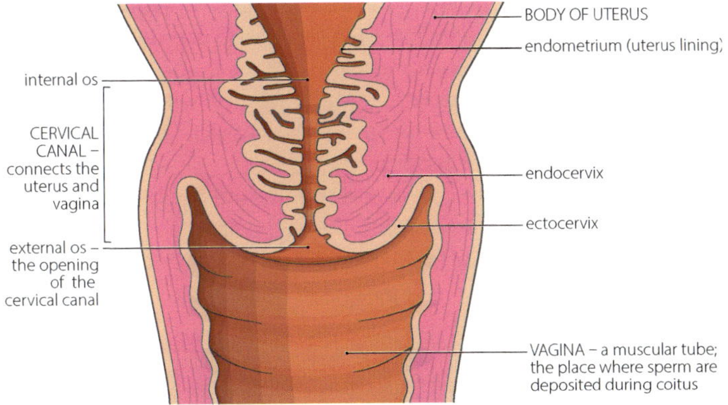

Figure 1.3: The cervix. Reproduced from *Anatomy and Physiology: an introduction for nursing and healthcare* (2020) with permission from Lantern Publishing Ltd.

- The ectocervix is lined with stratified squamous epithelium. The opening in the ectocervix is called the external os. This marks the transition from the ectocervix to the endocervical canal.
- The squamous epithelium of the ectocervix meets the glandular epithelium of the endocervix at the squamocolumnar junction (SCJ), also known as the transformation zone.

Cervical ectropion

- A cervical ectropion occurs when the glandular cells lining the endocervix are present on the outside surface of the cervix (the transformation zone). Glandular cells are red, so the area may look red.
- This condition is related to oestrogen, and is therefore common in young women, pregnant women and those taking the combined oral contraceptive pill (COCP).
- Usually there are no symptoms; however, some women notice an increase in vaginal discharge or experience intermenstrual vaginal bleeding or postcoital bleeding.
- A cervical ectropion may resolve on its own; with a change in contraception, for example. If the appearances are concerning, or it is causing symptoms and is not resolving, the woman can be referred to a colposcopy clinic for treatment, which may include diathermy or cryocautery.

1.1.5 The uterus

The uterus is a thick-walled muscular organ capable of expansion to accommodate a growing fetus. It has three parts:

- fundus – top of the uterus, above the entry point of the fallopian tubes
- body – usual site for implantation of a blastocyst
- cervix – lower part of uterus linking it with the vagina; the cervix is structurally and functionally different to the rest of the uterus.

Anatomical position

- The uterus is found in the centre of the female pelvic cavity, posterior to the bladder and anterior to the rectum.
- The posterior cul-de-sac, also known as the pouch of Douglas, or the rectouterine pouch, is the area between the uterus and the rectum.
    - Small amounts of fluid can accumulate here during ovulation and during a period. Other reasons for fluid accumulation here include pelvic abscesses, endometriosis, or metastases from gastrointestinal malignancies.
- The uterine position can vary:
    - An anteverted uterus tips forward towards the bladder, found in 70–80% of women.
    - A retroverted uterus, known as a tilted uterus, is a variation in which the uterus tilts backwards towards the spine. This position is less common and occurs in 20–30% of women. It is still considered a normal anatomical variation. Many women with a retroverted uterus have no symptoms but some may experience symptoms such as low back pain, dyspareunia, menstrual pain and difficulty inserting tampons.
    - The term 'flexion' refers to the angle between the cervix and the uterine body. Anteflexed means the uterus is bent forwards; retroflexed means it is bent backwards.
- Ligaments provide support, holding the uterus in place.

Myometrium and endometrium

The uterus consists of three layers:

- perimetrium – the outermost layer, lubricates the uterus to reduce friction
- myometrium – the muscular middle layer
- endometrium – the inner layer, or uterine lining. This has three layers: the stratum compactum, stratum spongiosum and stratum basalis.

1.1.6 The fallopian tube

- The fallopian tubes are muscular 'J-shaped' tubes, found in the female reproductive tract.
- They lie in the upper border of the broad ligament, extending laterally from the uterus, opening into the abdominal cavity, near the ovaries.
- The infundibulum is the funnel-shaped distal end of the fallopian tube. The fimbriae are finger-like projections at its margin that help capture the ovulated oocyte from the ovarian surface.

1.1.7 The ovary

- The ovaries are the female gonads. They are endocrine and reproductive organs, located in the ovarian fossae close to the fallopian tubes (see *Fig. 1.4*).

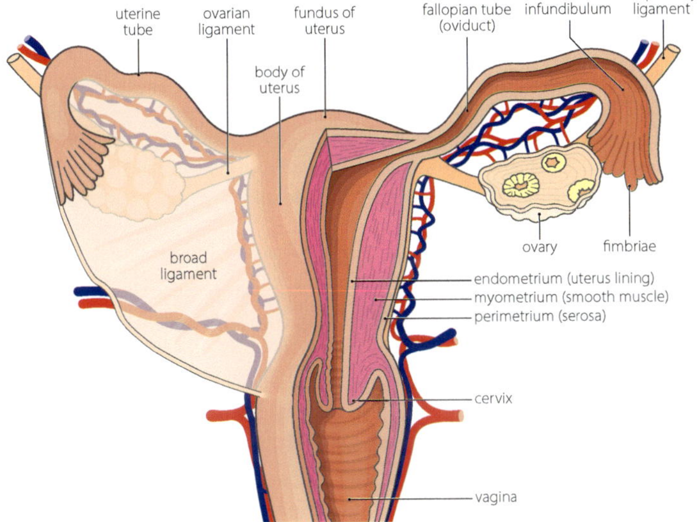

Figure 1.4: The female reproductive tract and the ovary. Reproduced from *Anatomy and Physiology: an introduction for nursing and healthcare* (2020) with permission from Lantern Publishing Ltd.

Ovarian structure

- An outer layer made of simple cuboidal epithelium – the germinal epithelium.
- A thick connective tissue capsule/collagen – the tunica albuginea.
- A cortex containing the ovarian follicles of different sizes and maturity.
- A central medulla, containing blood and lymphatic vessels; this region is also called the hilus.

Two functions of the ovary

Production of hormones

- The ovaries play a fundamental role in reproduction and in the production of hormones.
- At puberty the ovaries begin to produce hormones including oestrogen, testosterone and progesterone, in response to the pulsatile release of gonadotrophin-releasing hormone (GnRH) produced from the hypothalamus. GnRH stimulates the pituitary gland to release the gonadotrophins follicle-stimulating hormone (FSH) and luteinising hormone (LH).
- This activity creates the hypothalamic–pituitary–ovarian (HPO) axis.
    - The hypothalamus produces GnRH which acts on the cells in the anterior pituitary.
    - The anterior pituitary produces FSH and LH.

- FSH and LH act upon the ovary resulting in ovarian follicle maturation, ovulation and production of hormones including oestrogen, progesterone and testosterone.
- Negative feedback regulates the production and release of each hormone.

Production of oocytes

- An oocyte is the germ cell within the ovary.
- Oocytes begin to develop *in utero* and pause at the primordial follicle stage, until puberty occurs.
  - Primordial follicles consist of an oocyte surrounded by a single layer of granulosa cells.
  - These mature and grow in a process called folliculogenesis.
  - After puberty some of these follicles are recruited each month to mature further and become larger, hormone-producing follicles. One of these ultimately develops into a dominant Graafian follicle, in preparation for ovulation.

1.2 Hormones

- The sex steroid hormones oestrogen, progesterone and testosterone are produced in the ovary.
- The adrenal cortex produces steroid hormones.
  - It has three distinct functional and histological zones: the zona glomerulosa (outer layer), the zona fasciculata (middle layer) and the zona reticularis (inner layer). Each layer produces steroid hormones from the precursor cholesterol. The specific steroid hormone produced differs in each layer because of zonal-specific enzymes.
  - Glucocorticoids (such as cortisol) are produced in the zona fasciculata.
  - Mineralocorticoids (such as aldosterone) are produced in the zona glomerulosa.
  - Adrenal androgens: dehydroepiandrosterone sulphate (DHEAS), dehydroepiandrosterone (DHEA) and androstenedione are produced in the zona reticularis.
    - The androgen precursors, primarily DHEA, are released from the adrenal gland into the bloodstream and transported to the ovaries and peripheral tissues (such as skin, adipose tissue, brain and breast) where they are converted into active sex steroids, testosterone and oestrogen, by peripheral aromatisation.
- *Figure 1.5* shows some of the steps in the overall pathway of steroid hormone synthesis which can take place in the adrenal cortex, the ovary and some peripheral tissues, depending on the specific enzymes present. For example, the presence of the aromatase enzyme CYP19A1 in a cell means that conversion of androgens (such as testosterone and androstenedione) into oestrogens (such as estradiol and estrone) can occur. Other examples of enzymes in the pathway are 3 beta-hydroxysteroid dehydrogenase (3β-HSD) and 17 beta-hydroxysteroid dehydrogenase (17β-HSD).

1.2.1 Oestrogen

- Oestrogen is a hormone associated with the female reproductive organs. It is responsible for developing female sexual characteristics during puberty and has a role in regulating the menstrual cycle.
- Oestrogen levels fluctuate throughout life, naturally increasing during puberty and pregnancy, reducing after menopause and fluctuating throughout a natural menstrual cycle.
- Oestrogen moves through the blood and is active where oestrogen receptors are located.

Types of oestrogen

- To date, four oestrogens, estrone (E_1), estradiol (E_2), estriol (E_3) and estetrol (E_4), have been identified in humans. *Figure 1.5* summarises the steps in the synthesis of estrone, estradiol and estriol.
- Estrone (E_1):
  - Produced primarily in the ovaries, placenta, and in peripheral tissues (such as adipose tissue) through conversion of androstenedione.
  - The main type of oestrogen in postmenopausal women.

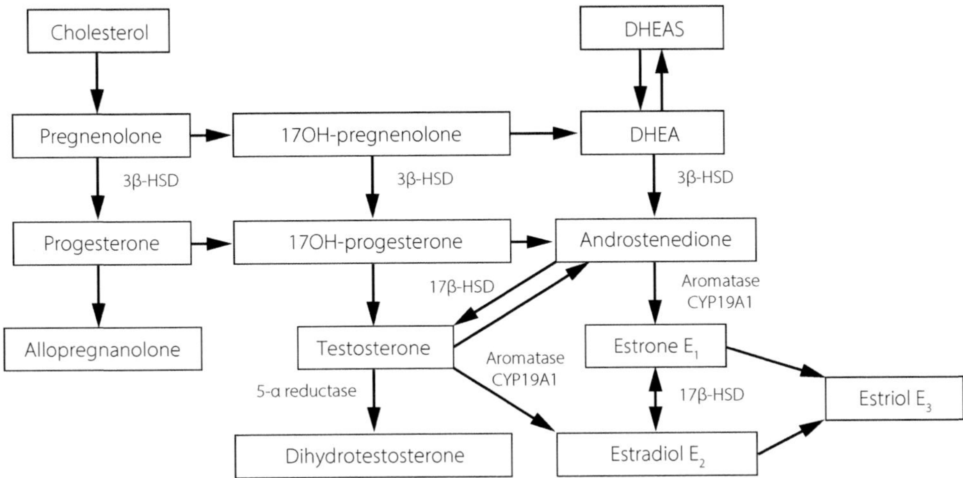

Figure 1.5: A summary of some steps in the pathway of steroid hormone synthesis.

- Estradiol (E_2):
  - E_2 is a common abbreviation for 17 beta-estradiol (17β-estradiol).
  - This is the predominant oestrogen produced by women of reproductive age.
  - It is produced primarily in the ovaries by aromatisation of testosterone, and acts as a circulating hormone, acting on distal tissues.
  - Small amounts of E_2 are produced in peripheral tissues, such as adipose tissue, where it is produced predominantly from adrenal precursors, and it acts locally.
  - It plays a major role in the development of secondary female sex characteristics, regulation of the menstrual cycle, and growth of the endometrial lining, from menarche to menopause.
  - Levels of E_2 fluctuate during the menstrual cycle.
- Estriol (E_3):
  - E_3 is the least potent oestrogen. It plays a greater role during pregnancy, when it is produced in large quantities by the placenta.
  - E_3 levels are negligible in non-pregnant women.
- Estetrol (E_4):
  - E_4 is a natural fetal oestrogen that is detectable only during pregnancy, and is exclusively produced by fetal liver.
- In premenopausal women, the ovaries produce two main oestrogens: estradiol (E_2) and estrone (E_1). Of these, E_2 is the predominant circulating oestrogen and is the most potent, due to its high affinity for oestrogen receptors. E_1 is less potent and circulates at lower levels, but serves as a reservoir that can be converted to E_2 within peripheral tissues such as the brain, bone, adipose tissue, muscle and heart. Interconversion between E_1 and E_2 occurs locally within tissues via 17β-hydroxysteroid dehydrogenase.
- After menopause, the ovaries no longer produce clinically significant amounts of oestrogen. It is instead derived from adrenal androgen precursors, such as androstenedione, which circulate in the bloodstream and are taken up by peripheral tissues. These androgens are converted by aromatase into estrone (E_1), the predominant postmenopausal oestrogen. E_1 is a weaker oestrogen but can be further converted within cells to estradiol (E_2) by 17β-hydroxysteroid dehydrogenase, providing local E_2 after menopause.
- After menopause, E_2 functions predominantly as an intracrine hormone, acting on receptors within the same cell and not being secreted, resulting in very low circulating serum concentrations.

- For people who have obesity, peripheral aromatisation of androgen precursors in the excess adipose tissue can result in higher levels of oestrogen. This may lead to abnormal uterine bleeding and increase the risk of endometrial hyperplasia and hormone-sensitive cancers (e.g. breast and endometrial).

Functions

- Oestrogen promotes proliferation of endometrial cells during the follicular phase of the menstrual cycle and plays a role in regulation of the HPO axis.
- Oestrogens also play an important role in breast development, the cardiovascular system, bone health, skin, hair, the brain, the musculoskeletal system, and the immune system.

Clinical uses of oestrogen include:

- Contraception: synthetic forms of oestrogen, such as ethinylestradiol, are used in combined hormonal contraceptives to prevent ovulation. Newer combined contraceptive pills now use estradiol or estetrol instead of ethinylestradiol.
- Hormone replacement therapy (HRT), also known as menopause hormone therapy (MHT): 17β-estradiol is the form of oestrogen most commonly used in HRT. It is referred to as a body-identical hormone because it is structurally identical to endogenous estradiol (E_2). It can be taken orally or transdermally.

1.2.2 Progesterone

- Progesterone is a hormone primarily produced in the ovaries, by the corpus luteum, after ovulation. It can also be produced by the placenta, adrenal glands and the brain.
- Progesterone has multiple physiological roles and serves as a precursor in the steroid hormone synthesis pathway.

Functions

- During the menstrual cycle, progesterone prepares the endometrium for implantation. It also plays a role in regulation of the HPO axis.
- Progesterone is essential for maintaining pregnancy. From around week 10, the placenta takes over from the corpus luteum as the primary source of progesterone, maintaining the endometrium, reducing myometrial excitability, and stimulating mammary development in preparation for lactation.
- Progesterone plays an important role in breast development, nervous system function and immune regulation.
- A metabolite of progesterone called allopregnanolone binds to gamma-aminobutyric acid (GABA) receptors and can exert calming, anxiolytic and neuroprotective effects. However, not all women experience this effect, and this is one proposed mechanism underlying premenstrual syndrome (PMS).
- Progesterone's effects on epilepsy are complex. While allopregnanolone may exert anticonvulsant properties by modulating GABAergic activity, fluctuations in progesterone levels throughout the menstrual cycle may also contribute to seizure exacerbation in women with catamenial epilepsy.

Clinical uses of progestogen

- The term *progestogen* refers to both the natural hormone progesterone and synthetic progestogens (also known as progestins), which are synthetic steroids designed to mimic the action of progesterone.
- Synthetic progestogens were originally developed because natural progesterone was poorly absorbed when taken orally, limiting its effectiveness for hormonal contraception and HRT. Progestins differ in chemical structure and are derived from either progesterone or testosterone.

- Scientists discovered that micronising progesterone and combining it with oil improved its oral bioavailability. Micronised progesterone is now available in formulations that can be taken orally or administered vaginally. Its clinical uses include fertility treatment, support of early pregnancy and HRT. It is not used as a contraceptive.
- Clinical uses of progestogens include the following:
  - All forms of hormonal contraception (synthetic progestogens).
  - HRT, alongside oestrogen, if endometrial protection is needed.
  - Management of endometriosis, amenorrhoea, abnormal uterine bleeding and endometrial hyperplasia.
  - To delay a period or induce a withdrawal bleed.
  - As a treatment in assisted reproduction, recurrent miscarriage and to maintain a pregnancy.
  - Prevention and treatment of some cancers.

1.2.3 Testosterone and androgens

- Although androgens are considered as the male sex hormones because of their masculinising effects, testosterone is an essential female hormone.
- Androgens in women:
  - Dehydroepiandrosterone sulphate (DHEAS)
    - Produced exclusively by the adrenal glands.
    - Serves as an important source of peripheral androgen production.
  - Dehydroepiandrosterone (DHEA)
    - Produced mainly by the adrenal glands and to a lesser extent by the ovaries.
    - Acts as a precursor to androstenedione, testosterone and oestrogens in peripheral tissues.
    - In both men and women, blood levels decline progressively from the age of 18 throughout the adult lifespan.
    - A 6.5mg vaginal pessary of DHEA is available for daily use for the treatment of genitourinary syndrome of the menopause (see *Section 6.7*). It is converted into oestrogen and testosterone locally in the vaginal tissues.
  - Androstenedione (A)
    - 50% produced by the adrenal gland and 50% by the ovary.
    - It is a precursor to both testosterone and oestrogen.
- The androgen precursors DHEAS, DHEA and androstenedione must be converted into testosterone to exert their androgenic effects.
  - Testosterone (T)
    - Testosterone is the most potent androgen and in women is secreted by the adrenal gland (25%) and the ovary (25%); the remaining 50% is produced from peripheral conversion of circulating androgen precursors.
    - Most circulating testosterone is bound to albumin or sex hormone-binding globulin (SHBG), which limits its biological activity. Testosterone exists in three forms: free (0.5–7.5%), loosely bound to albumin (30–45%), and tightly bound to SHBG (around 65%).
    - Women produce more testosterone than oestrogen, but women produce much less testosterone than men.
    - Circulating levels of pre-androgens and testosterone decline with age, beginning around 20 years old in the early reproductive years. By her mid-40s, a woman's levels of androstenedione, DHEA and testosterone are roughly half of those in her 20s.
    - Levels do not change significantly at the menopause transition.
    - There is a significant fall in SHBG during perimenopause; as a result, free androgen levels rise. This can contribute to scalp hair loss and unwanted facial hair growth.

        - There does not seem to be a correlation between female sexual desire and androgen levels, although for some women who experience hypoactive sexual desire disorder (HSDD), use of exogenous testosterone therapy can improve libido.
        - Having the ovaries removed surgically leads to a fall of approximately 50% in circulating testosterone levels.
    - Dihydrotestosterone (DHT)
        - Primarily a peripheral product of testosterone conversion, a small amount is made in the adrenal gland. It circulates in low concentrations in serum.
        - DHT is testosterone's more potent metabolite.
        - It cannot be aromatised.
- Androgen biosynthesis occurs in the adrenal gland and the ovary. DHEA and androstenedione can be converted in peripheral tissues such as the brain, bone and adipose tissue to either testosterone or estrone. Testosterone is converted in these cells to either estradiol by aromatisation or to DHT by hydroxylation.
- The ovaries continue being hormonally active, producing androgens for up to 10 years after the cessation of menstruation.

Measuring serum testosterone

- Measuring serum testosterone levels is indicated for a number of clinical reasons, including the investigation of menstrual irregularities, hirsutism, signs of virilisation in females, and in the management of HSDD.
- SHBG is often measured in conjunction with total testosterone.
- From these results the free androgen index (FAI) can then be calculated to give an estimate of bioavailable testosterone.
    - Free androgen index (FAI) = (total testosterone / SHBG) × 100%.
    - Samples should be collected early morning (8am to 11am).
    - Biotin is a common ingredient in multivitamins and hair loss supplements. Taking biotin can affect measurement of serum testosterone levels. If a patient is taking >5mg a day of biotin, collect the blood sample at least 8 hours after the last dose of biotin.
    - Changes in SHBG can cause shifts in free, bioavailable testosterone. Measuring SHBG can be helpful if androgen levels are normal but the patient is presenting with clinical symptoms which indicate an excess of androgens.
    - A high FAI suggests elevated levels of biologically active testosterone, potentially indicating conditions such as polycystic ovary syndrome (PCOS) or other hyperandrogenic conditions.
    - See *Section 7.18* for information about testosterone measurement and use for the treatment of hypoactive sexual desire disorder (HSDD).

Functions

- It has a critical role in folliculogenesis and fertility.
- Testosterone acts as a central neurosteroid. It affects a variety of functions in the body, including sexual desire. A sudden or gradual reduction may reduce sexual interest.
- The role of testosterone therapy to preserve musculoskeletal, cardiovascular and cognitive health is uncertain.

Clinical uses in of testosterone in women

- Testosterone replacement in menopause, off-label, can be prescribed to women who have HSDD which they find distressing, after a psychosocial approach has ruled out other causes. The BMS recommends that a trial of conventional HRT is given first.
- AndroFeme cream was approved by the UK regulator (MHRA) in 2025 specifically for postmenopausal women with HSDD. It is the first testosterone product licensed in the UK for use in women and is expected to become available in 2026. Being licensed does not

mean it will become available on the NHS, and currently this product is available as a private prescription.

1.2.4 Sex hormone-binding globulin

- Sex hormone-binding globulin (SHBG) is a protein made by the liver which binds tightly to testosterone, estradiol and DHT and transports them in the blood, regulating their bioavailability.
- SHBG levels are indicated in the investigation of hirsutism in women.
- Increased SHBG levels can be seen in anorexia, pregnancy, aging, growth hormone deficiency, androgen deficiency, hyperthyroidism, liver disease, hyperprolactinaemia, active porphyria and with oral oestrogens.
- Decreased SHBG levels can occur in obesity, hyperinsulinaemia, hypothyroidism and growth hormone excess, as well as with treatment using glucocorticoids, androgens or synthetic progestogens. It may also be familial. The drop of oestrogen levels after menopause leads to a decrease in SHBG, and an increase in unbound (active) testosterone and DHT.

1.2.5 Inhibin

- Inhibins A and B are protein hormones secreted by granulosa cells of the ovary. Inhibin B is produced by small antral follicles in the early follicular phase. Inhibin A is produced by the dominant follicle and later by the corpus luteum.
- Inhibins selectively suppress the secretion of FSH, and their levels fluctuate during the menstrual cycle.
- Oestrogens and inhibin B are both inhibitory factors for the secretion of FSH.
- At menopause as the ovarian follicular pool is exhausted, granulosa cells disappear, and inhibin A and B levels decline and FSH rises.

1.2.6 Growth factors

- Many growth factors form a network of interactions within the ovary and its compartments to regulate follicle development, steroidogenesis and ovulation.
- The best known are the insulin-like growth factors (IGFs).

1.2.7 Anti-Müllerian hormone

- Anti-Müllerian hormone (AMH) is a polypeptide secreted by granulosa cells of the pre-antral and small antral ovarian follicles. It is a marker of ovarian reserve.

1.3 Folliculogenesis

- The ovarian cortex contains follicles in various stages of development (primordial, primary, secondary and mature/Graafian). Each follicle houses an oocyte surrounded by granulosa cells and, as it matures, theca cells.
- Folliculogenesis is the process in which recruited primordial follicles grow and mature. Some develop into Graafian follicles with the potential to either ovulate its egg into the fallopian tube at ovulation to be fertilised; some die by atresia (degeneration).
- As follicles develop and mature, they are given different names corresponding to the phases of folliculogenesis.
- Primordial follicles are the first stage of follicular development. These start to develop in the ovary *in utero*, around the third month of gestation, and reach their maximum number during the fifth month of intrauterine life (about 6–7 million per ovary).
- The number of primordial follicles then falls steadily during the reproductive years due to ovulation and atresia (see *Box 1.1*).

BOX 1.1: Follicular number, depletion and age

- At birth: approximately 1–2 million primordial follicles.
- At puberty: 200 000–300 000.
- After menarche, approximately 500–1000 follicles are activated every month. They go through a phase of growth and then atresia. As oocyte numbers decline, so does their quality.
- At late 30s: 25 000 (critical threshold number). The age at which this number is reached varies from late 20s to 40s and can be associated with hormonal changes.
- Numbers rapidly decline after 40 years to around 1000 remaining at menopause.
- After menopause: few/none left.

1.3.1 Follicular maturation

- There are two distinct phases of ovarian follicle development.
- It takes approximately one year for a primordial follicle to fully mature before ovulation.

Pre-antral phase (primordial, primary, secondary, pre-antral)

This early stage of follicular development from primordial, to primary, to secondary to pre-antral follicles is not dependent on FSH or LH. It continues during all physiological circumstances including ovulation, pregnancy and periods of anovulation.

Primordial follicles

- These contain an immature oocyte arrested early in meiosis, surrounded by flattened granulosa cells and a basal lamina.

Primary follicles

- The oocyte grows and the flat cells that surrounded the oocyte in the primordial follicle now become cubic granulosa cells.

Secondary follicles

- The granulosa cell layers surrounding the oocyte and a zona pellucida surrounding the oocyte both increase in size and number.

Pre-antral follicles

- The granulosa cells further increase, and the oocyte is surrounded by theca cells.
- The main function of theca cells is to synthesise androgens that diffuse into the nearby granulosa cells for conversion to oestrogen.
- The granulosa cells acquire receptors for FSH, and follicular development from the early antral stage onwards becomes dependent on gonadotrophins.
- Granulosa and theca cells play important roles in female hormone regulation as they produce the hormones oestrogen and androgens, and these hormones in turn exert their effect on the developing follicles and form part of the HPO axis.

Antral phase (antral to Graafian follicle)

- Development of this stage of maturation of the follicle from an antral follicle to a Graafian follicle, in preparation for ovulation, is now dependent on FSH and LH.
- The antral follicle has a cavity filled with follicular fluid, known as the antrum.

- With the onset of puberty the HPO axis is activated. In the follicular phase of each menstrual cycle, due to the increase in the level of FSH, there is recruitment of several of these antral follicles to mature and continue their development to a Graafian follicle.
- The follicles that are more sensitive to FSH, rather than those less mature, are selected. In these follicles, the granulosa cells' aromatase activity will increase, converting androgens (produced by the theca cells) to oestrogens, prior to the LH surge. Inhibin will also be produced.
- As oestrogen and inhibin levels rise, they exert negative feedback on the anterior pituitary, causing a fall in the level of FSH. As FSH levels fall, many of the maturing follicles will be unable to continue their maturation. The follicles that are most sensitive to FSH, with a low threshold for a response to FSH, can continue to thrive and produce oestrogen and LH receptors.
- Many of the maturing follicles will enter atresia, and usually only one of them will be able to complete its development in each menstrual cycle and become the dominant follicle (see *Fig. 1.6*).

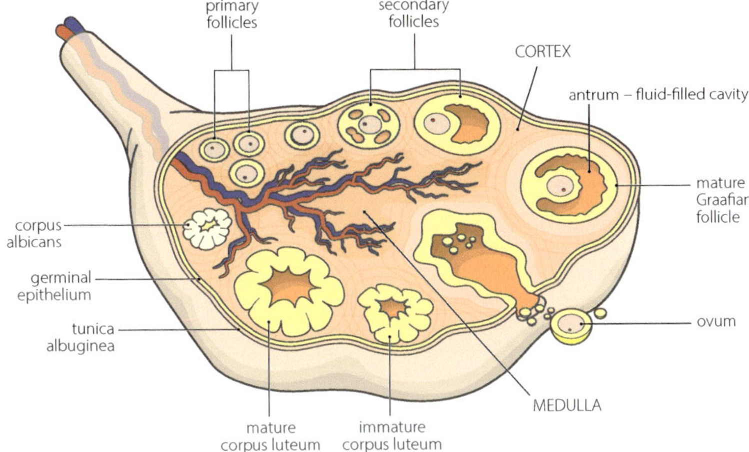

Figure 1.6: Maturation of follicles in the ovary. Reproduced from *Anatomy and Physiology: an introduction for nursing and healthcare* (2020) with permission from Lantern Publishing Ltd.

Graafian or pre-ovulatory follicle

- The Graafian or pre-ovulatory follicle is the fully developed follicle, which will lead to ovulation of the oocyte it contains.
- The preovulatory LH surge activates the Graafian follicle, generating a sequence of events including oocyte maturation and follicle rupture (release of the oocyte from the dominant follicle), referred to as ovulation.
- Luteinisation occurs and granulosa cells transition to become luteinised granulosa cells, developing LH receptors.
  - This is crucial: granulosa cells previously responded mainly to FSH; after the LH surge, they respond to LH.
  - This receptor switch allows them to start producing progesterone (instead of primarily oestrogen).

Corpus luteum

- After ovulation the remnants of the follicle (granulosa and theca cells) form the corpus luteum. The corpus luteum includes:
  - luteinised granulosa cells (from the follicle)
  - theca lutein cells (transformed theca cells).
- Together, these produce progesterone and some oestrogen.

- Progesterone peaks during this phase, preparing the endometrium for implantation.
- The corpus albicans is the fibrotic remnant of the corpus luteum that forms if pregnancy does not occur.

1.4 The menstrual cycle

- The female reproductive system goes through regular cyclical changes known as the menstrual cycle.
- Cyclical bleeding occurs because of hormonal changes throughout the month, which are controlled by the HPO axis.
- The purpose is to release an egg for possible fertilisation and to prepare the uterus for implantation.
- Periods start to occur at puberty, with menarche, and they stop at menopause, due to loss of ovarian follicular activity.

The menstrual cycle (see *Fig. 1.7*) comprises two distinct cycles: the ovarian cycle (changes in the ovaries) and endometrial cycle (changes in the endometrium).

- The phases of the ovarian cycle are the follicular phase, ovulation and the luteal phase.
- The phases in the endometrial cycle are the proliferative phase, the secretory phase and the menstrual phase.
- In the ovarian follicular phase, menstruation occurs and the endometrium then goes through a proliferative phase.
- In the ovarian luteal phase, the endometrium goes through the secretory phase in preparation for implantation.

1.4.1 The ovarian cycle

Follicular phase

- This phase varies in length and is the time of maturation of the ovarian follicles under the influence of FSH.
- It begins with the first day of menstruation and ends with ovulation.
- FSH levels rise during the follicular phase of the menstrual cycle, and this results in stimulation and maturation of ovarian antral follicles.
- As the recruited follicles mature, they produce 17β-estradiol and inhibin B, so the levels of these hormones rise. Most of the oestrogen is produced by the dominant follicle.
- As levels of 17β-estradiol and inhibin B rise, they provide negative feedback, causing FSH levels to reduce, and consequently there is less stimulation of the follicles, so the non-dominant follicles begin to degenerate.
- When inhibin and oestrogen levels reach their highest threshold level in the late follicular phase, their negative feedback function transforms into a positive feedback function which induces an LH surge.

Ovulation

- In late follicular phase, the high concentration of oestrogen switches from inhibiting GnRH release to stimulating it – a process known as positive feedback. Higher pulse frequency of GnRH leads to a rapid rise in the level of LH being released by the anterior pituitary gland. This occurs over a 24–48-hour interval and is called the LH surge. This stimulates changes in the Graafian follicle, resulting in ovulation. The remnant of the follicle is converted into the corpus luteum.
- Ovulation occurs 14 days before the next period is due. The exact day on which ovulation occurs will vary with the menstrual cycle, as the length of the follicular phase can vary.

- Towards the time of ovulation, the pH in the vagina becomes less acidic, the cervical mucus becomes more copious and less viscous, and the cervical os opens to help the sperm reach the oocyte.
- Ovulation can be suppressed – one recognised cause is RED-S (relative energy deficiency in sport); see *Section 2.6* on amenorrhoea.

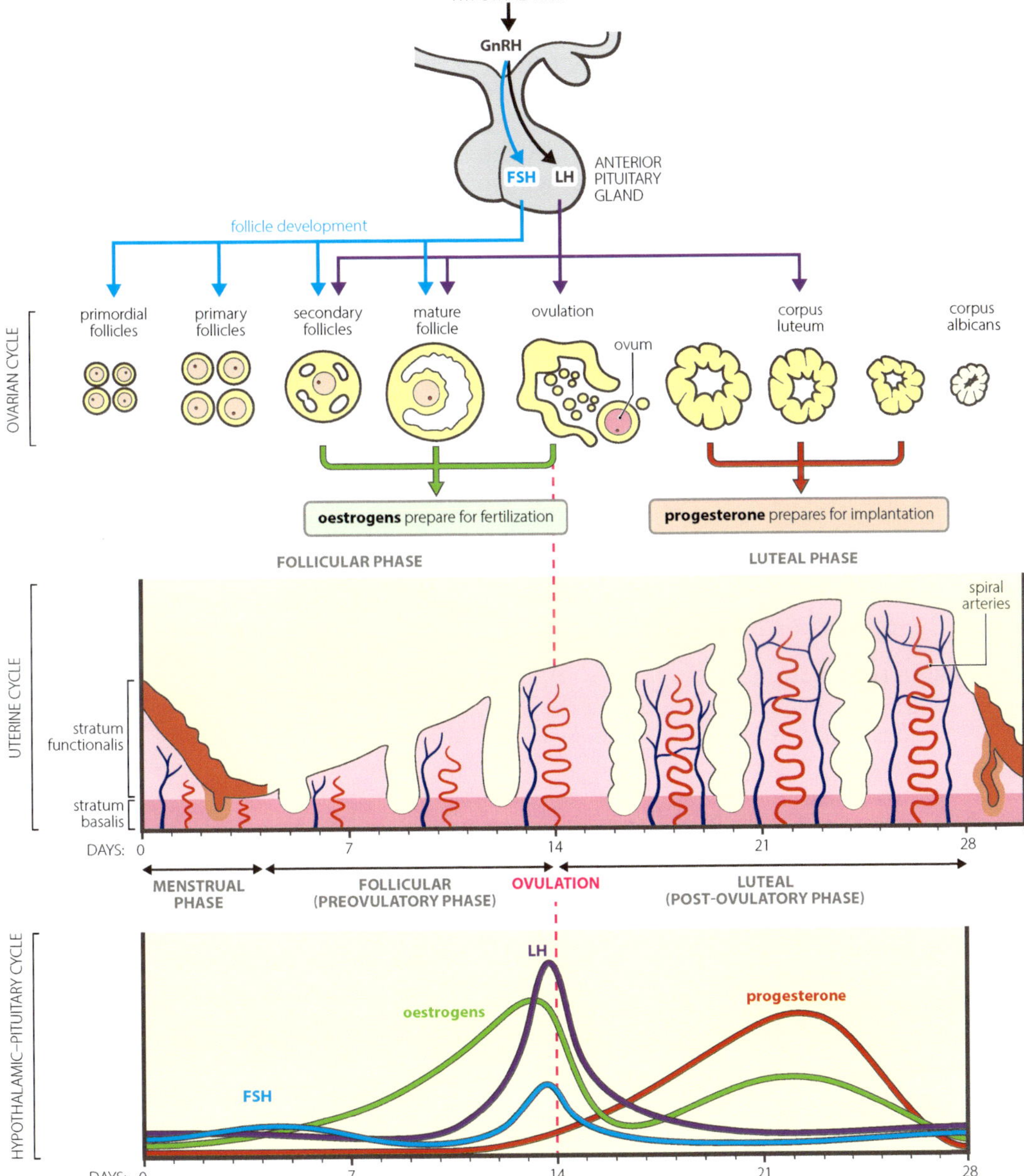

Figure 1.7: The menstrual cycle. Reproduced from *Anatomy and Physiology: an introduction for nursing and healthcare* (2020) with permission from Lantern Publishing Ltd.

Luteal phase

- This is the time after ovulation until the start of menstruation, lasting typically 14 days.
- Following ovulation, estradiol concentrations drop temporarily but are revived by production from the corpus luteum. The corpus luteum, left after ovulation, produces oestrogen, prompting endometrial growth, and progesterone, which is essential for endometrial maintenance.
- Through negative feedback progesterone also inhibits the hypothalamus and pituitary gland.
- In the absence of fertilisation, the corpus luteum can be sustained for 12–14 days. It then begins to regress and turn into fibrous tissue, and the remaining scar is known as a corpus albicans.
- Progesterone and oestrogen levels fall as the corpus luteum regresses.
- With the demise of the corpus luteum, oestrogen and progesterone concentrations fall rapidly to their lowest levels and no longer cause negative feedback, so the GnRH production in the hypothalamus resumes, and FSH begins to rise immediately preceding menstruation to prepare for the next follicular phase.
- The endometrium is no longer maintained by the progesterone, due to degeneration of the corpus luteum and is shed, resulting in menstruation.

Fertilisation

- Once ovulation occurs, if an egg has been fertilised by sperm in the fallopian tubes a zygote forms. Over the next 8–10 days the zygote will move into the uterus, where it implants and starts to develop into a fetus.
- Pregnancy starts at the point of implantation, but in practice the first day of the last menstrual period (LMP) is used as the starting point for calculating gestational age or dating the pregnancy.

1.4.2 The endometrial cycle

Changes in the endometrial layers throughout the menstrual cycle

- The endometrium has three internal layers:
  - stratum compactum
  - stratum spongiosum
  - stratum basalis.
- The deep stratum basalis changes little throughout the menstrual cycle and is not shed at menstruation.
- The endometrium proliferates in response to oestrogens and becomes secretory in response to progesterone. It is shed during menstruation and regenerates from cells in the stratum basalis layer.

The proliferative phase

- The endometrial proliferative phase begins at the end of menstruation and ends with ovulation.
- Oestrogen causes the endometrium to thicken; the endometrial stroma becomes thick and richly vascularised. The stratum compactum and stratum spongialis layers develop into the stratum functionalis. The endometrium is prepared for the secretory phase.

The secretory phase

- This is the time after ovulation when the endometrial glands become corkscrew-shaped and filled with glycogen, secreting a glycogen-rich secretion under the influence of progesterone secreted from the corpus luteum, in preparation for implantation of a fertilised zygote.

Menstruation

- Shedding of the uterine lining occurs if the egg is not fertilised, due to a fall in progesterone levels caused by the degeneration of the corpus luteum. The spiral arterioles in the stratum functionalis layer contract, resulting in ischaemia, and degeneration of the functionalis layer.
- The arteries rupture, and the rapid blood flow dislodges the necrotic functional layer, which is shed.
- The basal layer is unaffected, because it is supplied by straight arteries.

1.4.3 Normal menstrual cycle length and regularity

- This is covered briefly here, but refer to *Chapter 2, Menstrual disorders*, for more detail.
- The number of days in the menstrual cycle is calculated from the first day of the period to the day before the start of the next period.
  - The first day of active bright red bleeding and menstrual flow is considered day 1.
  - Spotting may occur in the days leading up to menstruation. When it does, it is typically brownish, sometimes greasy, and usually lasts for 1–2 days.
- Menstrual cycles usually occur every 21–35 days; the average length is 28 days.
- Normal menstrual cycles should have a consistent regularity, duration and volume of blood flow.
- Normal menstrual bleeding lasts 8 days or less (normally 3–7 days).
- It is normal for menstrual cycles to vary in length from month to month; this is called menstrual irregularity.

Menstrual cycle irregularities occur in about 14–25% of women of reproductive age. Cycles can be shorter or longer than average; bleeding can be irregular or can pause or stop. Some of the problems which can occur with the menstrual cycle include the following:

Amenorrhoea

- This is absence of menstrual bleeding.
- NICE CKS Amenorrhoea provides these definitions:
  - primary amenorrhea – periods have not started by age 15/16 years in girls with normal secondary sexual characteristics, or 13/14 years in girls with no secondary sexual characteristics
  - secondary amenorrhoea – the cessation of previously established menstruation for three cycles, or for ≥6 months.

Irregular menstrual cycles

- The international evidence-based guideline for the assessment and management of polycystic ovary syndrome (PCOS) states that irregular cycles are normal in the first year after menarche, as part of the pubertal transition. It defines irregular menstrual cycles as:
  - >1 to <3 years post menarche, cycles occurring <21 or >45 days
  - >3 years post menarche to perimenopause, cycles occurring <21 or >35 days, or having <8 cycles per year
  - >1 year post menarche, >90 days for any one cycle
  - menstrual chaos (a highly irregular menstrual pattern).
- When irregular menstrual cycles are present, a diagnosis of PCOS should be considered.

Anovulatory cycles

- This is when ovulation does not occur at the end of the follicular phase.
- If ovulation does not occur, there is no formation of a corpus luteum, and progesterone is not produced in significant amounts. Without progesterone, the endometrium cannot mature,

and there is no fall in progesterone to trigger the shedding at the end of the cycle. Meanwhile, oestrogen continues to stimulate the growth of the endometrium, causing it to thicken. Eventually the endometrium starts to break down and slough off, and this usually occurs irregularly, and menstrual flow can vary from light to very heavy.
- These types of cycles are common in the first 18 months after menarche and in the perimenopause. They are also associated with disorders which impact the HPO axis, such as PCOS, thyroid disorders and hyperprolactinaemia.

Intermenstrual bleeding

- Bleeding that occurs between the regular cyclical menstrual periods.
- It can be random or cyclical.
- Some women may have a regular light bleed at the time of ovulation each month which is normal for them and does not need to be investigated. Tracking their bleeding on a chart is helpful when considering this.

Postcoital bleeding

- Bleeding from the genital tract that occurs after sexual intercourse and is not related to menstruation.

Volume of menstrual flow

- This is subjective and can be classified as light, normal or heavy.
- As this is subjective NICE defines heavy menstrual bleeding as *"Excessive menstrual bleeding that interferes with a person's physical, social, emotional, and/or material quality of life"*.
- Helpful questions to ask when taking a history are:
  - What sort of sanitary protection do you need and how often do you change it?
  - Are you getting up at night to change sanitary protection?
  - What activities does your bleeding stop you doing?
- Consider in the history and examination if there are symptoms suggesting anaemia.
- It is vital to offer information and early treatment for women who experience heavy menstrual bleeding (either non-hormonal or hormonal) to prevent them from becoming anaemic. Refer to the NHS England leaflet about making a decision about managing heavy periods, available at: www.england.nhs.uk/wp-content/uploads/2023/11/PRN00250-dst-making-a-decision-about-heavy-preiods.pdf

Abnormal uterine bleeding

- Abnormal uterine bleeding (AUB) in women of reproductive age can occur for many reasons.

The International Federation of Gynecology and Obstetrics (FIGO) has developed a helpful classification system called the "PALM–COEIN" system (see *Fig. 1.8*), dividing causes into structural and non-structural.

- Structural causes include:
  - **P**olyps
  - **A**denomyosis
  - **L**eiomyomas
  - **M**alignancy/hyperplasia.
- Non-structural causes include:
  - **C**oagulopathy
  - **O**vulatory dysfunction, including endocrine and metabolic disorders affecting the HPO axis, such as PCOS, thyroid disorders, and elevated levels of prolactin, androgens or cortisol
  - **E**ndometrial dysfunction, including Asherman's syndrome and endometritis
  - **I**atrogenic causes
  - **N**ot otherwise classified.

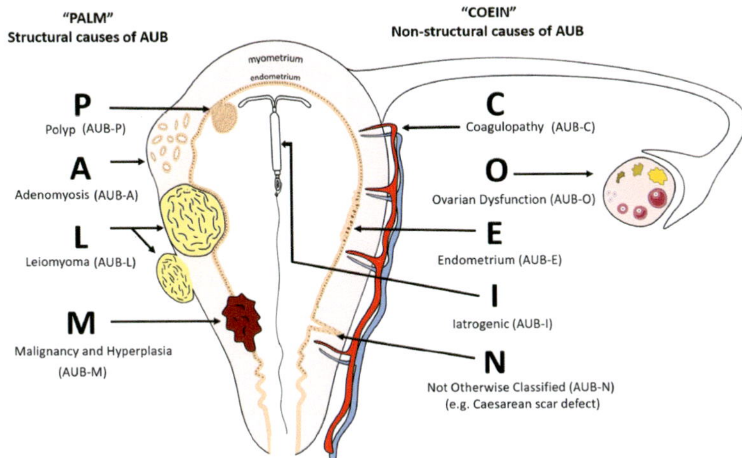

Figure 1.8: The FIGO classification of abnormal uterine bleeding. Reproduced under a CC-BY licence from Tsolova, A.O., Martínez Aguilar, R., Maybin, J.A. and Critchley, H.O. (2022) Preclinical models to study abnormal uterine bleeding (AUB). *EBioMedicine*, 84: 104238.

1.5 Puberty

- This describes the developmental changes a child undergoes to become sexually mature and physiologically ready for reproduction.
- It normally begins between the ages of 8 and 14 years in females and between the ages of 10 and 16 years in males.
- Precocious puberty is the appearance of secondary sexual characteristics before the age of 8 years in girls.

1.5.1 Hormonal changes

- During childhood, the levels of FSH and LH in the body are low. This is thought to be due to the slow cycling of the GnRH pulse generator in the hypothalamus. The onset of puberty involves the activation of the HPO axis.

1.5.2 Physical changes

- Female secondary sexual characteristics develop because of increasing oestrogen production.

Breast development

- The first sign of puberty in girls is the beginning of breast development (thelarche). This typically occurs at around age 9–10 years. Breast buds appear as small mounds with the breast and papilla elevated. Tanner staging is used to assess breast size/development, with stages from I–V.
- The breasts consist of lobulated glandular tissue embedded in adipose tissue, separated by fibrous connective tissue. Following the clearance of placental oestrogens after birth, the breasts are in a dormant stage until puberty. In this dormant stage, there are only lactiferous ducts with no alveoli.
- At puberty, the increase in ovarian oestrogens causes the development of the lactiferous duct system as the ducts grow in branches with the ends forming the lobular alveoli (small spheroidal masses). Mediated by progesterone, these lobules will increase in number through puberty.

- The breasts continue to increase in size following menarche due to increased fat deposition. Throughout the menstrual cycle, oestrogen and progesterone affect the breast size and composition.

Pubic hair

- The second sign of puberty in girls is usually the growth of hair on the mons pubis. The hair initially appears sparse, light and straight; however, throughout puberty, it becomes coarser, thicker and darker.
- Approximately 2 years after pubarche, hair begins to grow in the axillary area as well. In both sexes, hair growth is a secondary sexual characteristic mediated by testosterone.

Menarche

- Menarche is the first menstrual period and marks the beginning of the menstrual cycles.
- It normally occurs around 1.5–3 years after thelarche.
- Menarche is usually an anovulatory breakthrough bleed. The first years of menstruation can be anovulatory, resulting in an irregular cycle and heavier bleeds. Menarche and first ovulation can be years apart.
- Ovulation does not occur until full maturity has been reached and pulsatile secretion of GnRH has stabilised. This is usually between the ages of 10 and 16 years. Pregnancy can occur at this stage in sexually active teenagers. It is important to discuss contraception and sexually transmitted infections.
- It takes 8 years from menarche to reach reproductive maturity.

Growth spurt

- The pubertal growth spurt occurs because of an interaction between estradiol, testosterone, growth hormone (GH) and insulin-like growth factor 1 (IGF-1). GH levels will rise in puberty due to the increase in sex steroids and their positive effect on the pulsatile release of GH from the anterior pituitary gland.
- A rise in GH causes a rise in IGF-1, which causes growth via its metabolic actions (e.g. increases trabecular bone growth).

1.6 Menopause

Refer to *Chapter 6* for more detail about perimenopause and different types of menopause.

Menopause

- This is a retrospective diagnosis made 12 months after the final menstrual period, in the absence of any other physiological or pathological explanation for this.
- It marks the end of reproductive life and ovarian follicular activity.

The menopausal transition (the perimenopause)

- This is the time from the onset of menstrual cycle irregularity, through until 12 months after the last menstrual period. There can be symptoms of low oestrogen and of high oestrogen caused by erratic ovulation during this time, and hormones can fluctuate.

1.6.1 The stages of reproductive aging

The Stages of Reproductive Aging Workshop +10 (STRAW+10) criteria (see *Fig. 1.9*), based on menstrual bleeding patterns, represent a staging system for the menopause transition.

Final Menstrual Period (FMP)

Stages:	-5	-4	-3	-2	-1	0	+1	+2
Terminology:	**Reproductive**			**Menopausal Transition**			**Postmenopause**	
	Early	Peak	Late	Early	Late*		Early*	Late
				Perimenopause				
Duration of Stage:	variable			variable		(a) 1 yr	(b) 4 yrs	until demise
Menstrual Cycles:	variable to regular	regular		variable cycle length *(>7 days different from normal)*	≥2 skipped cycles and an interval of amenorrhea *(≥60 days)*	*Amen x 12 mos*	none	
Endocrine:	normal FSH		↑ FSH	↑ FSH			↑ FSH	

**Stages most likely to be characterized by vasomotor symptoms* ↑ *= elevated*

Figure 1.9: The Stages of Reproductive Aging Workshop +10 (STRAW+10) criteria. Reprinted from *Fertility and Sterility*, 76(5): Soules, M.R., Sherman, S., Parrott, E. *et al.*, Executive summary: stages of reproductive aging workshop (STRAW), pp. 874–8. Copyright 2001, with permission from Elsevier.

1.6.2 Hormonal changes in the menopause transition

- The decline in number of oocytes to a critical level (about 25 000) and a decline in ovarian follicular activity lead to the early changes in hormones, and consequently a change in the feedback mechanism between the ovary, pituitary and hypothalamus, leading to a rise in gonadotrophins.
- Inhibin B is produced by developing ovarian follicles. When the number, quality and activity of ovarian follicles declines, follicular phase inhibin B hormone concentrations decline, and as a result the FSH rises.
- This increase in FSH can maintain and even increase estradiol production during the perimenopause, stimulating ovarian folliculogenesis, which occurs at an accelerated rate up until menopause.
- The ovaries eventually become less responsive to FSH, due to a decrease in available binding sites, and a fall in follicle numbers.
- Follicles fail to reach full maturation and cycles can become anovulatory; consequently progesterone is not produced as it would be in an ovulatory cycle.
- Estradiol levels begin to fluctuate and eventually decrease to a level too low to stimulate the endometrium, and periods completely stop.
- When there is complete failure of follicles to develop, levels of estradiol remain persistently low and levels of FSH and LH remain high, due to a loss of negative feedback by estradiol.
- Testosterone levels decline gradually from a peak in the 20s, and reach their lowest level by around age 60, stabilising or rising slightly after that. Levels do not change significantly during the early menopausal transition, and this changes the ratio between the androgens and oestrogens, leading to symptoms of androgen excess in some women.

1.6.3 Menstrual changes in perimenopause

- Every woman will have a unique experience and hormone changes typically cause irregular menstrual cycles with shortening of the cycle length during the early perimenopause, followed by progressively longer gaps between periods with progression to late perimenopause.

- Some of this bleeding is the result of menstruation from ovulatory cycles.
- Other bleeds are from anovulatory cycles where endometrium has proliferated under oestrogen without the balance of progesterone from the corpus luteum after ovulation.
- Progesterone is required to support the endometrium, so that when ovulation does not occur the endometrial lining breaks down. This is termed breakthrough bleeding and can happen as frequently as every fortnight in some perimenopausal women.
- Some women experience menorrhagia in perimenopause. As with any woman with menorrhagia, it is important to take a history, perform an examination, arrange any necessary investigations and offer non-hormonal or hormonal pharmacological treatment at their consultation (see *Section 2.3*).
- As levels of oestrogen decrease, both types of bleeding will eventually stop.
- Menopause can be diagnosed retrospectively after 12 consecutive months without a period, with no other pathological or physiological cause.

1.7 Further reading

Ameer, M.A. and Peterson, D.C. (updated 2025) *Anatomy, Abdomen and Pelvis: Uterus*. StatPearls. Available at: www.ncbi.nlm.nih.gov/books/NBK470297

Cable, J.K. and Grider, M.H. (updated 2023) *Physiology, Progesterone*. StatPearls. Available at: www.ncbi.nlm.nih.gov/books/NBK558960

Chaudhry, S.R., Nahian, A. and Chaudhry, K. (updated 2023) *Anatomy, Abdomen and Pelvis, Pelvis*. StatPearls. Available at: www.ncbi.nlm.nih.gov/books/NBK482258

Cox, E. and Takov, V. (updated 2025) *Embryology, Ovarian Follicle Development*. StatPearls. Available at: www.ncbi.nlm.nih.gov/books/NBK532300

Davis, S.R. (2024) Testosterone and the heart: friend or foe? *Climacteric*, **27(1):** 53–9. Available at: https://doi.org/10.1080/13697137.2023.2250252

FIGO (undated) *Menstrual Disorders*. Available at: www.figo.org/figo-resources/menstrual-disorders

Gibson, E. and Mahdy, H. (updated 2023) *Anatomy, Abdomen and Pelvis, Ovary*. StatPearls. Available at: www.ncbi.nlm.nih.gov/sites/books/NBK545187

Guay, A. and Davis, S.R. (undated) *Testosterone insufficiency in women: fact or fiction?* Boston University School of Medicine. Available at: www.bumc.bu.edu/sexualmedicine/publications/testosterone-insufficiency-in-women-fact-or-fiction

Holesh, J.E., Bass, A.N. and Lord, M. (updated 2023) *Physiology, Ovulation*. StatPearls. Available at: www.ncbi.nlm.nih.gov/books/NBK441996

Homburg. R. (2014) *The Mechanism of Ovulation*. Available at: www.glowm.com/section-view/heading/The%20Mechanism%20of%20Ovulation/item/289

Nelson, L.R. and Bulun, S.E. (2001) Estrogen production and action. *Journal of the American Academy of Dermatology*, **45(3):** S116–24. Available at: https://doi.org/10.1067/mjd.2001.117432

NHS England (updated 2025) *Cervical screening: programme overview*. Available at: www.gov.uk/guidance/cervical-screening-programme-overview

Nucera, B., Rinaldi, F., Dono, F. *et al.* (2023) Progesterone and its derivatives for the treatment of catamenial epilepsy: a systematic review. *Seizure: European Journal of Epilepsy*, **109:** 52–9. Available at: https://doi.org/10.1016/j.seizure.2023.05.004

RCGP (2025) *Women's health toolkit: Menopause*. Available at: https://elearning.rcgp.org.uk/mod/book/view.php?id=12534&chapterid=832

Soules, M.R., Sherman, S., Parrott, E. *et al.* (2001) Executive summary: Stages of Reproductive Aging Workshop (STRAW). *Climacteric*, **4(4):** 267–72. Available at: https://doi.org/10.1080/cmt.4.4.267.272

Sundström-Poromaa, I., Comasco, E., Sumner, R. and Luders, E. (2020) Progesterone – friend or foe? *Frontiers in Neuroendocrinology*, **59:** 100856. Available at: https://doi.org/10.1016/j.yfrne.2020.100856

Talaulikar, V. (2022) Menopause transition: physiology and symptoms. *Best Practice & Research Clinical Obstetrics & Gynaecology*, **81:** 3–7. Available at: https://doi.org/10.1016/j.bpobgyn.2022.03.003

Thiyagarajan, D.K., Basit, H. and Jeanmonod, R. (updated 2024) *Physiology, Menstrual Cycle*. StatPearls. Available at: www.ncbi.nlm.nih.gov/books/NBK500020

Thompson, L. (updated 2022) *The Ovaries*. Available at: https://teachmeanatomy.info/pelvis/female-reproductive-tract/ovaries

University of Leeds (undated) *The Histology Guide*. Available at: www.histology.leeds.ac.uk/female/uterus.php

The Vulva Gallery (undated) *Anatomy*. Available at: www.thevulvagallery.com/anatomy

Chapter 2
Menstrual disorders

2.1 Introduction

- Menstrual health is a core aspect of women's wellbeing, influencing physical, emotional and social health throughout their reproductive life.
- In the UK, approximately 1 in 3 women suffer from heavy menstrual bleeding, 2 in 3 women will develop at least one fibroid in their lifetime and conditions such as endometriosis affect around 1 in 10 women of reproductive age.
- Menstrual disorders can lead to significant impacts on quality of life, including chronic pain, infertility, anaemia, mental health challenges, sexual problems, and limitations in daily activities and employment.
- Poor management can result in avoidable morbidity, impaired social participation and quality of life, and substantial economic costs due to time taken off from work. Research published in the Bupa Wellness Index in January 2024 found that 1 in 8 women in the UK had taken time off in the previous 12 months due to symptoms linked to their periods, but more than a third had given a different reason to their employer.
- Healthcare professionals are often the first point of contact for patients experiencing menstrual disorders, but many women feel their symptoms are dismissed or not taken seriously, with severe pain and heavy periods being normalised. It is important to be able to create a safe, empathetic and non-judgemental space for them to discuss these issues.
- For some conditions getting a diagnosis and treatment can take years. It is important for healthcare professionals to be able to identify, investigate and manage menstrual issues effectively to optimise women's health, alleviate symptoms, enhance their quality of life and reduce the socioeconomic burden associated with these conditions.

2.2 Normal menstruation

- Menstruation varies between individuals and each woman will have her own version of what normal is.
- Encouraging women to monitor their own cycles can help them to familiarise themselves with their own periods and then be able to report any changes.
- There are lots of mobile apps nowadays to make it easy to monitor cycles, e.g. Flo Period and Cycle Tracker.
- A lack of understanding of what constitutes a normal period or cycle can delay people from seeking help, especially if their female family members / friends suffer the same symptoms. It is important to educate women and have a reference point of what normal is:
  - **Normal cycle length:** typically can vary between 21 and 35 days. Average 28 days and can vary month to month.
  - **Normal duration of flow:** 2–7 days.
  - **Normal volume of blood loss:** around 30–40ml per cycle, which is about 2–3 tablespoons. Volume can vary through the period, being heavier on some days and then usually lighter towards the end or lighter at the start then getting heavier.

2.3 Heavy menstrual bleeding and other menstrual disorders

2.3.1 Heavy menstrual bleeding

Definition

- Heavy menstrual bleeding (HMB) is excessive menstrual blood loss that interferes with quality of life. Clinical volume (>80ml/cycle or 5 tablespoons) is less important than perceived impact on the woman.

- About 1 in 3 women will describe their periods as heavy, but some of these will have average blood loss. Some will describe their periods as normal but will actually have a heavy flow.
- Some women may pass clots >1cm in size, which indicates fast blood flow. These can cause pain when they are passed.
- Women use different sanitary products, and it can be hard to quantify how much blood is lost. Menstrual cups have measurements on them, so it is a little easier to work out how much is lost because this can be monitored. Regular tampons absorb about 5ml of fluid and superabsorbent about 10ml, but women do not usually wait until they are fully soaked to change them. The absorbency of pads can vary between products, but a normal pad absorbs 5ml of fluid and an extra-absorbent pad about 10ml. Some women use period pants, and this method is hard to quantify. Not all the fluid is blood so it can be hard to work out how much blood is actually lost.
- For practical purposes a period is considered heavy if a woman has one or more of these symptoms:
    - flooding through to clothes or bedding
    - needing to change sanitary towels / tampons frequently, e.g. every 1–2 hours
    - needing double sanitary protection (e.g. tampons and towels)
    - passing large blood clots >1cm in size.

Causes

- Unknown: in 4–6 out of 10 cases no cause is found, and it is then known as dysfunctional uterine bleeding.
- Structural causes: uterine fibroids, endometrial/cervical polyps and adenomyosis and infections, e.g. chlamydia, and endometrial cancer.
- Non-structural causes: coagulopathies, hypothyroidism.
- Iatrogenic causes: such as copper intrauterine device (IUD), medications such as warfarin and some chemotherapy drugs.

Assessment

- History: ask about nature of bleeding, frequency of sanitary product use, clots, flooding, pain, anaemia symptoms and impact on quality of life. Suggest keeping a menstrual diary if unsure.
- Vaginal examination: bimanual, speculum exam looking at the cervix and assess size and shape of uterus, swabs may be taken if infection suspected.
- Blood tests: full blood count (FBC), and if indicated ferritin, thyroid-stimulating hormone (TSH), coagulation screen.
- Pelvic ultrasound: if structural pathology suspected.
- Some women may need referral to secondary care where further tests such as endometrial sampling or hysteroscopy can assess the inside of the uterus, especially if you suspect fibroids, polyps or endometrial pathology.
- If there are any red flag symptoms, such as persistent or unexplained intermenstrual bleeding, unexplained postcoital bleeding, postmenopausal bleeding, persistent pelvic pain/masses or suspicion of a gynaecological cancer, then refer according to local guidelines to gynaecology or via the urgent care pathway (UCP) if needed. See *Section 2.4* for more information on these symptoms.

Management

- Provide women with information about HMB and all management options via NHS website, and discuss options with a view to shared decision-making.
- A very useful website to direct patients to is www.england.nhs.uk/wp-content/uploads/2023/11/PRN00250-dst-making-a-decision-about-heavy-preiods.pdf

- First-line: **levonorgestrel intrauterine device (LNG-IUD)** releases small amounts of progesterone that keep the endometrial lining thin. It can also double up as contraception or the progesterone part of HRT. In most women, bleeding becomes either very light or stops after 3–6 months, and period pains are usually reduced too. Sometimes the bleeding can persist and last longer than 6 months.
- Alternative treatments:
  - **Tranexamic acid:** works by reducing the breakdown of the blood clots. It can reduce the heaviness of the bleeding by almost half, but not the number of days of bleeding or pain. May cause stomach upset and must be avoided in people with clotting issues.
  - **Non-steroidal anti-inflammatory drugs (NSAIDs):** ibuprofen, mefenamic acid or naproxen. They reduce the high levels of prostaglandin in the womb lining which contributes to the heaviness and pain of periods. Can reduce blood loss by a quarter in most cases and can reduce pain, but they do not reduce the length of time of the bleeding. Can be taken with tranexamic acid. May cause dyspepsia so may need a proton pump inhibitor too.
  - **COCP:** this can reduce bleeding by a third in most women and help with pain as well as provide contraception. It can be used with NSAIDs in women who have a lot of pain. Taking packets back-to-back, in a tailored regime for 3 months followed by a short 4-day break, can reduce the frequency of periods, or it can even be taken continuously without a break (see *Section 3.4.10* for more information on how to do this).
  - **Progestogen-only pill (POP):** POPs can keep the lining of the womb thin and prevent ovulation. They can help stop or reduce heavy bleeding and be used for contraception. They may have side-effects such as breast tenderness, irregular bleeding, bloating or headaches.
  - **Cyclical progesterone:** sometimes used if other treatments have not helped or as a temporary measure to reduce very heavy bleeding. Used on days 5–26 of cycle or for short periods such as for 10 days, e.g. norethisterone.
- Surgical treatments are not first-line options but can be considered if other medical options have failed. They include:
  - **Endometrial ablation:** the uterine lining is removed, but this can affect fertility. May need to be repeated because it is not permanent. Inform women to avoid pregnancy post-procedure and use contraception.
  - **Myomectomy or endometrial artery embolisation:** used to remove fibroids if they are the cause of heavy bleeding.
  - **Hysterectomy:** used as a last option if medical therapy fails. May improve quality of life for women but will impact fertility, and the risks of having surgery must also be considered. Women who also have their ovaries removed before their menopause will be put into a surgical menopause and the implications of their surgery will need to be discussed before the operation. They may need to consider taking HRT after surgery (see *Section 6.10* for more guidance).

2.3.2 Dysmenorrhoea

Overview

- Dysmenorrhoea is painful cramping, usually in the lower abdomen, but it can radiate to the back or inner thighs, which occurs shortly before and/or during menstruation.
- It can be associated with other non-gynaecological symptoms such as vomiting, nausea, diarrhoea, fatigue, irritability, dizziness and headaches.
- The prevalence rates vary in different studies and can range between 16% and 91% in women of reproductive age.

- It can be really debilitating, impact quality of life, and lead to restrictions of daily activities and absence from school and work.

Types

Primary

- This is pain without any identifiable pelvic pathology and is caused by the production of uterine prostaglandins that cause uterine contractions and pain.
- It usually begins 6–12 months after menstruation first starts.
- Risk factors include earlier age of starting menstruation, nulliparity, HMB and a family history of dysmenorrhoea.

Secondary

- This is caused by underlying pathology due to conditions such as endometriosis, fibroids or pelvic inflammatory disease (PID), or can rarely be caused by an IUD *in situ*.
- Ectopic pregnancy or gynaecological cancers are rare causes and need prompt referral.
- Pain can start after several years of painless periods. The pain may occur at other times in the cycle but is exacerbated by the periods.
- There may be other symptoms present such as dyspareunia, intermenstrual or postcoital bleeding and vaginal or cervical discharge, together with pelvic pain.

Management

- **First-line:** NSAIDs (e.g. mefenamic acid) to reduce prostaglandin production and reduce pain, or paracetamol. Other options for pain management include applying heat in the form of patches or a hot water bottle, or transcutaneous electrical nerve stimulation (TENS).
- **Hormonal options:** if not considering pregnancy, then options such as the COCP or intrauterine devices such as the LNG-IUD can be considered and can also provide contraception. A newly launched pill containing the progesterone dydrogesterone (Nalvee 10mg) can also be effective for pain relief.
- **Referral:** if pain is severe, unresponsive to treatments after 3–6 months, or suggestive of endometriosis or other causes of secondary dysmenorrhoea, then refer to secondary care for further investigations and management.

2.3.3 Irregular menstrual cycles

Normal cycles can vary between 21 and 35 days, so anything outside of this can be considered irregular.

Common causes

- PCOS: oligomenorrhoea and anovulation, hyperandrogenism, polycystic ovaries (see *Section 2.9*).
- Thyroid dysfunction.
- Around puberty or perimenopause.
- Early pregnancy.
- Stress and anxiety.
- Losing or gaining weight.
- Exercising too much.

Management

- Address any underlying cause.
- Consider doing a pregnancy test.
- Consider COCP for cycle regulation if desired.
- Consider a progesterone; dydrogesterone (Nalvee 10mg) is licensed for the treatment of irregular cycles.

- Consider starting metformin in PCOS if insulin resistance is present (see *Section 2.9*).
- Treat any underlying thyroid issue.
- Consider HRT if perimenopausal (see *Chapters 6* and *7* for details of perimenopause and HRT).
- If there are fertility issues, consider referral to a fertility clinic (see *Chapter 5*).

2.3.4 Menstrual health and contraception

- Hormonal contraceptives can regulate, lighten or stop periods.
- LNG-IUD is both a contraceptive and therapeutic for HMB and dysmenorrhoea.
- Discuss dual benefits when initiating contraception; see *Chapter 3* for more information.

2.3.5 Premenstrual syndrome and premenstrual dysphoric disorder

- Recurring psychological and/or physical symptoms during the luteal phase, usually resolving with menstruation.
- These topics are covered in more detail in *Chapter 8*.

2.4 Non-menstrual bleeding

Types

This is when bleeding occurs outside of the normal menstrual cycle. There are three types:

- intermenstrual bleeding (IMB)
- postcoital bleeding (PCB)
- postmenopausal bleeding (PMB).

Causes

- Cervical ectropion, polyps, fibroids and infection.
- Endometrial hyperplasia or endometrial cancer.
- Genitourinary syndrome of the menopause – generally due to vaginal atrophy (in PMB).
- Due to contraception use – also termed breakthrough bleeding.

Investigations

- Speculum and bimanual exam.
- Check cervical smear history.
- Consider pelvic ultrasound scan if unsure of cause.
- Careful questioning on contraceptive use and compliance.

Management

- Treat any underlying cause.
- Gynaecology referral may be needed for further investigation.
- Referral under UCP if red flags: PCB or IMB in women >40 years, or any PMB.

2.5 How to delay a period

- There may be different reasons for women wanting to delay their period, such as holidays, exams, a special event or for religious reasons.
- It may also be requested by transgender and gender-diverse individuals who have a negative association or may experience distress with periods.
- There are different methods that can be used, and it is important to understand when the delay needs to start, so that treatment can be commenced at an appropriate time.
- Despite the use of medications to delay periods sometimes these methods can fail to stop the bleeding, and it is important for women to be aware of this.

2.5.1 Methods

- **Medroxyprogesterone acetate:** can be used in women with a high risk of venous thromboembolism (VTE) because it has a minimal effect on liver synthesis of clotting factors. Oral formulations of 10mg three times a day starting three days before the period is due, is the recommended dose. A bleed will start 2–3 days after stopping it. It may cause breakthrough bleeding and is not a form of contraception. It may inhibit ovulation so it can take time for fertility to return to normal. Depot formulations can also be used as injections every 12 weeks, but can take a long time to work so are not generally used.
- **Norethisterone:** 5mg TDS, starting 3 days before expected period for up to 14–28 days. Menstruation will occur 2–3 days after stopping the tablets. Women need to be informed that using norethisterone in this way is not for contraception and other methods should be used. Avoid in women with a high risk of VTE because in the liver part of the dose can be converted to ethinylestradiol, which can increase coagulation factor production.
- **COCP:** continue active pills without taking the 7-day break. Vaginal ring can also be used continuously as well as patches without a break.
- **POP:** these pills are taken daily and can cause irregular bleeding, making it hard to stop the bleeding when needed. Additional progesterone in the form of norethisterone or medroxyprogesterone acetate can be used on top for short periods.

2.6 Amenorrhoea

Overview

- This is the absence of menstruation.
- It can be normal, such as during puberty, pregnancy, lactation and post menopause.
- It is pathological when someone has not menstruated for at least 3 cycles or for more than 6 months. It occurs in about 3–4% of women.
- Prolonged amenorrhoea associated with oestrogen deficiency can increase the risk of osteoporosis/fractures and cardiovascular disease.
- Amenorrhoea causes anovulatory cycles and can impact fertility.
- Amenorrhoea can cause psychological distress due to altered self-image and loss of self-esteem. Many women have concerns about loss of fertility, loss of femininity or unwanted pregnancy. The diagnosis of some underlying conditions, e.g. developmental delay, can be traumatic.

Classification

- **Primary amenorrhoea:** this is when no periods have started by the age of 15 with normal secondary sex characteristics, or by age 13 without secondary sex characteristics.
- **Secondary amenorrhoea:** cessation of periods for more than 3 cycles or >6 months after established menstruation.

Causes

- Pregnancy: always needs to be excluded.
- Hypothalamic amenorrhoea: triggered by eating disorders, stress, weight loss, excessive exercise.
- Pituitary causes: prolactinoma.
- Ovarian causes: premature ovarian insufficiency (POI), PCOS.
- Uterine causes: Asherman's syndrome (scarring or adhesions in the uterus that can affect menstruation, fertility and pregnancy). Outflow tract obstructions.
- Genetic and congenital conditions.

Investigations

- History:

  - For **primary amenorrhoea** ask about:
    - pubertal development, sexual history and contraception, past medical history and family history
    - for prolactinoma – headaches, visual disturbance or galactorrhoea
    - for hypothalamic amenorrhoea – lifestyle factors such as stress, exercise, depression, body mass index (BMI)
    - for Kallmann's syndrome – anosmia
  - For **secondary amenorrhoea** ask about:
    - contraception use, plus thyroid and other endocrine issues and past medical history and family history
    - for POI – hot flushes and vaginal dryness
    - for prolactinoma – headaches, visual disturbance, galactorrhoea
    - for PCOS – acne, hirsutism, weight gain
    - for hypothalamic amenorrhoea – stress, depression, weight loss/gain, exercise levels
    - medication for drugs that increase prolactin, e.g. antipsychotics; illicit drug use, e.g. cocaine or opioids which can cause hypogonadism.
- Pregnancy test, FSH, LH, estradiol, TSH, prolactin, total testosterone, coeliac screen.
- Pelvic ultrasound if PCOS or Asherman's syndrome suspected.
- Magnetic resonance imaging (MRI) pituitary if hyperprolactinaemia.

Management

- For primary amenorrhoea:
  - Refer to secondary care for specialist investigations and management.
  - Refer girls with no menstruation by age 15, with normal secondary sexual characteristics or no menstruation by the age of 13 and no signs of secondary sexual characteristics.
  - Refer to a gynaecologist with a specialist interest in adolescent gynaecology or paediatric endocrinologist if any developmental, thyroid or excess androgen issues.
- For secondary amenorrhoea refer to gynaecology:
  - Elevated FSH and LH levels (and <40 years of age to consider a diagnosis of POI).
  - Recent history of uterine or cervical surgery, or severe pelvic infection.
  - Infertility.
  - Suspected PCOS where the diagnosis is unclear or where there are complications that cannot be managed in primary care.
- For secondary amenorrhoea refer to endocrinology:
  - Hyperprolactinaemia.
  - Low FSH and LH.
  - An increased testosterone level not explained by PCOS.
  - Features of Cushing's syndrome or late-onset congenital adrenal hyperplasia.
- Women with secondary amenorrhoea due to PCOS, hypothyroidism, menopause or pregnancy should be managed in primary care, where appropriate.
- Amenorrhoea caused by weight loss, excessive exercise, stress or chronic illness may be managed in primary care after an endocrinologist has assessed and excluded other hypothalamic or pituitary causes (such as a tumour). However, if an eating disorder is suspected, a prompt referral should be made to an age-appropriate community eating disorders service.
- Consider bone protection when the amenorrhoea has been ongoing >6 months in a woman with osteoporosis risk factors; >12 months in otherwise healthy young women; and anyone with POI. HRT/COCP is considered first-line treatment for osteoporosis for women under the age of 60 before bisphosphonates. Also discuss lifestyle measures such as weight-bearing exercise, adequate calcium intake, vitamin D supplementation, smoking cessation and limiting alcohol.

2.6.1 Relative energy deficiency in sport (RED-S)

- RED-S is a syndrome resulting from insufficient energy intake relative to the demands of exercise, affecting multiple body systems that can impact female (and male) athletes.
- It was previously known as female athlete triad – amenorrhoea, low energy availability and osteoporosis. RED-S reflects the wider impacts this condition can have on impaired metabolic rate, menstrual function, bone health, immunity, protein synthesis, cardiovascular health and psychological health.
- It can affect exercisers of any activity, age group or level of competition.

Pathophysiology

- The core problem is low energy availability (energy intake minus exercise energy expenditure), leading the body to downregulate non-essential functions to conserve energy.

Prevalence

- It is common in sports emphasising leanness (e.g. running, gymnastics, cycling) but can occur across all levels of activity. Studies suggest up to 45% of female athletes may be at risk.

Diagnosis

- No single test confirms RED-S; it is a clinical diagnosis based on symptoms, energy imbalance, and exclusion of other causes.
- History: ask about menstrual irregularities (amenorrhoea, oligomenorrhoea), recurrent injuries (stress fractures), gastrointestinal symptoms, fatigue, reduced performance, disordered eating behaviours.
- Physical examination: low BMI or unexpected weight loss, signs of hormonal deficiency, bone tenderness or fracture history.
- Investigations: FBC, urea and electrolytes (U&Es), liver function tests (LFTs), ferritin, thyroid function tests, prolactin, estradiol, FSH, LH, vitamin D, bone density scan (dual-energy X-ray absorptiometry; DEXA) if stress fractures or amenorrhoea >6 months, electrocardiogram (ECG) if bradycardia suspected.

Management

Multidisciplinary approach required, involving GP, dietitian, sports physician, psychologist/psychiatrist as necessary.

Key principles

- Energy restoration: increase caloric intake and reduce exercise intensity if necessary.
- Nutritional counselling: focus on balanced diet rich in calcium and vitamin D.
- Menstrual health: monitor for resumption of periods; hormonal contraception should not be used solely to induce withdrawal bleeds, because it masks underlying energy issues.
- Bone health: supplement vitamin D and calcium and consider bisphosphonates in severe osteoporosis under specialist advice.
- Psychological support: address disordered eating and body image issues, using cognitive behavioural therapy (CBT) if needed.
- Monitoring: regular menstrual tracking and repeat DEXA scanning annually in severe cases.
- Return to sport: guided by symptom resolution and energy balance restoration. RED-S CAT provides a framework (see https://bjsm.bmj.com/content/bjsports/49/7/421.full.pdf) to grade risk and guide safe return-to-play decisions.
- For more information direct to RED-S website, https://red-s.com.

2.7 Endometriosis and adenomyosis

2.7.1 Endometriosis

- Endometriosis is a chronic systemic inflammatory condition where tissue similar to endometrial tissue is found outside of the uterus and can cause damage to surrounding areas. It is a condition where there is no cure, and the cause is still unknown.
- It can be found in the pelvis around the outside of the uterus, ovaries, fallopian tubes, bowels, bladder and rarely in surgical scars, umbilicus, diaphragm or the lungs.
- Endometriosis is a long-term condition that has significant physical, psychological, sexual and social impacts. It can also impact fertility. This makes it an important condition not to miss.
- 1 in 10 women will be diagnosed with endometriosis, which is similar to the prevalence of diabetes – which shows how common it can be. However, unlike diabetes there are long delays in establishing a diagnosis of endometriosis, with the average wait being 7–9 years. Vague and variable symptoms that overlap with other conditions, lack of specific tests, limited expertise in some healthcare professionals, long NHS waiting times and dismissal of symptoms and normalisation of pain have been put forward as some of the reasons for the delay.
- The exact cause of endometriosis is still unknown, but a combination of several factors may be implicated, such as retrograde menstruation, genetic predisposition, lymphatic or circulatory spread, immune dysfunction, environmental causes and metaplasia. More research is needed in this area.

Symptoms

- You should suspect endometriosis in women and girls under the age of 17 who have one or more of the following symptoms:
  - chronic pelvic pain that can radiate to back and thighs
  - period-related pain (dysmenorrhoea) affecting daily activities and quality of life
  - deep pain during or after sexual intercourse
  - period-related or cyclical gastrointestinal symptoms, in particular, painful bowel movements (dyschezia)
  - period-related or cyclical urinary symptoms; in particular, blood in the urine or pain passing urine
  - infertility in association with one or more of the above.
- However, they may have multiple other symptoms associated with the pain, such as fatigue, nausea, vomiting, bloating and heavy, prolonged periods and/or irregular periods. Rare symptoms may include shoulder tip pain, cyclical cough, haemoptysis, chest pain and cyclical scar swelling/pain.
- Pain and symptoms diaries (such as the one in the endometriosis tool kit from www.menstrualhealthproject.org.uk) can really help diagnose and aid discussions with doctors.

Diagnosis

- It can be hard to diagnose endometriosis in primary care because there are no simple blood tests, and it does not always show up on pelvic ultrasound scans. The symptoms can also overlap with other conditions such as irritable bowel syndrome, chronic cystitis, pelvic inflammatory disease, adenomyosis, ovarian cysts, fibromyalgia or other musculoskeletal or neuropathic pain syndromes.
- Pelvic and abdominal exams can be offered to identify abdominal masses and pelvic signs, such as reduced organ mobility and enlargement, tender nodularity in the posterior vaginal fornix, and visible vaginal endometriotic lesions.
- Clinical suspicion from cyclical pain with any positive findings on exam and the impact the symptoms have on a woman's life should prompt a referral to an endometriosis clinic.

- Pelvic ultrasound scans can be of limited value for diagnosis but can pick up cysts on the ovaries (endometriomas) and should be done to rule out other causes of pain.
- Pelvic MRI scans may be of more benefit for more extensive disease but are done in secondary care. It is important to note that a normal scan does not rule out the diagnosis.
- The gold standard for diagnosing endometriosis and treating at the same time is a diagnostic laparoscopy.

Management

- There is no cure for endometriosis and the treatments and surgery are there to reduce the severity of the symptoms and improve quality of life for women living with the condition.
- For first-line management of pain in endometriosis are NSAIDs and/or paracetamol, and these are advised for 3 months. If this is not effective, then for moderate–severe pain consider alternative analgesia including codeine, dihydrocodeine or tramadol. For severe pain consider morphine, oxycodone, buprenorphine or fentanyl. In some cases, the endometriotic patches may infiltrate nerve endings and so neuropathic painkillers may be helpful. If pain is difficult to manage then consider an early referral to a pain management clinic whilst trying different medication.
- COCPs or POPs can be used to manage the symptoms of endometriosis by preventing bleeding and ovulation, and they can also reduce pain. Combined hormonal contraception (CHC) pills can be used continuously in a tailored regime, off-licence, without the pill-free breaks. Progesterone can suppress the growth of the endometrial tissue and reduce inflammation. Oral hormonal contraceptives, implant (IMP), depot medroxyprogesterone acetate (DMPA) or the 52mg LNG-IUDs can be used. Dydrogesterone (Nalvee 10mg) has recently been licensed for endometriosis pain management.
- If these hormonal treatments are not effective, then referral to an endometriosis clinic is recommended.
  - This is where additional hormonal treatments such as GnRH agonist injections may be used. These treatments act on the pituitary gland to suppress oestrogen and progesterone production from the ovaries. While they are being taken, they can induce a temporary menopause. They may be used for short periods to suppress pain and inflammation prior to surgery. Add-back HRT can be given alongside, to prevent or reduce side-effects associated with the menopause, if needed, making treatment more tolerable.
  - Oral GnRH antagonists approved by the Medicines and Healthcare products Regulatory Agency (MHRA) are now available. These can help to manage the pain and some of the other symptoms associated with endometriosis and can also be used to reduce heavy bleeding related to uterine fibroids. Some formulations are now available combined with oestrogen and a progestogen (HRT). These treatments offer greater convenience and flexibility compared to injectable forms of GnRH agonists. This is the direction in which management of endometriosis is now moving.
- Surgical procedures used in endometriosis include diagnostic laparoscopies, where the endometrial tissue is excised or ablation is used. Sometimes further surgery, such as hysterectomy with bilateral oophorectomy, may be needed depending on the severity of the symptoms. Post surgery, hormonal treatments as above may be used to prolong the effects of the surgery.
- Those with extensive disease, such as on the bladder or bowel, will need referral to a specialist endometriosis clinic, where they will have access to a gynaecologist, nurse specialist, bowel surgeon, bladder surgeon and pain management specialist in the same clinic.
- Most women with endometriosis will be able to conceive naturally, but those who are struggling or experience a delay should be referred to a multidisciplinary clinic where there is input from a fertility specialist and access to fertility treatments.

2.7.2 Adenomyosis

- Adenomyosis occurs when endometrial tissue is found within the uterine myometrium.
- No clear cause is known. It is a benign condition but can cause troublesome symptoms in some women, such as pain and HMB.
- It affects 15% of women in their 40s to 50s, and 15% of cases will also have endometriosis present.
- It often coexists with HMB, dysmenorrhoea and dyspareunia of other aetiology. There may be some problems associated with fertility in some cases.
- Some women have no symptoms, and it is sometimes just picked up on a pelvic scan.

Diagnosis

- Pelvic ultrasound or MRI. On the scan you can usually see an enlarged uterus with a thickened myometrium containing glandular irregularities.
- A diagnosis can only be confirmed histologically after a hysterectomy.

Management

- Treatment depends on the type and severity of the symptoms.
- Use simple analgesia such as NSAIDs/paracetamol to manage pain initially, or stronger analgesia if this does not help. Tranexamic acid may help reduce heavy bleeding.
- A 52mg LNG-IUD is usually the first-line treatment. Other options include combined contraceptive pills / patches or POPs.
- Hormonal therapy with GnRH analogues may relieve symptoms prior to considering surgery.
- Uterine artery embolisation can be considered, but fertility may be affected.
- An abdominal or vaginal hysterectomy is usually recommended if symptoms persist.

2.8 Fibroids

Overview

- Uterine fibroids (leiomyoma) are benign uterine tumours. They are caused by a proliferation of smooth muscle cells and fibroblasts that form hard, round, whorled tumours in the wall of the uterus.
- They can be single or multiple and vary in size, ranging from a few mm up to 30cm.
- They occur in women of reproductive age because growth of the fibroid is related to oestrogen and progesterone.
- Risk factors associated with fibroids are increasing age, early menarche, nulliparity, older age at first pregnancy and obesity/diabetes/hypertension. They occur more frequently in women from black and Asian backgrounds or in those with a first-degree relative with fibroids.
- They can grow anywhere in the endometrium and can be classified as:
    - **submucosal** – extend into the uterine cavity and cause heavy bleeding, pain and fertility issues
    - **intramural** – remain within the wall of the uterus and cause pain or heavy bleeding
    - **subserosal** – protrude from the uterus externally and are usually asymptomatic. This type are only symptomatic when large, due to pressure symptoms on adjacent structures.

Symptoms

- Fibroids can cause heavy menstrual bleeding, which can be severe and lead to iron-deficiency anaemia.
- Dysmenorrhoea, back and pelvic pain and dyspareunia which may impact sexual function.
- Depending on the size of the fibroid, some women may have pressure symptoms on nearby structures such as the bladder, causing recurrent urine infections, urinary frequency, urinary retention and hydronephrosis. If there is pressure on the bowel, this can cause bloating and constipation.
- Infertility may occur if the fibroid distorts the uterine cavity and interferes with implantation.

- Problems during pregnancy and delivery – rarely causes miscarriages, fibroid vascular infarction (acute pain following rapid growth of a fibroid), fetal malpresentation, higher risk of caesarean delivery and preterm delivery.
- Rarely torsion of a pedunculated fibroid.
- Haemoperitoneum – from rupture of a fibroid or a blood vessel overlying it.

Diagnosis

- On abdominal or pelvic exam, a large, firm, irregular, non-tender mass may be felt on the uterus or in the lower abdomen.
- Transvaginal ultrasound can help to diagnose the number, size, location and type of fibroids.
- FBC and ferritin if iron deficiency is suspected in cases of HMB.

Management

- If the fibroids are confirmed by ultrasound scan and are asymptomatic, they do not require treatment or follow-up. Offer review if any symptoms change or there are new symptoms.
- For symptomatic fibroids, medical management involves the use of NSAIDs and tranexamic acid or cyclical progesterone or hormonal contraception to manage pain and heavy bleeding. An LNG-IUD is also recommended.
- If symptoms are not well controlled, fibroids are growing rapidly, fertility is impacted or if fibroids are >3cm, then consider referral to a gynaecology clinic for further management such as GnRH analogues for preoperative size reduction. There are also newer oral GnRH antagonists that can be used to shrink fibroids.
- The selective progesterone receptor modulator ulipristal acetate has been granted restricted use for intermittent treatment of moderate–severe symptoms before menopause, if unsuitable for surgery or uterine artery embolisation.
- Surgical options include myomectomy, endometrial ablation, uterine artery embolisation, hysterectomy.
- Direct women towards the British Fibroid Trust for more information (www.britishfibroidtrust.org.uk).

2.9 Polycystic ovary syndrome

Overview

- Polycystic ovary syndrome (PCOS) is a common endocrine disorder affecting reproductive-aged women and is diagnosed using the Rotterdam criteria which require two out of three of the following diagnostic criteria:
  - hyperandrogenism with clinical features such as acne and hirsutism or high testosterone on a blood test
  - ovulation disorder that presents as oligomenorrhoea or amenorrhoea
  - polycystic ovaries on ultrasound scanning.
- Due to the different combinations of diagnostic criteria there are different phenotypes that can arise: phenotype A, with all three criteria; phenotype B, with hyperandrogenism and ovulatory dysfunction but normal ovaries on the scan; phenotype C, with hyperandrogenism, polycystic ovaries but regular cycles; and phenotype D, with ovulatory dysfunction, polycystic ovaries and no hyperandrogenism. It is best to think of PCOS as a spectrum and not discrete diseases, as phenotypes can change over time, e.g. with age, weight, treatments.
- However, in adolescents and younger patients, caution is advised before making this diagnosis. During the years following menarche, features such as irregular cycles and multifollicular ovaries can be physiological, making early diagnosis challenging. Therefore, a diagnosis of PCOS should not be based on ultrasound findings alone in those who have not yet reached reproductive maturity (typically within 8 years post-menarche). In this group,

clinical and biochemical features should guide assessment, and a cautious, symptom-focused approach to management is recommended.

- The cause is unknown and likely to be multifactorial, with both genetic and environmental factors playing a part. The prevalence can vary but it is thought to affect 1 in 10 women, and 50% may not have any symptoms.
- It is related to abnormal hormone levels in the body, including high levels of insulin.
- Many women with PCOS are resistant to the actions of insulin and so the body produces higher levels (hyperinsulinaemia) to overcome this.
- 65–80% of women with PCOS will have insulin resistance. Insulin resistance can affect body fat, by promoting fat storage and making fat loss more difficult, particularly around the abdomen. This can lead to further raised levels of insulin and weight gain.
- The hyperinsulinaemia can lead to reduced production of SHBG in the liver. SHBG is a protein that binds to testosterone, making it inactive. With a lower level of SHBG, more unbound active testosterone is available in the blood, even though the total testosterone levels may be normal or just moderately raised.
- The high insulin levels also increase androgen production, which stops follicular development and causes anovulation. This can lead to menstrual disturbances as well as clinical symptoms such as acne and hirsutism.
- Serum LH levels are raised in 40% of women with PCOS and when they rise above the FSH levels, the ovaries tend to produce more androgens than oestrogen.
- Women with PCOS may also have high levels of oestrogen, because the ovaries continue to produce oestrogen despite no ovulation. The unopposed oestrogen can cause the endometrial lining to develop hyperplasia, especially if the interval between periods is more than 3 months.
- Prolactin levels can be raised in some women with PCOS.
- Due to the hormonal changes, women with PCOS are at risk of:
  - type 2 diabetes mellitus (T2DM), hypertension and high cholesterol leading to heart disease
  - depression and anxiety disorders due to the symptoms of the condition
  - sleep apnoea due to excess weight
  - non-alcoholic fatty liver disease due to excess androgens
  - they may also be at risk of endometrial cancer due to the very irregular periods and continued oestrogen production.

Symptoms

Symptoms can vary from very mild to symptoms of severe hyperandrogenism and menstrual disturbances. They usually start in the late teens or early 20s.

- Irregular periods or amenorrhoea.
- Hirsutism on the face, chest, back or buttocks.
- Acne or oily skin.
- Weight gain.
- Thinning hair or hair loss from the head.
- Difficulty getting pregnant due to the irregular cycles or no ovulation.

Investigations

Blood tests should be undertaken once the patient has been off all hormonal contraception for at least 6 weeks.

- Testosterone can be normal or moderately raised.
- SHBG can be low or normal.
- LH/FSH – LH can be raised and is usually higher than FSH.
- TSH – should be normal, but if abnormal consider hypothyroidism as the diagnosis.
- Prolactin – may be mildly elevated.
- Screen for diabetes/heart disease – check HbA1c, lipids, BMI, blood pressure (BP), smoking status.

- Pelvic ultrasound – 20 or more follicles in one ovary or ovarian volume of >10cm. Note that polycystic ovaries do not have to be found on the scan to make the diagnosis, and finding polycystic ovaries on the scan does not confirm the diagnosis. 20–30% of women just have an incidental finding of polycystic ovaries on scan with no hormonal changes or symptoms, and they do not need any treatment.

Management

PCOS is a chronic condition that has no cure, and the aim of treatment is to manage the symptoms and reduce the risk of T2DM and heart disease.

- Lifestyle modification for weight loss. Weight loss of just 5% can lead to significant improvements in PCOS.
- COCP or LNG-IUS for cycle regulation and reducing the risk of endometrial cancer, especially if there is amenorrhoea of >3 months.
- Consider gynaecology referral if there are any suspicious symptoms or endometrial thickening, or no response to treatments.
- For acne consider topical retinoids, topical antibiotics and/or oral antibiotics. Consider oral contraceptive pills to help with acne.
- For excess hair, contraceptive pills may help or offer eflornithine cream to slow down the growth of unwanted facial hair (note that this may not be available on the NHS in some places). Some women opt for laser hair removal, and this may be available in some parts of the UK on the NHS. Other options include anti-androgens such as spironolactone or minoxidil for scalp hair loss.
- Referral to an endocrinologist to consider metformin for insulin resistance and in those women with a BMI of >25 (off-licence use); it may also be used when trying to get pregnant. If not considering pregnancy, then contraception must be used.
- There is not enough evidence to recommend the use of inositol supplements.
- Referral for fertility planning – consider early referral and clomiphene to increase ovulation; laparoscopic ovarian drilling may be recommended to destroy the tissue in the ovaries that produces excess androgens. Occasionally other drugs such as letrozole or gonadotrophins may be used, which may overstimulate the ovaries. If these do not work, then *in vitro* fertilisation (IVF) will be offered.
- Direct women towards support groups for women with PCOS:
  - PCOS Challenge: the National Polycystic Ovary Syndrome Association (https://pcoschallenge.org)
  - Verity (www.verity-pcos.org.uk).

2.10 Conclusion

Healthcare professionals have a critical role in menstrual health through early recognition, patient education and appropriate referral. They should:

- Provide a safe, non-judgemental space to discuss menstrual concerns and reassure women they have been heard, and their symptoms are taken seriously.
- Encourage period tracking to assist diagnosis and pick up changes to their normal cycles.
- Offer evidence-based treatments and shared decision-making.
- Look out for red flags that may need referral such as intermenstrual or postcoital bleeding, postmenopausal bleeding, persistent pelvic pain or masses, suspicion of malignancy or complex endocrine pathology.
- Ask about the impact on sexual function and refer appropriately.
- Liaise with secondary care where appropriate and refer if symptoms persist despite medical treatments.

2.11 Further reading

Bupa (2024) *The Bupa Wellbeing Index 2024: the impact of stigmas to women's health*. Available at: www.bupa.co.uk/~/media/Files/MMS/cli-03158.pdf

NHS (reviewed 2022) *Irregular periods*. Available at: www.nhs.uk/conditions/irregular-periods

NHS England (updated 2023) *Making a decision about: managing heavy periods*. Available at: www.england.nhs.uk/wp-content/uploads/2023/11/PRN00250-dst-making-a-decision-about-heavy-preiods.pdf

NHS Specialist Pharmacy Service (updated 2025) *Delaying periods*. Available at: www.sps.nhs.uk/articles/choosing-a-medicine-to-delay-periods

NICE (updated 2021) *Heavy menstrual bleeding* [NG88]. Available at: www.nice.org.uk/guidance/ng88

NICE (revised 2023) *CKS: Dysmenorrhoea*. Available at: https://cks.nice.org.uk/topics/dysmenorrhoea

NICE (revised 2023) *CKS: Fibroids*. Available at: https://cks.nice.org.uk/topics/fibroids

NICE (revised 2024) *CKS: Amenorrhoea*. Available at: https://cks.nice.org.uk/topics/amenorrhoea

NICE (updated 2024) *Endometriosis* [NG73]. Available at: www.nice.org.uk/guidance/NG73

NICE (revised 2025) *CKS: Polycystic ovary syndrome*. Available at: https://cks.nice.org.uk/topics/polycystic-ovary-syndrome

Menstrual Health Project (2025) *Endometriosis diagnostic toolkit* (including pain and symptoms journal for patients). Available at: https://menstrualhealthproject.org.uk/toolkits/endometriosis-diagnosis-toolkit

Mountjoy, M., Sundgot-Borgen, J., Burke, L. *et al.* (2015) RED-S CAT: relative energy deficiency in sport (RED-S) clinical assessment tool (CAT). *Br J Sports Med*, **49**: 421–3. Available at: https://bjsm.bmj.com/content/bjsports/49/7/421.full.pdf

Mountjoy, M., Ackerman, K.E., Bailey, D.M. *et al.* (2023) 2023 International Olympic Committee's (IOC) consensus statement on Relative Energy Deficiency in Sport (REDs). *Br J Sports Med*, 57(17); erratum in 58(3). Available at: https://bjsm.bmj.com/content/57/17/1073

RCOG Patient information leaflets: www.rcog.org.uk/for-the-public/browse-our-patient-information

RED-S website: https://red-s.com

Teede, H., Tay, C.T., Laven, J. *et al.* (2023) *International evidence-based guideline for the assessment and management of polycystic ovary syndrome 2023*. Available at: www.monash.edu/__data/assets/pdf_file/0003/3379521/Evidence-Based-Guidelines-2023.pdf

Women and Equalities Committee (2024) *Women's Reproductive Health Conditions*. Available at: https://publications.parliament.uk/pa/cm5901/cmselect/cmwomeq/337/report.html

Chapter 3
Contraception

Access the UKMEC 2025 either by scanning the QR code above, or visiting www.cosrh.org/Common/Uploaded%20files/documents/UKMEC_2025.pdf

3.1 Introduction

Being able to make a conscious decision on whether and when to have children is important to women. It is essential for all women to have access to a full range of contraceptive methods and sexual and reproductive health services throughout their lives. They need to be provided with clear advice about which contraceptive methods are suitable for them, considering efficacy, non-contraceptive benefits, risks and possible side-effects.

3.1.1 Methods of contraception

These are the contraceptive methods available in the UK:

- Emergency contraception (EC) includes the copper IUD (Cu-IUD) and oral hormonal emergency contraceptives.
- Combined hormonal contraception (CHC) includes pills (COCP), transdermal patches (CTP) and vaginal rings (CVR).
- Progestogen-only pills (POP).
- Progestogen-only injectables (DMPA).
- Progestogen implants (IMP).
- Copper intrauterine contraceptives (Cu-IUD).
- Levonorgestrel intrauterine devices (LNG-IUD, formerly known as the intrauterine system or IUS).
- Diaphragms, cervical caps.
- Male and female condoms.
- Natural fertility awareness.
- Male and female sterilisation.

3.1.2 UK Medical Eligibility Criteria for Contraceptive Use (UKMEC) 2025

- The UKMEC helps health professionals by providing guidance on the safety of contraceptive methods, using medical conditions and patient characteristics.
- It does not address the use of contraceptives for non-contraceptive benefits or consider how effective the contraceptive methods are. Clinical judgement is also required, particularly when prescribing for women with multiple medical and social factors.
- It includes four risk categories (see *Table 3.1*), which are applicable to each contraceptive method. Initiation (I) of a method is sometimes classified differently to continuation (C) of the method.
- The UKMEC was updated in 2025. The UKMEC 2025 supersedes the third edition of the UKMEC in 2016 (updated in 2019).
- Multiple topics were reviewed and a summary of the UKMEC 2025 key changes can be found at: www.cosrh.org/Common/Uploaded%20files/documents/UKMEC_2025_Summary_Tables.pdf
- Changes include:
  - Caution / apply clinical judgement if there are multiple risk factors (>1 risk factor) for a condition such as VTE or cardiovascular disease (CVD), or if there are multiple UKMEC 2 or 3 conditions affecting the same risk.
  - The addition of new conditions: multiple sclerosis, chronic kidney disease and sickle cell trait.
  - Some conditions have been updated: evidence shows an increased risk of VTE with DMPA use in the general population; this evidence has been applied to the MEC and some conditions have changed category to reflect the increase in clot risk; anxiety and 'mood disorders' has replaced 'depression'.
  - Other changes include: clarification around use of e-cigarettes; the addition of NICE classification of blood pressure (BP); a change in the definition of past/current breast cancer; the addition of high-risk human papillomavirus (HPV) to cervical intraepithelial neoplasia (CIN) and updates in sexually transmitted infections (STI) and HIV.

Table 3.1: UKMEC risk categories and their definitions

UKMEC Category	Definition	Do you recommend this?
1	A condition where there is no restriction for use of the method.	Yes
2	A condition where the advantages of using the method generally outweigh the theoretical or proven risks.	Probably yes
3	A condition where the theoretical or proven risks usually outweigh the advantages of using the method. The provision of a method requires expert clinical judgement and/or referral to a specialist contraceptive provider, since the use of the method is not usually recommended, unless other more appropriate methods are not available or not acceptable.	Probably not
4	A condition which represents an unacceptable health risk if the method is used.	No

Adapted from the UK Medical Eligibility Criteria for Contraceptive Use (UKMEC 2025) © The College of Sexual & Reproductive Healthcare 2025.

Example of UKMEC

- If a patient is seeking advice about a contraceptive method and has a history of headache and migraine attacks, which contraceptive methods can you safely consider, and how can the UKMEC help you to decide?
- *Table 3.2* shows an example. All contraceptive methods in all categories of headache or migraine, as shown in the left-hand column of the table, are a UKMEC 1 or 2 (where the advantages of using them generally outweigh any risks), except the CHC methods. The CHC methods are a UKMEC 1, 2, 3 or 4 depending upon the type of headache or migraine, and whether the method is being initiated (I) or continued (C).
- If a woman develops migraine without aura whilst she is using CHC, continuation of the CHC method becomes a UKMEC 3 (a condition where the risks usually outweigh the advantages), so all other safer methods should be considered.
- If a woman has migraine with aura, use of CHC would be a UKMEC 4. This would represent an unacceptable health risk, and another safer method should be used.

Table 3.2: An example of use of the UKMEC from the summary table (amended September 2019) to guide contraceptive choice in a patient with migraine

<table>
<tr><th>Headaches</th><th>Cu-IUD</th><th>LNG-IUD</th><th>IMP</th><th>DMPA</th><th colspan="2">POP</th><th colspan="2">CHC</th></tr>
<tr><td rowspan="2">Non-migrainous</td><td rowspan="2">1</td><td rowspan="2">1</td><td rowspan="2">1</td><td rowspan="2">1</td><td colspan="2" rowspan="2">1</td><td>I</td><td>C</td></tr>
<tr><td>1</td><td>2</td></tr>
<tr><td rowspan="2">Migraine without aura at any age</td><td rowspan="2">1</td><td rowspan="2">2</td><td rowspan="2">2</td><td rowspan="2">2</td><td>I</td><td>C</td><td>I</td><td>C</td></tr>
<tr><td>1</td><td>2</td><td>2</td><td>3</td></tr>
<tr><td>Migraine with aura at any age</td><td>1</td><td>2</td><td>2</td><td>2</td><td colspan="2">2</td><td colspan="2">4</td></tr>
<tr><td>History (≥5 years ago) of migraine with aura, at any age</td><td>1</td><td>2</td><td>2</td><td>2</td><td colspan="2">2</td><td colspan="2">3</td></tr>
</table>

Reproduced under licence from CoSRH 2025.

The UKMEC can be found on the CoSRH website in two useful resources: the UKMEC full book and the UKMEC summary table (see www.cosrh.org/Public/Standards-and-Guidance/uk-medical-eligibility-criteria-for-contraceptive-use-ukmec.aspx).

3.1.3 Effectiveness of contraceptive methods

The effectiveness of each method of contraception varies, as shown in *Table 3.3*.

Table 3.3: Percentage of women experiencing an unintended pregnancy within the first year of use

Method of contraception	Typical use	Perfect use
No method	85%	85%
Implant	0.1%	0.1%
LNG-IUD	0.1–0.4%	0.3%
Cu-IUD	0.8%	0.6%
Progesterone-only injectable (DMPA)	4%	0.2%
Combined hormonal pill, patch or vaginal ring	7%	0.3%
Progestogen-only pill	7%	0.3%
Female diaphragm plus spermicide	17%	16%
Male condom	13%	2%
Fertility awareness methods	2–23%	0.4–5.0%
Female sterilisation	0.5%	0.5%
Vasectomy	0.15%	0.1%

Information adapted from UKMEC 2025 at www.cosrh.org/Common/Uploaded%20files/documents/UKMEC_2025.pdf

3.2 The contraceptive consultation

- Educating and empowering women to choose the most acceptable and suitable method of contraception for their lifestyle should increase the chances of ongoing and correct use of the method. Use an empathetic, non-judgemental, shared decision-making approach, ascertaining the woman's ideas, concerns and expectations.
- Ideally, explore what the patient wants from her contraception while you take the contraceptive history (see *Table 3.4* and *Section 3.2.4*).

3.2.1 Taking a contraception history

It is important to take a detailed history to ensure safe, effective prescribing of all contraceptive methods.

Table 3.4: Medical history-taking in a contraceptive consultation

Age	For contraceptive purposes some methods of contraception should be stopped at 50 years, for example CHC and injectable contraceptives
Consent	Consider 'Gillick competence' for those aged <16, and safeguarding / issues and consent for all women (*see Section 13.1*)
Menstrual cycle details	Last menstrual period (was it normal?) Length and regularity of cycles (longest and shortest) IMB or PCB, their frequency, duration and associated symptoms, such as pain HMB Dysmenorrhoea

Table 3.4 *cont'd*	
History of gynaecological conditions	Such as ovarian cysts, endometriosis, adenomyosis, pelvic infection
Cervical screening history	If appropriate
Obstetric history	Previous pregnancies – planned and unplanned Number of children, mode of delivery, problems during pregnancy or delivery Breastfeeding history Miscarriages, pregnancy terminations, ectopic pregnancies
Sexual history	Any sexual problems Symptoms of STI, including change in vaginal discharge, dysuria, abdominal pain, skin changes or rash; suggest screening if risk factors are present Do not assume that if someone has a stable partner, they do not also have other partners; questions can include: *"How many sexual partners have you had in the last year?"* *"Do you use condoms – always, sometimes or never?"*
Past medical history (not an exhaustive list)	Epilepsy, diabetes, hypertension, CVD, VTE, cerebrovascular disease, migraine ± aura, gynaecological or non-gynaecological cancers
History of mental health problems	Can include previous mood change with hormonal contraceptives, history of postnatal depression (PND) or PMS, so caution can be taken with choice of contraception Refer to *Chapter 8* Refer to the National Association for Premenstrual Syndromes (NAPS) Guidelines on premenstrual syndrome: www.pms.org.uk/app/uploads/2018/06/guidelinesfinal60210.pdf
Medication	Include: • liver enzyme inducers • weight loss injections, such as GLP-1 agonists • herbal remedies / over-the-counter (OTC) medications, such as St John's Wort
Family history (include age at diagnosis)	Myocardial infarction (MI) Cardiovascular event (CVE) VTE Breast cancer and ovarian cancer (referral to secondary care or for genetic screening may be required, depending upon the family history) • Breast cancer family history: refer to NICE guidance CG164 • Ovarian cancer family history: refer to NICE guideline NG241 • NICE recommends that those with first-degree relative with ovarian cancer and/or a second-degree relative with ovarian cancer should be referred to genetic services who will assess eligibility for genetic testing
Check allergies	Lactose: all combined oral contraceptives (COCs) and POPs contain lactose (usually only a problem with severe lactose intolerance) Peanuts: some desogestrel (DSG) POPs contain soya bean oil and may cause cross-reaction in individuals allergic to peanuts (see https://bnf.nice.org.uk/drugs/desogestrel) The brand Cerelle does not contain soya bean oil

cont'd

Table 3.4 *cont'd*

Social history	Smoking – cigarettes per week, use of e-cigarettes Alcohol use – per week Domestic violence Female genital mutilation Religious and/or cultural beliefs that may affect contraceptive choice
Explore other concerns; apart from preventing a pregnancy, what else does she want from her contraception?	These are examples: • Does she want to have regular periods or no periods? • Lighter or less painful periods? • Less acne? • Less premenstrual syndrome (PMS)

3.2.2 Assessing competence – Fraser guidelines and Gillick competency

- When deciding if a child is mature enough to make their own decisions about matters that affect them, practitioners often refer to whether the child is *Gillick competent* or meets the *Fraser guidelines.*
- Both Gillick competency and the Fraser guidelines come from a 1980s legal case that considered whether doctors could give contraceptive advice or treatment to young people under 16 without their parents' consent.
- The Fraser guidelines continue to apply to advice and treatment about contraception and sexual health. Gillick competency is often used in a wider context to help assess whether a child has the maturity to make their own decisions and fully understand the consequences (see *Section 13.1*).
- The legal age for consent in the UK is 16, but surveys suggest that about 30% of young people have had sex by this age.
- It is legal to advise and supply contraception without parental consent if the child is deemed to be competent to consent. Those under the age of 13 are not considered capable of consenting to sexual activity. Those aged 14 and 15 may be able to consent if competence can be demonstrated.
  - Young people over the age of 16 (including those with a disability) are presumed to be competent to consent to medical treatment including contraception, unless otherwise demonstrated.
  - If they are under the age of 16, competence to consent must be demonstrated. They must have sufficient understanding and maturity to understand what is being proposed and why, and to understand the benefits, risks and alternatives and the consequences of treatment. They must be able to retain the information for long enough to use it and consider it to arrive at a decision. It is considered good practice to follow the Fraser Guidelines. These guidelines advise that the clinician can provide advice and treatment to a young person, if the young person:
    - understands the professional's advice
    - cannot be persuaded to tell their parents or to allow the doctor to tell them
    - is very likely to begin or to continue having sexual intercourse, with or without contraceptive treatment
    - is likely to suffer damage to their physical or mental health unless they receive advice or treatment.
  - The advice or treatment must also be in the person's best interests.
- A confidential sexual health service is essential for the welfare of children and young people.
- Via the NHS app patients have access to their consultations, and when the child is between 11 and 16 parents may be allowed proxy access to their child's online services. Young people

with capacity have the legal right to access their own health records and can allow or prevent access by others, including their parents.

- Managing sensitive information documented during a consultation may result in the need to redact the information so that it remains confidential to the young person. Redacting information may be necessary in other situations, such as in cases of domestic violence or if any information could be harmful to the patient. More information can be found at: www.england.nhs.uk/long-read/redacting-information-for-online-record-access/#:~:text=Individual%20words%2C%20sentences%2C%20or%20paragraphs,such%20as%20post%2Dcoital%20contraception
- When working with young people, consider safeguarding and the possibility of physical, sexual and emotional harm, including coercion and/or exploitation. If a child or young person is involved in abusive or seriously harmful sexual activity, you must act quickly to protect them, by sharing relevant information with appropriate people or agencies, such as the police or social services. You should usually share information about sexual activity involving children under 13, who are considered in law to be unable to consent. If you do not disclose, you should discuss your decision with a named or designated professional or a lead clinician and record your reasons for it.
- Refer to :
  - The CoSRH *Contraceptive Choices for Young People guideline*
  - The General Medical Council (GMC) publication, *0–18 Years: guidance for all doctors.*

3.2.3 Patient information

- There are many myths surrounding contraception, and patients are likely to have questions which should be addressed during the consultation (see *Section 3.2.4* for examples of common questions women may ask).
- It is also helpful to offer patients information to read before and after the consultation to help guide them to make the right choice for them, such as:
  - Brook: Sexual health and wellbeing website (www.brook.org.uk)
  - CoSRH: Contraception choices (www.contraceptionchoices.org).

3.2.4 Common questions asked by patients

These are examples of common questions women may ask, and examples of simple answers.

How do contraceptives work?

- They work in four ways:
  - Block the sperm from reaching the egg, e.g. barrier methods; the POP and LNG-IUDs thicken the cervical mucus.
  - Disable sperm before they reach the egg, e.g. a spermicide, ideally with a barrier method.
  - Suppress ovulation because pregnancy requires an egg and a sperm, e.g. hormonal contraceptives (such as the IMP, CHC, DMPA and some POPs) prevent eggs being released from the ovary.
  - Prevent the fertilised egg from implanting, e.g. the IUDs.

Is it harmful if contraception stops my periods?

- Periods can stop because use of hormonal contraception provides a constant stable level of hormones.
- A menstrual period occurs because of the rise and fall of hormones produced by the brain and the ovary which cause an egg to be released each month and the lining of the womb to become thickened. If you do not become pregnant, that lining is shed as a bleed (a menstrual period), each month. A constant stable level of hormones means ovulation does not occur (the egg is not released), the endometrium (lining of the womb) remains thin

(blood does not build up inside) and consequently there is no regular menstrual period. Future fertility is not affected by this.

Should I take a break from contraception to check my body is still working properly?

- There is no medical need to do this.
- Contraceptives work by suppressing or stopping ovulation and as soon as the contraception is stopped, the body's own natural menstrual cycle can return. Sometimes there is a delay, for example if injectable contraceptives are used there can be a delay in the return to fertility, and it can take several months for ovulation and normal menstrual cycles to resume.

3.2.5 Short-acting and long-acting contraception methods

Short-acting, reversible contraceptives

- CHC methods and POPs which need to be taken regularly.
- Pills must be taken orally, daily, at the same time of day. Combined contraceptive patches are changed weekly and contraceptive rings changed after 3 weeks.

Long-acting, reversible contraceptives (LARC)

- This is a collective term for DMPA, IMP and all types of IUD.
- These are administered every 13 weeks (DMPA), 3 years (IMP) and every 3–10 years for the IUDs depending upon which IUD is used, at what age it is fitted and what its indication for use is. For example, a 52mg LNG-IUD can be used for 5 years for endometrial protection as part of HRT (as recommended by the CoSRH), but if fitted under the age of 45, solely for contraceptive purposes it can be used for up to 8 years.
- LARCs have lower failure rates compared with oral hormonal contraceptive pills.

3.2.6 Examples of questions to ask patients to help contraceptive choice

These questions can help you guide women to some suitable contraceptive options. Safety of prescribing of these options can be considered alongside their medical history and UKMEC guidance.

- *"Are you good at remembering to take something at the same time every day?"*
  - Yes: consider a short-acting method such as a COC or POP.
  - No: consider the CTP or CVR, or a LARC method.
- *"Do you want protection from sexually transmitted infections?"*
  - Yes: add a barrier method alongside another method.
- *"When do you want to think about contraception?"*
  - Only before sex: consider a barrier method, diaphragm or cap.
  - Routinely: consider a short-acting method such as CHC or a POP.
  - Rarely: a LARC may be best.
- *"Are you happy to use hormonal contraceptives?"*
  - Yes: any hormonal method is an option.
  - No: reduces choice to a Cu-IUD, barrier methods, diaphragm or cap, natural fertility methods and sterilisation.
- *"Do you want to control when you have your period?"*
  - Yes: use of the CHC means it is easy to control when a period comes; a period will come when the method is stopped for a break.
- *"Do you want lighter periods or reduced bleeding?"*
  - Yes: CHC, POP, LNG-IUD, DMPA and IMP can all make periods lighter (CHC best if used continuously, although this is off-licence).
  - *Table 3.7* shows expected bleeding patterns in women in the first 3 months, and in the longer term, for different methods. It is important to advise women of the expected

bleeding pattern of their chosen method, as this is a reason many women stop using hormonal contraception.

- *"Do you want to stop your periods completely?"*
  - Yes: some hormonal contraceptive methods can have this effect. About half of users of the DMPA will not have a period after 1 year and amenorrhoea is possible with longer duration use of 52mg LNG-IUDs.
  - Periods can be delayed by continuous use of CHC methods.
- *"Do you want less period pain?"*
  - Yes: CHC, POP, LNG-IUD, DMPA and IMP can reduce period pain.
- *"Do you want less premenstrual syndrome (PMS)?"*
  - Yes: hormonal contraception (CHC, POP, IMP and DMPA) works by levelling out hormones and so can be helpful for reducing PMS.
  - The Royal College of Obstetricians & Gynaecologists (RCOG) Green-top guideline 48 states that some women find using the COCP helps PMS symptoms, and recommends newer generation pills containing drospirenone, as these have been shown to improve PMS symptoms and are considered as first-choice treatments.
- *"Do you want to improve acne?"*
  - Yes: consider a CHC method, ideally a less androgenic 3rd or 4th (new) generation progestogen (see *Section 3.3*), or the drospirenone POP may be helpful.
- *"Are you open to having something fitted inside your womb?"*
  - Yes: a Cu-IUD or an LNG-IUD may be suitable (see *Section 3.8*).
  - No: explore why this is and, if possible, show the types of IUD and try to clarify any misunderstandings they may have.
- *"Are you open to having an implant inserted underneath the skin in your arm?"*
  - Yes: consider IMP.
- *"Are you open to having an injection regularly?"*
  - Yes: consider an injectable method and advise about the possibility of self-administering this; advise about the delayed return to fertility (for up to 12 months).
- *"Do you want the best method for preventing a pregnancy?"*
  - Yes: if an unplanned pregnancy would be a problem, LARC methods are the best options, as they are the most effective.
- *"Might you want to become pregnant soon after stopping a method of contraception?"*
  - Yes: avoid injectable methods because they can delay the return to fertility by up to 12 months.

3.2.7 Starting a contraceptive method

- Refer to the UKMEC and CoSRH website for advice on starting each individual contraceptive method, switching contraceptives, how long the method takes to become effective, and licensing guidance. Ensure there are no allergies.

Options for starting a method include:

- Waiting until the first day of the next period, when the method will be effective immediately.
- Quick-starting contraception involves starting a method of contraception at any time in the cycle the woman requests it, and using additional contraception until the method becomes effective.
  - If pregnancy can be excluded, all methods of contraception can be quick-started.
  - If pregnancy cannot be excluded (and a pregnancy test is negative):
    - Note that pregnancy cannot be excluded until ≥21 days after the last episode of unprotected sexual intercourse.
    - Emergency contraception (EC) may be required.
    - If a woman does not want to delay starting contraception the CHC, POP, DMPA or IMP can be started (DMPA is considered less suitable).
    - A pregnancy test is needed 3 weeks after the method is commenced.

  - The Cu-IUD can be quick-started if indications for EC are met.
  - Quick-starting after using hormonal EC:
    - After using levonorgestrel EC (LNG-EC), the CHC, POP, IMP (and DMPA) can be quick-started immediately.
    - After using ulipristal acetate EC (UPA-EC), wait 120 hours before quick-starting a hormonal contraceptive (to avoid progestogens displacing UPA from the receptor).
    - Consider that ulipristal acetate (UPA) works by binding to progestogen receptors (and recent use of progestogen may reduce the effectiveness of UPA-EC).
- Using a bridging method of contraception:
  - This is where one method of contraception is used short-term, until the chosen method can be provided, e.g. the use of the POP until an IUD can be fitted.
- Switching methods of contraception:
  - See CoSRH guidance on switching or starting methods of contraception.

3.2.8 Advice to include when prescribing a method of contraception

Your advice when prescribing should include:

- The efficacy of the chosen method (and that contraceptive effectiveness relies on correct use).
- How to use the chosen method.
- When to start it in the cycle and how long before it becomes effective.
- Bleeding pattern to be expected in the short and long term; see *Table 3.7*.
- Benefits, risks and possible side-effects.
  - Include information about breast cancer with hormonal contraceptives, as in *Section 3.2.23*.
- Advice about use of medications that could interact with the chosen method (for example weight loss medications and enzyme-inducing drugs including St John's Wort).
- Timing of check-ups or replacement of the method.
- Safety-netting: when to seek advice, for example, if they develop migraine whilst using a CHC method.
- That an annual contraceptive review is required, which should include measurement of BMI and BP, and medical history, drug history, method adherence and satisfaction.
- If using oral contraceptives, advise how often they should be taken (e.g. standard or tailored use of CHC), what constitutes a late or missed pill for the product they are taking (see *Section 3.2.9*).
- If using CHC, give advice about VTE, major surgery, periods of immobility or time at altitude, and how to seek medical advice.
- If using a LARC method, advise when and how to arrange a replacement or the next dose and that the method may not be effective if it is replaced later than advised, and emergency contraception may be required.

3.2.9 Incorrectly taken oral hormonal contraceptive pills

- Absorption of oral hormonal contraceptives and efficacy of the method can be reduced if the pills are not taken correctly (late or missed pills and vomiting or diarrhoea).
- Refer to the Summary of Product Characteristics (SPC) for the method used to advise how to correctly take it, as the rules are different depending on which type of oral contraceptive pill is taken (for example, some pills have a 12-hour window and some a 24-hour window in which to remember to take them).
- Direct the patient to find the patient information leaflet for their contraceptive method, online, by searching the medicines A–Z on the eMC website, www.medicines.org.uk/emc/browse-medicines. This will give them information about how to take the pill and what to do if the pill is taken late or if there is vomiting or diarrhoea, any of which could affect the effectiveness of the pill.
- If pills are missed or late, or there is vomiting or diarrhoea, there may be a need for EC and use of a bridging method, such as a barrier method, until the chosen method becomes effective again (see *Section 3.12*).

- Advise that CTPs and CVRs also need to be used correctly and replaced as advised, in order to provide effective contraception. Refer to the individual product guidance for advice.
- Consider changing to a LARC if there are frequent missed or late pills, patches or rings.
- Refer to:
  - The individual specific product licence for advice on the eMC website.
  - CoSRH Clinical Guidance: *Drug interactions with hormonal contraception.*
  - CoSRH CEU Guidance: *Recommended actions after incorrect use of combined hormonal contraception.*
  - CoSRH Guideline: *Progestogen-only pills.*
  - NICE CKS: *Progestogen-only pill.*
  - NICE CKS: *Combined oral contraceptive.*

3.2.10 Contraceptive choices for women over 40 years

- Effective contraception (see *Table 3.5*) is needed to prevent an unintended pregnancy.
- Women over the age of 40 have an age-related increased background risk of cardiovascular disease and obesity, and of breast and most gynaecological cancers, which may affect their choice of contraception.

Table 3.5: Contraceptive methods suitable for women over 40 years

Contraceptive method	Suitable for
Implant, POP, IUS, all IUDs	Any age – can be continued until age 55 No evidence that they increase the risk of VTE, MI or stroke and do not affect bone mineral density (BMD)
CHC methods, pill, patch and ring	Up to age 50 (for non-smokers) and then switch to a non-hormonal or progestogen-only method Up to age 35 (for smokers) and then switch to a non-hormonal or progestogen-only method Consider VTE risk when choosing a COC; choose a pill with a lower VTE risk first-line (see *Table 3.8*)
DMPA	Up to age 50 (may be continued beyond 50 years on an individual basis after appropriate discussion of risks and benefits) DMPA is a UKMEC 3 if there are multiple risk factors for CVD (such as smoking, diabetes, hypertension, obesity and dyslipidaemias), current and history of ischaemic heart disease or stroke. Remember that evidence shows an increased risk of VTE with DMPA use, so some conditions have changed in UKMEC 2025 to reflect this increase in risk. Risk is likely to be lower than the VTE risk associated with CHC.
Fertility awareness	Methods are less reliable with age, as cycles change and it becomes more difficult to predict ovulation
Diaphragm	Any age, but can be less reliable if there is a prolapse
Non-hormonal	Age <50 – can stop contraception 2 years after LMP Age >50 – can stop contraception 1 year after LMP

3.2.11 Overweight, obesity and contraception

- Weight should be discussed sensitively, and with permission.
- Consider carefully the choice of contraception for those with a BMI ≥30kg/m^2, due to the increased risk of VTE and hypertension, and breast and endometrial cancer.
- All IUDs, IMP and POP are safe to use in women who are overweight or obese. A double dose of POP is not recommended.

- CHC use is a UKMEC 2 for use by women with BMI 30–34kg/m^2 and UKMEC 3 for women with BMI ≥35kg/m^2. Evidence suggests that the effectiveness of the COCP and CVR are not affected by body weight, but the CTP may be less effective in women who weigh ≥90kg.
- DMPA use in women with a BMI 30–34.9kg/m^2 is a UKMEC 1 and for women with a BMI ≥35kg/m^2 is a UKMEC 2. Use of DMPA becomes a UKMEC 3 when obesity is one of multiple risk factors for cardiovascular disease (such as smoking, diabetes and hypertension). DMPA can cause some weight gain, especially if used in women <18 years who have a BMI ≥30kg/m^2.
- Emergency hormonal contraception varies in effectiveness with body weight / BMI:
    - LNG-EC may be less effective at >70kg or BMI ≥26kg/m^2.
    - Consider a Cu-IUD or UPA-EC. If these are not suitable a double dose (3mg) of LNG-EC can be used, but the effectiveness of this is unknown.
    - UPA may be less effective at >85kg or BMI >30kg/m^2. Double dose of UPA-EC is not recommended.
- Refer to the CoSRH Overweight, obesity and contraception guideline.

3.2.12 Weight loss treatments and contraception

Use of glucagon-like peptide-1 receptor agonists (GLP-1 agonists)

- Incretin therapies are not recommended during pregnancy, so women who are using a GLP-1 agonist should use an effective method of contraception if they are at risk of pregnancy.
- Women using tirzepatide and an oral hormonal contraceptive should switch to a non-oral contraceptive method, or add a barrier method of contraception, for 4 weeks after initiation of tirzepatide, and for 4 weeks after each dose increase. There is no need to add a barrier method of contraception when using semaglutide, dulaglutide, exenatide, lixisenatide or liraglutide, as there is currently no evidence that these drugs reduce the effectiveness of oral hormonal contraceptives.
- It is not known if oral EC is affected by GLP-1 agonists. The Cu-IUD is the most effective method of emergency contraception.
- There is no evidence to suggest that GLP-1 agonists affect non-oral methods of contraception.
- GLP-1 agonists can cause side-effects such as diarrhoea and vomiting, which could also affect absorption of the pill. If vomiting occurs within 3 hours of taking the contraceptive pill, or severe diarrhoea occurs for more than 24 hours, women should follow CoSRH recommendations for missed or late pills. Refer to: www.cosrh.org/Common/Uploaded%20files/documents/drug-interactions-with-hormonal-contraception-5may2022.pdf
- Preconception advice for women planning a pregnancy and taking GLP-1 agonists should be given as follows. Because there is *insufficient safety data and potential risk* to the fetus, contraception should be used while taking them and during a 'wash-out' period before conception.
    - Exenatide: discontinue 12 weeks before attempting to conceive.
    - Semaglutide: discontinue ≥2 months before attempting to conceive.
    - Tirzepatide: discontinue ≥1 month before attempting to conceive.
- Refer patients to the CoSRH patient information leaflet: *GLP-1 agonists and contraception.*

Bariatric surgery

- Women planning bariatric surgery need to discuss their contraceptive needs prior to the operation.
- The effectiveness of oral hormonal contraceptives could be reduced by bariatric surgery, and non-oral methods should be considered.
- Prior to planned major surgery or an expected period of limited mobility, stop CHC and switch to an alternative contraception for at least 4 weeks.
- After bariatric surgery refer to UKMEC for appropriate methods.
- Refer to the CoSRH Overweight, obesity and contraception guideline.

3.2.13 Prescribing in other groups

- Guidance for managing contraception in other groups (such as those with breast cancer, after pregnancy, young people, transgender and non-binary people) can be found at the CoSRH guidelines: *Contraception for specific populations.*

3.2.14 Non-contraceptive benefits of contraceptive methods

- When choosing a method of contraception always consider the non-contraceptive effects that may benefit each patient (see *Table 3.6).*
- Contraceptive methods which suppress ovulation, for example, can benefit patients with endometriosis, recurrent ovarian cysts, menstrual migraine, epilepsy and other medical conditions affected by fluctuating hormones. They can also be helpful to relieve ovulation pain and in the management of premenstrual syndrome / premenstrual dysphoric disorder (PMDD).

Table 3.6: Other benefits of contraceptive methods

Benefit	Type of contraception
Less period pain and lighter periods	Hormonal contraception methods (IMP, DMPA, LNG-IUD, CHC and POP) can reduce period pain and make periods lighter
Cycle control	Tailored use of CHC can give a controlled cycle, or amenorrhoea
Stop the period	47% of users of DMPA will have no periods after the first year 25% of IMP users will have no periods and more than 50% will have light frequent bleeding
Treat PMS	Refer to *Chapter 8* The RCOG guidelines recommend use of a combined new generation CHC pill containing drospirenone, cyclically or continuously (see *Section 3.4.3)**
Endometriosis	Hormonal treatment can reduce endometriosis-related pain: CHC (particularly continuous regimes), POP, DMPA, IMP or an LNG-IUD
Acne	Consider a CHC method, with a 2nd, 3rd or 4th (new) generation progestogen The drospirenone POP may be helpful Co-cyprindiol (cyproterone acetate with ethinylestradiol) (not first-line)
PCOS management Refer to the PCOS guidelines†	The COCP could be used (consider UKMEC) for management of hirsutism and/or irregular menstrual cycles Although there are no specific guidelines, a COCP with drospirenone may be helpful Co-cyprindiol is licensed as a treatment for severe acne or moderately severe hirsutism, but not for first-line use (it provides effective contraception for such women, but it should not be used solely as a contraceptive) Endometrial protection in PCOS: for prolonged amenorrhoea (less than one period every 3 months once pregnancy has been excluded) a cyclical progestogen is required to induce a withdrawal bleed every 3 months; this is not necessary if a hormonal contraceptive method is being used

*RCOG Premenstrual Syndrome Management (Green-top Guidelines No.48)

†International Evidence-based Guideline for the assessment and management of polycystic ovarian syndrome 2023

3.2.15 Contraception after having a baby

- This should be discussed with women during their antenatal appointments, so they are aware of their choices and when the method can be started.
- A woman can get pregnant 21 days after having a baby, even if she has not had a period, or is breastfeeding.
- Breastfeeding, otherwise known as the lactational amenorrhoea method, is 98% effective as a contraceptive method, but only if the woman fulfils all three of the following:
    - Exclusively breastfeeding, with no use of formula milk.
    - Less than 6 months postnatal.
    - Amenorrhoeic.
- The IMP, DMPA, POP and condoms can be started immediately after birth.
- LNG-IUDs and the Cu-IUD can be fitted within 48 hours of delivery. After 48 hours, insertion should be delayed until 4 weeks after giving birth.
- Both types of emergency oral hormonal contraception pills are safe in the immediate postnatal period but are not needed until 21 days after birth. The Cu-IUD is safe to use for EC from 28 days after childbirth.
- All women should have a risk assessment for VTE postnatally. CHC or DMPA should not be used by women who have risk factors for VTE within 6 weeks of childbirth (including immobility, BMI ≥30kg/m^2, postpartum haemorrhage, post-caesarean delivery, pre-eclampsia or smoking).
- Refer to UKMEC 2025 for safe prescribing in postpartum categories: 0 to <3 weeks; 3 to <6 weeks; 6 weeks and over, and breastfeeding.
- The diaphragm is not recommended in the first 6 weeks after childbirth.
- After miscarriage or termination of pregnancy, fertility can return immediately so advise about contraception.
- Refer to the CoSRH Guideline: *Contraception after pregnancy.*

3.2.16 Contraception and breastfeeding

- The IMP, DMPA, POP and all IUDs can be used, and have no adverse effects on lactation, infant growth or development.
- Both forms of oral emergency contraception, LNG-EC and UPA-EC, can be used. While small amounts of UPA are found in breast milk, no adverse effects on the infant have been found, so breastfeeding does not need to be interrupted.
- Women who are breastfeeding should wait until 6 weeks after giving birth before starting a CHC method.

3.2.17 Problematic bleeding on hormonal contraception

- Women over 40 with a significant change in their bleeding pattern should have appropriate gynaecological assessment and investigation, whether they are using a contraceptive method or not.
- When prescribing a method of contraception, advise women about the bleeding pattern to be expected both initially and in the long term, as shown in *Table 3.7.*
- Many women stop using contraceptive methods because they do not understand how their bleeding pattern will be affected.

History

Clinical history-taking in women with problematic bleeding on hormonal contraception (HC) should include:

- Current method of contraception, duration of use and compliance.
- Use of any medications (including OTC preparations) which may interact with the contraceptive method.

Table 3.7: Expected bleeding pattern after commencing hormonal contraception (adapted from the CoSRH)

Contraceptive method	Expected bleeding patterns in the first 3 months	Expected bleeding patterns in the longer term
CHC	20% have irregular bleeding	Irregular bleeding usually settles
POP	Bleeding is unpredictable	Bleeding may not settle with time After 12 months of DSG-POP use, over a 3-month period: • 50% of women will have no bleeding or infrequent bleeding • 40% of women will have 3–5 episodes of bleeding or spotting • 10% of women will have 6 or more episodes of bleeding/spotting • 20% of women will have episodes of bleeding lasting longer than 2 weeks (prolonged bleeding)
DMPA	Bleeding is common and can be spotting, heavy, light or prolonged 10% of women have no bleeding	Rates of amenorrhoea increased with duration of use; 50% or more have amenorrhoea at 12 months
IMP	Bleeding disturbances are common	As a guide: • 20% of women are amenorrhoeic • 30% of women have infrequent bleeding • <10% of women have frequent bleeding • 20% of women have prolonged bleeding
52mg LNG-IUD	Frequently bleeding and spotting is common in the first few months after insertion	Bleeding decreases over time with all doses of LNG-IUD At 12 months of use of 52mg LNG-IUD there is about a 90% reduction in menstrual blood loss Infrequent bleeding is common and some women will be amenorrhoeic At 3 years 24% are amenorrhoeic, in comparison to 12.7% with a Jaydess and 18.9% with a Kyleena

- Illness/condition that may affect absorption of orally administered hormones.
- Cervical screening history: arrange one if it is due.
- Risk of STIs, e.g. age <25 years / new sexual partner or >1 partner in last year.
- Bleeding pattern before starting hormonal contraception, since starting, and currently.
- Other symptoms suggestive of an underlying pathology, such as abdominal pelvic pain, postcoital bleeding, dyspareunia, or heavy menstrual bleeding.
- Do a pregnancy test if there is possibility of pregnancy.

Examination

- An examination may not be needed if a woman using hormonal contraception for <3 months has problematic bleeding (could consider up to 6 months with LNG-IUD and IMP) if there are no risk factors for STI, no symptoms suggesting underlying pathology and she is up to date with cervical screening. Offer a follow-up assessment if the bleeding doesn't settle or other symptoms occur. You can consider medical management to manage the bleeding.
- Women do need a speculum examination to visualise the cervix:
  - For persistent bleeding beyond the first 3 months of use (6 months with LNG-IUD and IMP).
  - For new symptoms or a change in bleeding after at least 3 months of use.
  - If a woman has not participated in the cervical screening programme.

- If requested by a woman.
- After a failed trial of the limited medical management available.
- If there are other symptoms such as pain, dyspareunia or postcoital bleeding. These symptoms would also warrant bimanual examination.

Referral

- If the examination above is abnormal, refer / manage appropriately.
- If the assessment/examination are normal, in women who have used hormonal contraception for >3 months and who have ongoing, persistent bleeding; new symptoms (including pain, dyspareunia, heavy bleeding), a change in bleeding pattern, failed medical treatment or are not having cervical screening, consider pathology such as endometrial cancer, endometrial polyp, fibroid or ovarian cyst. In those aged ≥45 years, or aged <45 years (with risk factors for endometrial cancer) refer for endometrial assessment (e.g. ultrasound scan, biopsy or hysteroscopy) depending on age and the likelihood of pathology.
- Women who use an LNG-IUD with pain, discharge or non-visible threads in addition to bleeding require investigation to exclude expulsion, perforation or infection.

Medical management of problematic bleeding on hormonal contraception

- Consider why the bleeding occurs:
  - With CHC, as long as there is no underlying pathology, poor compliance or drug interactions, unscheduled bleeding may be related to the dose of oestrogen, the type of oestrogen and progestogen, the regime and the routine of administration. Ethinylestradiol provides greater endometrial stabilisation than estradiol, resulting in improved cycle control.
  - With progestogen-only methods unpredictable bleeding can be caused by endometrial changes (such as a thin endometrium with an unstable surface; disturbed angiogenesis with thin-walled, distended, fragile superficial microvessels, and down-regulation of steroid receptors). This results in bleeding through spontaneous breakdown of tissue and/or defective repair.
- CHC users:
  - Continue with the same pill for 3 months as bleeding may settle.
  - Consider increasing the dose of ethinylestradiol (EE) to 35μg; this may help to achieve good cycle control. Anecdotally a 30mcg EE/gestodene pill or a 35mcg EE/norgestimate pill may be helpful. Other options include a CVR, or a progestogen method such as DMPA if suitable, as >50% are amenorrhoeic at 12 months.
- POP users:
  - Bleeding may settle with time; if pathology has been excluded, continue for at least 3–4 months.
  - There is no evidence that changing to a different POP will improve bleeding patterns, but it can be helpful in some women. Anecdotally, changing from an anovulatory POP to a traditional POP may give a more regular frequency of bleeding, and changing from a traditional POP to an anovulatory POP may result in more infrequent bleeding and/or amenorrhoea over time. A drospirenone (DRSP) POP may give less unscheduled bleeding and less prolonged bleeding than a DSG POP.
- DMPA/IMP/LNG-IUD users:
  - A COCP with 30–35mcg ethinylestradiol and levonorgestrel or norethisterone can be used cyclically or daily for up to 12 weeks (off-licence).
  - Reducing injection interval of DMPA is not likely to help, but, off-licence, consider reducing the injection interval down to 10 weeks when starting injectables to prevent bleeding problems, and in long-term users to control problematic bleeding.

    - Mefenamic acid 500mg 2–3 times daily, or tranexamic acid 1g four times daily can be used for up to 5 days to reduce a bleeding episode, but this will not help with long-term bleeding.
    - If using a Jaydess or Kyleena IUD consider changing to a 52mg LNG-IUD. If there is problematic bleeding in LNG-IUD users there is little point in giving more progestogen orally, as the intrauterine levels of LNG are about 800 times higher than those achieved by a POP.
    - With the IMP anecdotally consider one DSG POP daily, or therapeutic doses of progestogen for 3 months. It may be helpful to change to implant, if it was fitted for more than 2 years.
    - If the bleeding is not settling and is unacceptable, consider a different method of contraception.
- Follow-up should be offered in the event of persisting bleeding, other symptoms or concerns.
- CoSRH Clinical Guideline: *Problematic bleeding with hormonal contraception.*

3.2.18 When can contraception be stopped?

- All women can stop using contraception at the age of 55 as spontaneous conception after this age is exceptionally rare, even in women who still have menstrual bleeding.
- If a woman has her last natural period before the age of 50, she needs to continue using contraception for two more years. If she has her last natural period over the age of 50, she needs to continue using contraception for one more year.
- Women over 50 years who are amenorrhoeic due to their contraception (e.g. POP/IMP/LNG-IUD) can have their FSH level tested to check menopausal status. If the FSH is >30IU/L, they can stop using contraception after one more year of use. If preferred, they can continue until age 55, then stop.
- Women using CHC or HRT have suppressed levels of estradiol and gonadotrophins, and measuring these hormones is not recommended to check menopause status and when to stop contraception. CHC could be stopped and an FSH tested after 6 weeks.
- If a 52mg LNG-IUD is inserted at ≥45 years, and is not being used as part of HRT, it can be used for contraception until the age of 55 (see *Section 3.8*).

3.2.19 Hormone replacement therapy (HRT) and contraception

- Contraception does not affect the onset or duration of menopausal symptoms, but may mask them.
- HRT is a treatment used to help menopause symptoms, but it does not provide contraception, unless a 52mg LNG-IUD is used. A separate contraceptive method is required for sexually active women who are not yet postmenopausal.
- Measurement of FSH to assess menopausal status is largely unreliable whilst taking HRT or CHC.
- Generally, if HRT is started in a woman who still requires contraception, a contraceptive method should be continued until the age of 55.
- A 52mg LNG-IUD is effective and licensed to provide endometrial protection from the stimulatory effects of oestrogen replacement therapy for 5 years (CoSRH approved).
- POP, implants and DMPA are not licensed for endometrial protection as the progestogen part of HRT. With use of a POP, it is important to note that:
    - There is lack of evidence for the use of desogestrel 75mcg as the progestogen part of HRT. If desogestrel 75mcg is used as a contraceptive in women who take HRT, a progestogen such as micronised progesterone 100mg daily, or 200mg for 12–14 days a month should be taken alongside it, to provide endometrial protection.

    - The British Menopause Society *HRT preparations and equivalent alternatives* practical guide states that use of 150mcg desogestrel (two 75mcg tablets daily), off-licence, is effective as the progestogen component of HRT, with no increase in risk of endometrial hyperplasia.
    - This guide also states that drospirenone 4mg (Slynd) can be used, off-licence, daily as an alternative for women who have side-effects with other HRT preparations. One active hormonal tablet can be taken daily and the four hormone-free (placebo) pills in each pack can be discarded.
    - Refer to https://thebms.org.uk/wp-content/uploads/2024/02/15-BMS-TfC-HRT-preparations-and-equivalent-alternatives-JAN2024-B.pdf (page 3).
- All progestogen-only methods of contraception are safe to use alongside HRT.
- CHC methods cannot be used alongside HRT. CHC can be considered in eligible women under 50 years as an alternative to HRT for relief of menopausal symptoms.

3.2.20 Drug interactions

Always ask about use of prescription, non-prescription and recreational drugs, and herbal preparations and dietary supplements when providing contraception.

- It could be that a drug taken reduces the effectiveness of a contraceptive method.
    - The most significant pharmacokinetic interaction affecting hormonal contraception occurs with drugs which stimulate hepatic cytochrome P450 enzymes (such as enzyme-inducing drugs) and increase the clearance of contraceptive hormones. This can reduce the effectiveness of CHC, POPs, the IMP and oral EC.
    - Women using an enzyme-inducing drug should be offered a reliable method of contraception that is not affected by the enzyme inducer, such as an LNG-IUD, Cu-IUD or DMPA.
- Further examples include:
    - A contraceptive method which reduces the effectiveness of a drug taken alongside it: as an example of this, CHC induces glucuronidation of lamotrigine and reduces lamotrigine exposure, which could reduce seizure control.
    - The effect of one drug influences another: for example, progestogen-only contraception could reduce the effectiveness of UPA-EC because of opposing action on progestogen receptors.
    - The POP drospirenone is an aldosterone antagonist and has potassium-sparing properties. It is not recommended to be used alongside potassium-sparing diuretics. Angiotensin-converting enzyme (ACE) inhibitors and angiotensin II receptor antagonists could also potentially increase risk of hyperkalaemia.
    - St John's wort, which is a herbal medicine traditionally used to relieve low mood and anxiety, can decrease the effect of all hormonal contraceptives, except intrauterine devices for which there is no data. Women taking hormonal contraception to prevent pregnancy should not take herbal products that contain St John's wort.
- Useful sources to review interactions are:
    - CoSRH Clinical Guidance: *Drug interactions with hormonal contraception.*
    - The *BNF.*

3.2.21 Contraception for women using known teratogenic drugs

- Consider any use of teratogenic drugs and advise women about the importance of using highly effective contraception.
- An example is topiramate, a drug which has enzyme-inducing activity at higher doses and is a teratogen. Recommended contraceptive options to be used alongside topiramate are a Cu-IUD, LNG-IUD and DMPA (a barrier method can be added).
- Useful sources to review interactions are:

- CoSRH CEU Statement: *Contraception for women using known teratogenic drugs or drugs with potential teratogenic effects.*
- Detailed information regarding teratogenic drugs or drugs with potential teratogenic effects is available from the UK teratology information service (UKTIS) website.

3.2.22 Contraception for trans men and non-binary people

- Trans and non-binary people who were assigned female at birth (AFAB) can get pregnant if a sperm meets an egg.
- It is possible to become pregnant on masculinising hormones, even if periods have stopped. If the patient is planning to become pregnant, stop masculinising gender-affirming hormones.
- Contraception methods suitable for people taking masculinising hormones include condoms, POP, IMP, LNG-IUDs, Cu-IUDs, DMPA, diaphragm, EC and sterilisation.
- Refer to the CoSRH CEU Statement: *Contraceptive choices and sexual health for transgender and non-binary people.*

3.2.23 Breast cancer risk and hormonal contraception

- There is a small increased risk of breast cancer associated with current or recent use of all forms of hormonal contraception; this risk reduces with time after the hormonal contraception is stopped.
- Current data suggests that all hormonal methods of contraception carry a small (20–30%) increased risk of breast cancer diagnosis over a 15-year period of time (5 years of use of the method, and an excess risk 10 years after stopping). This can be explained to women in relation to their baseline risk, which differs depending on age:
  - Age 16–20: an extra 8 cases per 100 000 users.
    - a 0.084% baseline incidence (<1:1000) which increases to 0.093%.
  - Age 25–39: an extra 265 cases per 100 000 users.
    - age 25–29: incidence increases from a baseline of 0.50% to 0.57%.
    - age 35–39: incidence increases from a baseline of 2% (1:65) to 2.2%.
  - Refer to the CoSRH response to a new study on use of combined and progestogen-only hormonal contraception and breast cancer risk.
- Risk must be balanced against the benefits of use of hormonal contraceptives. The COCP also has the benefit of long-lasting reduced risk of ovarian, endometrial, and possibly colorectal cancer.
- Advise women to be breast aware.
- To advise women about contraception if they have, or have had breast cancer, refer to: CoSRH CEU Guidance: *Supporting contraceptive choices for individuals who have or have had breast cancer.*

3.2.24 Risk of intracranial meningioma

- The CoSRH has released statements about the increased risk of meningioma in patients using cyproterone acetate, nomegestrol acetate and medroxyprogesterone acetate (MPA) and desogestrel.
- It advises that patients with meningioma or a history of meningioma should not use cyproterone acetate, Zoely (estradiol 1.5mg, nomegestrol acetate 2.5mg), MPA or desogestrel.

3.3 Progestogen choice in contraception

- Progestogens can be divided into two types: natural and synthetic.
- Progesterone (produced from the ovary) is the only natural progestogen.
  - Micronised progesterone capsules are available to be taken as part of body-identical HRT, but do not provide contraception.

  - All hormonal methods of contraception contain a synthetic progestogen. There are many different types.
- Synthetic progestogens, also known as progestins, are synthetic steroids designed to mimic the actions of progesterone.
- Synthetic progestogens bind to the progesterone receptor, but they also bind to other steroid receptors where they have either agonist or antagonist effects (which explains why they might have side-effects; see *Box 3.1*).

3.3.1 Synthetic progestogen classification

- Progestogens can be classified in two ways: generationally or based on structural properties.

Generationally

- Traditionally, synthetic progestogens have been classified by the decade of their introduction or 'generation'.
  - First: norethisterone (NET), medroxyprogesterone acetate (MPA) and norgestrel.
  - Second: levonorgestrel (LNG).
  - Third: desogestrel, gestodene, norgestimate.
  - Fourth or newer: drospirenone, dienogest, nomegestrol acetate (designed to have minimal androgenic or oestrogenic actions and to be closer in activity to natural progesterone).

Structurally

- Progestogens vary in their chemical structures and pharmacological properties depending on whether they are derived from progesterone (pregnanes) or testosterone (estranes and gonanes).
- Progesterone and its synthetic analogues are less androgenic than testosterone analogues.
  - Progesterone-derived progestogens
    - e.g. dydrogesterone, medroxyprogesterone acetate, cyproterone acetate and nomegestrol acetate
  - Testosterone-derived progestogens
    - e.g. norethisterone, norgestrel, levonorgestrel, desogestrel, norgestimate and gestodene
    - Dienogest is a hybrid progestogen. It is derived from testosterone but, like drospirenone, has no androgenic effect. It does, however, have partial anti-androgenic activity. It can be used in the management of endometriosis.
- Drospirenone is one of the new generation progestogens but differs from the others as it is derived from spironolactone. It is an anti-mineralocorticoid steroid with no androgenic effect and a partial anti-androgenic effect.
- Dydrogesterone is referred to as a retroprogesterone, and has a similar structure to progesterone. Dydrogesterone is more readily absorbed from the digestive tract than progesterone, and has a higher affinity for the progesterone receptor compared to progesterone, allowing it to be effective at lower doses.
  - It is available as a stand-alone product, Nalvee 10mg. It is also available as an oral tablet in fixed combination doses with estradiol, in the Femoston range of HRT.
  - Dydrogesterone can be used to manage conditions such as dysmenorrhoea, endometriosis, irregular menstrual cycles, secondary amenorrhoea and PMS, and it can be used as the progestogen part of HRT.
  - At therapeutic doses it does not prevent ovulation or have contraceptive effects. It is being discussed in this section as we discuss progestogens and their uses.
- More information on use of all progestogens can be found on the electronic medicines compendium: www.medicines.org.uk/emc

BOX 3.1: Side-effects of progestogens in relation to physiological activity

- Progestogenic activity: breast tenderness, change in bowel activity, bloating, increased appetite, tiredness, mood changes, skin changes
- Androgenic activity: oily skin, acne, hirsutism, weight gain, mood changes
- Glucocorticoid activity: mood swings, increased appetite, water retention
- Mineralocorticoid activity: water retention, bloating

3.3.2 Indications for use of synthetic progestogens

- As well as providing contraception, progestogens can also be used to treat a variety of conditions either on their own, or in combination with oestrogen.
- *Table 3.8* provides details of the activity of different progestogens on receptors. This can explain how different progestogens can be beneficial to manage different conditions such as heavy periods, acne or PMS.

Table 3.8: Indications for use of synthetic progestogens and summary of characteristics

Generation	Progestogen	Physiological activity + weak ++ moderate +++ strong	Good for these conditions*
1st	MPA	Androgenic ++ Glucocorticoid +	Irregular or missed periods
	NET	Progestogenic ++ Androgenic +	Menorrhagia Adenomyosis
2nd	LNG	Progestogenic +++ Androgenic +++	Menorrhagia Adenomyosis
3rd	Desogestrel/etonogestrel	Progestogenic +++	Dysmenorrhoea Endometriosis
	Norgestimate/norelgestromin	Progestogenic ++ Androgenic +	Moderate acne
	Gestodene	Progestogenic +++ Androgenic +	Dysmenorrhoea
4th/new	Drospirenone	Anti-androgenic Anti-mineralocorticoid	Acne, PCOS, PMS
	Dienogest	Anti-androgenic	Endometriosis
	Nomegestrol	Anti-oestrogenic (targeted at the endometrium) Anti-androgenic (partial)	Menorrhagia, PCOS, PMS
	Dydrogesterone	Progestogenic +++ No oestrogenic, androgenic or corticoid effects	Dysmenorrhoea, endometriosis, PMS, irregular menstrual cycles, dysfunctional uterine bleeding, secondary amenorrhoea Does not provide contraception

Adapted from Chakrabarti, R. and Chakrabarti, R. (2021) Prescribing the oral contraceptive pill: key considerations for primary care physicians. *BJGP, 71(712): 522–4.*

*The indications for use apply whether the progestogen is used in a POP or in combination with oestrogen in a CHC method.

3.4 Combined hormonal contraception

3.4.1 Mechanism of action

- The primary mechanism of action of the combined oral contraceptive pill is prevention of ovulation through negative feedback on the hypothalamic–pituitary axis, suppressing FSH release and preventing the LH surge.
- Other effects include thickening of cervical mucus, which inhibits sperm penetration; suppression of endometrial growth, making the endometrium less receptive; and alterations in tubal motility.
- Refer to:
  - NICE CKS: *Contraception – combined hormonal methods.*
  - NICE CKS: *Combined vaginal ring.*
  - NICE CKS: *Combined transdermal patch.*
  - CoSRH Guideline: *Combined hormonal contraception.*

3.4.2 Available forms of combined hormonal contraception

- Combined oral contraceptive pills (COCP), combined transdermal patches (CTP) or combined vaginal rings (CVR).
- Combined hormonal contraceptives contain two hormones, an oestrogen and a progestogen.

3.4.3 Types of combined oral contraceptive pill (COCP)

- The majority of COCPs contain variable doses of the synthetic oestrogen ethinylestradiol (EE), as the oestrogen component, combined with one of a variety of synthetic progestogens.
- COCPs containing 17β-estradiol and estetrol have now been introduced.
  - These types of oestrogens are structurally identical to that naturally occurring in the human body (see *Chapter 1*), and are combined with a synthetic progestogen to provide contraception.
- Newer combined oral contraceptives incorporate newer progestogens (see *Section 3.3*) and, in some formulations (17β-estradiol and estetrol), resulting in different hormonal and side-effect profiles. Examples are:
  - Estradiol valerate plus dienogest (Qlaira).
  - Estradiol hemihydrate plus nomegestrol acetate (Zoely).
  - Estetrol plus drospirenone (Drovelis).
  - Ethinylestradiol plus drospirenone (Eloine).

Monophasic and multiphasic pills

- Monophasic pills contain the same fixed amount of oestrogen and progestogen in each pill in the packet:
- Most monophasic COCPs are available in packs containing 21 active pills only. The 21/7 method involves taking active pills for 21 days followed by a 7-day break. This is the standard, widely-known way to take the pill. It creates the appearance of a cycle, even though ovulation is suppressed, with the 7-day break leading to a withdrawal bleed. This is not a true menstrual period, but a withdrawal bleed caused by temporarily stopping the hormones in the COCP.
- Some brands of COCP are available as everyday (ED) pills. There are 28 pills in each packet; some are active pills and some are placebo pills. A pill is taken every day in order, with no break. These preparations can be considered for patients with compliance issues who might forget to restart the next pill packet after a break, potentially impacting efficacy.
  - Examples include Microgynon 30 ED which has 28 pills in each packet (21 active and 7 placebo) and Zoely (24 active and 4 placebo).

- Multiphasic pills contain varying amounts of oestrogen and progestogen and may contain placebo pills in the pack. For example, Qlaira (which contains estradiol valerate plus dienogest) is quadriphasic, which means there are four hormone doses over the cycle. Phasic pills need to be taken in the correct order.

Combined transdermal patch (CTP)

- The ethinylestradiol plus norelgestromin CTP is replaced every 7 days for 3 weeks followed by a patch-free week.

Combined vaginal ring (CVR)

- The ethinylestradiol plus etonogestrel CVR is replaced every 21 days followed by a ring-free week.

3.4.4 Advantages of combined hormonal contraception

- CHC is a short-acting method of contraception, which is easy to use.
- In addition to the benefits, including cycle control and reduction of heavy bleeding, CHC offers non-contraceptive benefits, as shown in *Table 3.6*.
- CHC can be used in perimenopause to suppress ovarian function, provide contraception and relieve menopausal symptoms (refer to UKMEC).
- Reduced incidence of endometrial cancer, ovarian cancer (this risk reduction increases with length of CHC use and persists many years after stopping) and possibly colorectal cancer.
- Qlaira is licensed as a COCP, primarily for the treatment of heavy menstrual bleeding in women who desire contraception.

3.4.5 Disadvantages of combined hormonal contraception

- A small increase in incidence of CIN and cancer of the cervix after 5 years of use; women should all participate in cervical screening.
- Current CHC use is associated with increased risk of VTE, MI and ischaemic stroke.
- Increased risk of VTE; the risk varies between different pills (*Table 3.9*) and the woman's individual risk factors, e.g. smoking and obesity. VTE and CVD risks increase with increasing EE doses. Long-term safety data for new formulations of COCP containing estradiol and estetrol is limited, but their VTE risk might be similar to COCs containing levonorgestrel.
- Women should be advised to stop CHC and to switch to an alternative contraceptive method at least 4 weeks prior to planned major surgery or expected period of limited mobility.
- Advise to reduce periods of immobility during travel (long duration travel is a weak risk factor for VTE) and to consider an alternative method if spending time at high altitude.

Table 3.9: Risk of developing a VTE in a year with CHC

Women not using a combined hormonal pill/patch/ring and who are not pregnant	About 1–5 out of 10 000 women (increases with age)
Women who are pregnant or in the immediate postpartum period	About 29 out of 10 000 women
Women using a CHC containing levonorgestrel, norethisterone or norgestimate	About 5–7 out of 10 000 women
Women using a CHC containing etonogestrel or norelgestromin	About 6–12 out of 10 000 women
Women using a CHC containing drospirenone, gestodene or desogestrel; co-cyprindiol is associated with a similar VTE risk	About 9–12 out of 10 000 women
Women using a CHC containing dienogest or nomegestrol acetate	Not yet known

Data taken from MHRA website; SPC for estradiol valerate and dienogest and SPC for estradiol hemihydrate and nomegestrol acetate.

3.4.6 Starting CHC

- Read alongside *Section 3.2.7.*
- The COCP can be started on day 1 of the menstrual cycle, and no additional contraception is required.
- If the COCP is started on days 2–5 of the menstrual cycle, no additional contraception is required unless the woman is starting Qlaira (use condoms for the first 9 days) or Zoely or Drovelis (use condoms for the first 7 days).
- If the COCP is quick-started at any other time in the menstrual cycle, and it is reasonably certain she is not pregnant, advise use of condoms for the first 7 days (9 days for Qlaira).
- Refer to NICE CKS: *Contraception – combined hormonal methods* for information about how to start each CHC (pill and patch) and what to do if switching from another method of contraception.
- Advise about options for tailored regimes such as tricycling / continuous use which are supported by the CoSRH, but off-licence.
- Discuss eligibility criteria – advise to seek review if risk increases, such as weight gain or she starts smoking.
- The pill should be taken at the same time every day.

3.4.7 Incorrect use of CHC (late or missed pills, ring or patch)

- See *Section 3.2.9.*
- Missed pill advice depends on the specific combined oral contraceptive formulation, so ensure the woman is given correct advice about the timing of taking or replacing her CHC product (pill, patch or ring).
- COCPs should be taken at the same time daily. For Zoely (estradiol and nomegestrol acetate), pills taken less than 24 hours late do not reduce contraceptive efficacy, but if taken more than 24 hours late, missed pill advice should be followed. For Qlaira (estradiol valerate and dienogest), missed pill advice applies if a pill is taken more than 12 hours late. Standard ethinylestradiol-containing COCPs, and Drovelis (estetrol and drospirenone), follow the 24-hour missed pill rule.
- If the hormone-free interval has been extended, this may affect contraceptive efficacy.
- Refer to NICE CKS: *Contraception – combined hormonal methods* for missed pill advice.
- Consider the need for emergency contraception.

3.4.8 Vomiting and diarrhoea in women taking a COC

- Efficacy of CHCs can be affected by vomiting or severe diarrhoea. If vomiting occurs within 3 hours of taking a COCP, another pill should be taken as soon as possible.
- If vomiting continues or severe diarrhoea occurs, follow missed pill advice.
- Refer to the NICE CKS: *Contraception – combined hormonal methods* for missed pill advice. Keep taking pills as usual, and consider the need for condoms and emergency contraception.

3.4.9 Seek urgent review

- Advise women when review is needed, and to report the following:
  - Symptoms of VTE such as calf pain, swelling or redness, chest pain or shortness of breath.
  - Breast lump or breast changes.

  - New-onset migraine.
  - Persistent or heavy unscheduled vaginal bleeding.
  - Development of new diagnoses that may contraindicate the CHC, e.g. hypertension, BMI ≥35kg/m^2, VTE or stroke.

3.4.10 Tailored pill regimes

- As discussed, the traditional regime for CHC use has been a 21/7 regime where the CHC is taken for 21 days followed by a 7-day hormone-free interval (HFI), but symptoms during the HFI can be a problem for some women.
- Tailored regimes can reduce the frequency of withdrawal bleeds and therefore reduce symptoms during the HFI, but unscheduled bleeding is common.
- Such regimens are as safe and as effective for contraception as standard 21/7 regimens and are off-licence but supported by the CoSRH (see *Table 3.10*).
- Tailored regimes should not be used with multiphasic pills.

Table 3.10: Indications for use according to CHC regime

Regime	Pattern of CHC use	Indications
Standard use	21 days on pill, 7 days off pill	Women who are symptom-free in the HFI and want to have a regular bleed
	CTP changed every 7 days for 21 days followed by a patch-free week	
	CVR inserted into the vagina and remains in place for 3 weeks followed by a ring-free week	
Tailored use, shortened HFI	24 days on pill, 4 days off pill	Women who want to have a shorter regular bleed
	3 patches or 1 ring used followed by 4 days off	
Extended use	3 months on pill (3 packs in a row), 4 or 7 days off pill	Women with severe dysmenorrhoea or mood swings before or during their periods, e.g. those with endometriosis and PMS
	CTP changed every week for 9 weeks followed by 4 or 7 days off	
	CVR changed every 3 weeks for 9 weeks followed by 4 or 7 days off	
Continuous flexible	The CHC method can be used flexibly with continuous use for a minimum of 21 days. If troublesome bleeding occurs for 3–4 days the CHC can be stopped for an interval of 4–7 days, and then it can be used for at least another 21 days before a method-free interval is taken	Women with severe dysmenorrhoea or mood swings before or during their periods, e.g. those with endometriosis and PMS
Continuous	Continuous use with no pill-free days	Women with severe dysmenorrhoea or mood swings before or during their periods, e.g. those with endometriosis and PMS May be associated with unscheduled bleeding

3.4.11 Possible side-effects of CHC and how to manage them

- Side-effects of hormonal contraception can be caused by:
  - Oestrogen – bloating, breast swelling and tenderness, decreased sex drive, stimulation of growth of fibroids, headaches, irregular bleeding, mood swings, nausea and vomiting and vaginal discharge.
  - Progestogen – acne (especially the older generation of progestogens), anxiety, bloating, breast tenderness and swelling, effect on sex drive, headaches, hirsutism, irregular bleeding and mood swings.
- The UKMEC 2025 update states that there is not consistent evidence that hormonal contraceptives worsen or improve anxiety or mood (affective) disorders in those with pre-existing conditions. When starting hormonal contraception, clinicians should provide individualised counselling and advise patients to monitor their mood, seeking follow-up with their healthcare provider if they notice a deterioration.

How to manage some common side-effects

- Mood changes – take a full history and do a risk assessment.
  - Consider previous sensitivity to progestogens, history of premenstrual syndrome and postnatal depression.
  - Ask about suicidal ideation.
  - Change the progestogen and consider use of drospirenone.
  - Review and signpost to supportive agencies.
- Loss of libido – CHC can affect libido in some women; encourage perseverance for 3 months.
  - Take medical and psychosexual history, explore relationship issues.
  - Change progestogen to a more androgenic progestogen such as norethisterone or levonorgestrel.
  - Consider a COCP with a lower dose of oestrogen (20mcg EE), to reduce the effect on SHBG.
  - Change to a progestogen-only or non-hormonal method.
- Water retention – take history and exclude pathology.
  - Encourage perseverance for 3 months.
  - Reduce oestrogen content to a 20mcg EE or change to a COCP containing drospirenone which has anti-mineralocorticoid activity.
  - Change to a progestogen-only or non-hormonal method.

3.5 Progestogen-only pills

- This type of pill contains a progestogen and is also known as the 'mini pill'.
- Refer to:
  - NICE CKS: *Progestogen-only pill*
  - CoSRH Guideline: *Progestogen-only pills*

3.5.1 Mechanism of action

- The mechanism of action depends upon the type of progestogen used.
- The contraceptive effect of desogestrel (DSG) and drospirenone (DRSP) POPs relies primarily on inhibition of ovulation.
- Levonorgestrel (LNG) and norethisterone (NET) POPs (often referred to as 'traditional' POPs) do not reliably inhibit ovulation and exert their contraceptive effect using their impact on cervical mucus, the endometrium and tubal motility.

3.5.2 Available forms of POP

- The three types of POP which can be taken orally, daily, at 24-hour intervals with no break are:

  - Desogestrel 75mcg POP.
  - Levonorgestrel 30mcg POP.
  - Norethisterone 350mcg POP.
- Drospirenone 4mg POP is taken orally daily at 24-hour intervals and, unlike the other POPs, each pack contains 28 tablets: 24 active tablets and four inactive tablets, so giving a hormone-free interval, during which some users will have a scheduled bleed.
  - DRSP is a potent progestogen with a similar pharmacological profile to progesterone. It has anti-mineralocorticoid and mild anti-androgenic activity.
  - It is an aldosterone antagonist and so there is potential risk of hyperkalaemia in susceptible individuals. Its use with ACE inhibitors and angiotensin receptor antagonists could increase risk of hyperkalaemia.
  - Consider safety of prescribing in those with renal impairment. In women with significant risk factors for chronic kidney disease (CKD), particularly in those over 50 years, consider measuring renal function and BP before initiating treatment. The UKMEC 2025 update under the category of CKD states that DRSP should not be used in individuals with severe renal insufficiency or acute renal failure, and should be used with caution in individuals at risk of hyperkalaemia.

3.5.3 Advantages of POPs

- Ideal for women with oestrogenic side-effects when using CHC.
- Can be taken by those with medical conditions where CHC is contraindicated, such as migraine with aura, hypertension, history of VTE.

3.5.4 Disadvantages of POPs

- Side-effects such as irregular bleeding, breast tenderness, headache or mood changes.

3.5.5 Starting the POP

- See *Section 3.2.7.*
- Traditional POP and DSG POP can be started on days 1 to 5 of a natural menstrual cycle without the need for additional contraceptive precautions. If started at any other time in the cycle, then additional use of a barrier method is needed for 2 days.
- DRSP POP can be started on day 1 only of a natural menstrual cycle without the need for additional contraceptive precautions. If the DRSP POP is started at any other time, then additional use of a barrier method is needed for 7 days.

3.5.6 Incorrect use of POPs

- See *Section 3.2.9* for information on missed or late pills.
- Traditional POP (LNG and NET) – considered missed if taken more than 3 hours late (i.e. more than 27 hours since the last pill).
- Desogestrel POP – considered missed if it is taken more than 12 hours late (i.e. more than 36 hours since the last pill).
- Drospirenone POP – considered missed if it is taken more than 24 hours late (i.e. 48 hours since the last pill).
- Follow missed pills rules if the pill is taken incorrectly. Refer to NICE CKS: *Progestogen-only pill.*

3.5.7 Vomiting and diarrhoea

- The efficacy of the POP may be reduced by vomiting or severe diarrhoea. If vomiting occurs within 2 hours of pill taking, another pill should be taken as soon as possible. If this replacement pill is taken >3 hours late for traditional POPs, >12 hours late for desogestrel POP,

or >24 hours late for drospirenone POP, missed pill advice should be followed. If vomiting continues or there is severe watery diarrhoea, each day should be managed as a missed pill. Condoms should be used during the illness and for 48 hours afterwards for traditional and desogestrel POPs, and for 7 days afterwards for drospirenone POP.
- Consider the need for emergency contraception. Missed pill rules for each individual product can also be found in NICE CKS: *Progestogen-only pill.*

3.6 Injectable contraception

- This section will discuss Depo-Provera (DMPA 150mg) and Sayana Press (DMPA 104mg) but not norethisterone enanthate, which is used infrequently in the UK.
- Refer to:
  - NICE CKS: Progestogen-only injectables
  - CoSRH Guidance: Progestogen-only injectable contraception.

3.6.1 Mechanism of action

- Inhibits ovulation by suppressing LH and to some extent FSH. Alters cervical mucus, preventing sperm penetration into the upper genital tract, induces endometrial atrophy, and modifies sperm function and motility.

3.6.2 Available forms of injectable contraception

- **Depo-Provera**
  - Depot medroxyprogesterone acetate (DMPA) 150mg (as aqueous suspension); should be shaken vigorously prior to use.
  - Given as a deep intramuscular injection every 13 weeks (approved by the CoSRH but outside the product licence for DMPA which is 12 weeks ± 5 days), in the upper outer quadrant of the gluteal region, lateral thigh or deltoid muscle of the arm.
- **Sayana Press**
  - DMPA 104mg (as aqueous suspension); should be shaken vigorously prior to use.
  - Given subcutaneously every 13 weeks in anterior thigh or lower abdomen.
  - It is licensed for pharmacy or self-administration, with appropriate training, so patients can do this themselves.

3.6.3 Advantages of injectable contraception

- This is an effective long-acting method of contraception which has non-hormonal benefits, as shown in *Table 3.6*.
- Can be used by women with sickle cell disease, and may reduce the severity of a sickle cell crisis but is UKMEC 2 (use caution if other UKMEC 2 for VTE).
- Not affected by enzyme-inducing drugs.

3.6.4 Disadvantages of injectable contraception

- The UKMEC 2025 states that five studies have shown an increased risk of VTE with DMPA use when compared to those who do not use hormonal contraception. This evidence has been reflected across the MEC. Some conditions have changed from 1 to 2, or 2 to 3, to reflect increase in risk. Risk is likely to be lower than the VTE risk associated with CHC.
- Weight gain is common; adolescents with a BMI ≥30kg/m^2 are more likely to gain weight. Those who gain more than 5% of their body weight in the first 6 months are likely to experience further weight gain.
- Other side-effects include acne, decreased libido, mood swings, headache, hot flushes, vaginitis and injection site reactions.

- BMD can reduce while using an injectable method, but recovers when it is stopped.
- The delay in return to fertility for approximately 12 months (but can be up to 18 months) may make it less suitable for those who wish to conceive soon.
- There is a weak association between cervical cancer and use of DMPA for 5 years or longer, so encourage women to attend cervical screening.
- See *Section 3.2.11* on use in obesity.

3.6.5 Starting injectable contraception

- Read in conjunction with *Section 3.2.7* for a basic introduction to starting contraception.
- Both injections need to be given every 13 weeks, with a review every 2 years to assess continuation of treatment.
- If more than 14 weeks has elapsed since the last injection, the risk of pregnancy needs to be assessed. EC and/or bridging contraception may be required.
- If under 18 years old, other contraceptive options should be considered first.
- If over 50 years old, discuss discontinuation.

3.6.6 Managing prolonged bleeding with DMPA

- Exclude other causes for bleeding, and manage as described in *Section 3.2.17.*

3.7 Contraceptive implant

- A highly effective method of contraception providing long-acting, reversible contraception for 3 years. Nexplanon (etonogestrel implant) should be inserted subdermally in the inner upper arm, avoiding the biceps–triceps sulcus. The insertion site is located 8–10cm above the medial epicondyle, then 3–5cm posteriorly over the triceps, perpendicular to the sulcus.
- In January 2026 the FDA approved 5-year use for Nexplanon for contraception. This is not yet the case in the UK.
- Refer to:
  - NICE CKS: *Progestogen-only implant.*
  - CoSRH Guideline: *Progestogen-only implant.*

3.7.1 Mechanism of action

- The main mechanism is inhibition of ovulation by suppressing LH, altering cervical mucus, altering the genital tract environment, reducing sperm penetration and transport, and inducing endometrial atrophy; it may also modify sperm function and motility.
- Ovarian activity is not completely suppressed; serum estradiol levels fluctuate but are not suppressed below levels typically seen during the follicular phase of natural menstrual cycles.

3.7.2 Advantages of contraceptive implant

- Effective LARC.
- There is no limit to the number a woman can use consecutively.
- Effectiveness is not affected by body weight.

3.7.3 Disadvantages of contraceptive implant

- May cause side-effects including headache and acne.
- Irregular, unpredictable bleeding is common and bleeding pattern can change over time, but the average number of days of bleeding/spotting is usually less than that of a normal menstrual cycle.
- Requires a minor surgical procedure with risk of bruising and infection. Other risks such as intravascular insertion, nerve damage and distant migration are rare.

- The contraceptive effectiveness of the IMP can be reduced using enzyme-inducing drugs, for the duration of their use and for 28 days after stopping them, so another reliable contraceptive method that is not affected by enzyme-inducing drugs should be used.
- Patients can feel very anxious about having a procedure to fit and remove. It is important to use adequate local anaesthetic and advise about analgesia which can be taken afterwards if needed.

3.7.4 Starting the IMP

- See *Section 3.2.7.*
- If the IMP is put in during the first 5 days of the menstrual cycle, it is effective immediately.
- If it is put in on any other day of the menstrual cycle, additional contraception such as condoms should be used for 7 days.
- Refer to CoRSH Guideline for detail about insertion and removal. The IMP should only be inserted and removed by a qualified health professional with training in this technique.
- Advise the patient how to feel for the implant (it should always be palpable) and when to return for replacement.

3.7.5 Routine follow-up

- Women can be advised to return if they have concerns, cannot feel the implant, have pain over the implant site or have any signs of infection.

3.7.6 Managing side-effects and bleeding

- See *Section 3.2.17.*

3.8 Intrauterine contraception

- Intrauterine devices (IUDs) are long-acting, reversible contraceptives (LARC) with licensed durations of use ranging between 3 and 10 years, depending on the device used.
- There are two types:
  - Levonorgestrel intrauterine devices (LNG-IUDs).
  - Copper IUDs – all Cu-IUDs in the UK have a copper surface area ≥300mm^2.
- All IUDs are suitable for most women, including adolescents and those who are nulliparous or have never been sexually active, provided appropriate counselling and STI risk assessment are undertaken.
- Refer to:
  - NICE CKS: *Levonorgestrel intrauterine device.*
  - NICE CKS: *Copper intrauterine device.*
  - CoSRH Guideline*: Intrauterine contraception.*

3.8.1 Levonorgestrel intrauterine device

Mechanism of action

- Alters the cervical mucus and utero-tubal fluid, inhibiting sperm penetration and migration.
- Down-regulates oestrogen and progesterone receptors in the endometrial tissue, making it less sensitive to circulating oestrogen, consequently preventing endometrial proliferation and causing atrophic changes, making it unsuitable for implantation.
- In a small number of users ovulation may be suppressed in the first year, but serum estradiol levels are not reduced.

Available forms of LNG-IUD

- *Table 3.11* shows the different LNG-IUDs and their product licences. Three strengths of LNG-IUD are available:

Table 3.11: Current CoSRH guidelines for different LNG-IUD products

Hormone LNG-IUD	Dose LNG	Contraception fitting <45 years	Contraception fitting ≥45 years	Endometrial protection as part of HRT
Jaydess	13.5mg	3 years	3 years	Not suitable
Kyleena	19.5mg	5 years	5 years	Not suitable
Mirena	52mg	8 years	until 55 years	Can be used for 5 years
Levosert Benilexa	52mg	8 years	until 55 years	Can be used for 5 years

- 13.5mg LNG-IUD (Jaydess).
- 19.5mg LNG-IUD (Kyleena).
- 52mg LNG-IUD (Mirena, Levosert and Benilexa).

Advantages of LNG-IUDs
- Highly effective long-acting method of contraception.
- Effective for contraception 7 days after fitting.
- Any 52mg LNG-IUD can be used for endometrial protection as part of HRT for 5 years.
- A 52mg LNG-IUD reduces menstrual loss by up to 90% after 6 months of use. Effective for 5 years for menorrhagia (can be left for up to 8 years if still effective).

Disadvantages of LNG-IUDs
- Irregular/prolonged bleeding is common and tends to decrease over time.
- LNG-IUDs cannot be used as emergency contraception.
- Can cause progestogenic side-effects, such as acne, breast tenderness, headache and mood changes, which tend to improve with time.
- Incidence of ovarian cysts may be increased with LNG-IUD use, but it does not seem to be clinically significant, and history of PCOS or ovarian cysts is not a contraindication.
- Requires a procedure to fit, which can be painful.

Bleeding with an LNG-IUD *in situ*
If the bleeding pattern changes and an LNG-IUD is in place, consider the cause for this and arrange an examination and appropriate investigations. Causes (the 5Cs) include:
- Conception (pregnancy).
- Compliance (is the IUD in the right place, has there been a perforation, or has it moved or been expelled?).
- Chlamydia (or another STI).
- Cervix (examine and ensure the cervical screening is up to date).
- Cancer (vulva, vagina, cervix, endometrial, ovarian).

See *Section 3.2.17* for advice on management of problematic bleeding, once pathology has been excluded.

3.8.2 Copper intrauterine device

- If fitted under the age of 40, it can be left in place for 5–10 years, depending upon the type of device fitted.
- A Cu-IUD with copper surface area ≥300mm^2 inserted at ≥40 years can be used for contraception until the menopause, or until age 55.

Mechanism of action
- The main mode of action of Cu-IUDs is the inhibition of fertilisation through the effect of copper on the ovum and sperm.
- Copper in the cervical mucus inhibits the passage of sperm into the uterus.

- Cu-IUDs cause an inflammatory response within the endometrium, which could impair implantation.

Advantages of Cu-IUD

- A highly effective method of contraception and EC.
- Effective immediately after insertion.

Disadvantages of Cu-IUD

- Associated with heavier periods and intermenstrual bleeding. This can be significant, and this method is less suitable for women with menorrhagia.
- Heavy periods may settle with time. Bleeding can be managed with the use of tranexamic acid or mefenamic acid, or a 3-month trial of COCP if there are no contraindications.

3.8.3 Fitting and removal of Cu-IUD and all LNG-IUDs

- Clinicians offering any IUD insertion should be appropriately trained.
- Check there are no allergies, or contraindications such as distortion of the uterine cavity (UKMEC 3), infection such as current pelvic inflammatory disease (UKMEC 4).
- Seek advice from cardiology for women with some cardiac diseases, such as a pre-existing arrhythmia or postural orthostatic tachycardia syndrome (POTs) with history of syncope, as fitting in a hospital setting may be advised.
- Seek advice from Haematology for women with inherited bleeding disorders, and consider risk of bleeding in those on anticoagulants.
- Discuss risk of expulsion (1 in 20); perforation (1–2 in 1000); infection (<1%) and expected bleeding pattern. Advise to feel for the threads within the first 6 weeks after insertion, and then monthly.
- Can be inserted at any time during the menstrual cycle, providing that pregnancy can be reasonably excluded. The cervix is softer in the first week of the cycle, and it can be easier to fit an IUD then.
- IUDs fitted within 48 hours of delivery of a baby have a higher expulsion rate (review at the postnatal check).
- Take a sexual history prior to IUD insertion and offer screening to women at risk of STIs. Screening can be performed at the time of insertion of the device.
- When removing IUDs, check and document that the device is complete.
- Cervical screening should be postponed for 12 weeks after a gynaecological procedure, including fitting of an IUD, so the cells can regenerate.
- Patients can feel very anxious about having a procedure to fit and remove an IUD.
  - Advise women that most IUD insertions are associated with mild to moderate pain or discomfort, but that pain can range from none at all to severe.
  - For some women, fitting can cause dizziness or a vasovagal reaction.
  - It is important to advise about appropriate and adequate analgesia, to be used before, during and after fitting.
  - There is no single analgesic approach proven to be better. Options such as a paracervical block, intracervical local anaesthetic injection, 10% lidocaine spray applied to the cervix and external os 3 minutes before the procedure, or EMLA cream applied to the tenaculum site and into the cervical canal may help reduce insertion-related pain. Taking naproxen 1 hour prior to the procedure may help with both insertion and post-insertion pain, and NSAIDs can be helpful in managing pain after insertion.
  - Offer a chaperone, or a supportive relative to accompany them. Support and encourage women to tell you if they are experiencing pain or discomfort, and reassure them that the procedure can be paused or stopped at any time. They can be given a word to say, such as 'stop' or ask to raise a hand if they want to pause the procedure.

- There should be a referral process for circumstances where a patient requests an analgesia option that the clinician is unable to provide.
- See the CoSRH statement: *Pain associated with insertion of intrauterine contraception.*

3.8.4 IUD missing threads

- Missing threads could be due to pregnancy, expulsion, perforation or just retraction.
- Advise thread checks and the need for additional effective contraception or EC.
- If the ultrasound scan shows a correctly-sited IUD, offer reassurance that the device can be left *in situ* until it would usually be removed or replaced.

3.8.5 Malpositioned IUD

- A malpositioned IUD is likely to be less effective, so consider pain or bleeding, or an IUD in the cervical canal or >2cm from the fundus as a reason to replace it.
- Consider the need for EC, alternative contraception and a pregnancy test.

3.9 Barrier methods

These include male and female condoms, diaphragms and cervical caps. Anyone using a barrier method needs to be informed of the efficacy of the method, in comparison with other more effective methods. They must be advised how to use them correctly, factors which affect their efficacy, and when STI testing, use of EC and post-exposure prophylaxis following sexual exposure (PEPSE) to human immunodeficiency virus (HIV) may be needed.

- For more detailed information refer to: CoSRH Guideline: Barrier methods for contraception and STI prevention (www.cosrh.org/Common/Uploaded%20files/documents/ceuguidancebarriermethodscontraceptionsdi.pdf).

3.9.1 Mechanism of action

- To act as a barrier to ejaculate, pre-ejaculate and cervicovaginal secretions.

3.9.2 Types of barrier method

- Male condoms (latex, non-latex and deproteinised latex varieties).
- Female condoms (nitrile or latex).
- Diaphragms (latex, silicone).
- Cervical cap (silicone).
- Dams (latex, non-latex).

3.9.3 Condoms

- Male condoms fit over an erect penis, and female condoms are worn inside the vagina.
- Check the use by date and safety markings on the packet to ensure they meet the recommended standards for strength and quality.
- Those with a latex allergy should use non-latex condoms.
- For use of lubricants with condoms see *Section 3.9.6.*

Advantages of condoms

- Both male and female condoms are >94% effective at preventing a pregnancy, but only when used consistently and correctly.
- Consistent and effective use of condoms is the most effective means of protecting against HIV and other STIs.
- Can be used as a primary method of contraception, or while a chosen method becomes effective, or in the long term to provide double contraception.

Disadvantages of condoms

- Ill-fitting condoms can be associated with breakage, so advise that different sizes and shapes are available.

3.9.4 Diaphragms and caps

- Both the cervical cap and diaphragm (see *Table 3.12*) cover the cervix, and spermicide should be applied to the device before it is inserted.
- The diaphragm is available in a single size and the cap in several sizes. An examination may be required to ensure correct fit by an experienced clinician.

Advantages

- When used consistently, correctly and with spermicide, diaphragms and cervical caps are estimated to be between 92% and 96% effective at preventing pregnancy.
- They are a choice for women who prefer a method without hormones.
- They can be inserted with spermicide any time before intercourse, but spermicide should be reapplied if the diaphragm or cap has been in place for longer than 3 hours and sex is to take place, or if sex is repeated with the device in place.

Disadvantages

- They must be left in place for at least 6 hours after the last episode of intercourse.
- They do not protect against HIV and other STIs. They provide a physical barrier to sperm reaching the cervix, but they do not prevent exposure of the vaginal mucosa to semen or exposure of the penis to cervicovaginal secretions.
- They must be correctly fitted.
- Caps and diaphragms should not be left in place for longer than recommended by the manufacturer, or used during menstruation.

Table 3.12: Diaphragms and caps

	Presentation	Brand	Size
Diaphragm	Silicone – flexible rim	Caya	One size (fits women who require 65–80mm diaphragm)
Cap	Silicone	Femcap	22mm, 26mm and 30mm

3.9.5 Dental dam

- A thin square piece of latex or polyurethane used during oral sex to help prevent the transmission of STIs. It creates a barrier between the mouth and the partner's genitals or anus, essentially acting like a condom for oral sex.
- They are not a contraceptive method.

3.9.6 Lubricants for sexual intercourse

- Avoid oil-based lubricants with latex condoms, diaphragms and caps.
- Some low-dose localised vaginal oestrogen products can damage latex condoms (and potentially latex diaphragms and caps), such as estriol 0.03mg pessaries, estriol 0.01% cream and prasterone (DHEA) pessaries, so advise to use an alternative localised oestrogen product. For more information on localised oestrogen refer to *Section 7.7.*
- There is an increased risk of the condom slipping off if a lubricant is applied to the penis or if the lubricant is applied inside the condom.

3.10 Fertility awareness

This involves working out when a woman is likely to ovulate, and using a condom or avoiding having sex at this time in the cycle.

- It has a high risk of failure, so should not be used when pregnancy would be a problem, particularly by those for whom pregnancy would be high risk.
- Women should receive support and instruction from a trained practitioner.
- It may be suitable for women who have a regular menstrual cycle, but is not suitable for those with irregular periods.
- Methods include:
  - measuring basal body temperature
  - keeping a record of menstrual cycles over a 12-month period to calculate the longest and shortest cycle
  - noticing monthly changes in cervical mucus
  - the use of devices or apps to track the fertile phase.
- Refer to: CoSRH Clinical Guideline: Fertility awareness methods.

3.11 Male and female sterilisation

Vasectomy for men and laparoscopic sterilisation for women are permanent methods of contraception, suitable for those who do not ever wish to have children or have completed their family. Reversal of both often fails and is generally not available on the NHS.

- Vasectomy is carried out under local anaesthetic and the surgeon cuts both vas deferens tubes and seals the ends. This stops the sperm from leaving the body. It takes about 30 minutes, and the patient can go home about an hour later. A semen analysis is done at 12 weeks to check the vasectomy has been fully effective. The vasectomy should not be relied on for contraception until the surgeon has confirmed that this result does not contain any sperm. It does not affect sexual drive or the ability to achieve an erection. The amount of ejaculate is unchanged, only sperm are absent.
- Female sterilisation is traditionally done by laparoscopic surgery under general anaesthetic. A clip (or other device) is placed onto both fallopian tubes to prevent the egg and sperm meeting. It does not affect ovulation and has no effect on the menstrual cycle. There is no evidence it affects sexual desire.
- Counselling should include:
  - Advantages and disadvantages.
  - Ensuring both partners do not want children.
  - Identify reasons for a sterilisation request.
  - Current contraception.
  - Other methods of contraception to consider.
  - Menstrual history.
  - Past medical and surgical history.
  - Risk factors for surgery.
  - Failure rate.
  - Irreversibility and possible regret.
  - Time until procedure is effective.
  - Details of the procedure.
  - No protection against STIs.
- Refer to: CoSRH Guideline: Male and female sterilisation (www.cosrh.org/Public/Documents/cec-ceu-guidance-sterilisation-cpd-sep-2014.aspx).

3.12 Emergency contraception

3.12.1 Types of emergency contraception

- There are three types of emergency contraception (EC):
  - Cu-IUD
  - Two types of oral emergency contraception:
    - Ulipristal acetate (UPA-EC)
    - Levonorgestrel (LNG-EC).
- Refer to:
  - NICE CKS: *Emergency hormonal contraception.*
  - CoSRH Guideline: *Emergency contraception.*
- EC should be taken as soon as possible after unprotected sex or after failure of the current method of contraception.
- Pregnancy risk is greatest in the 6 days leading up to and including the day of ovulation, but always offer EC if there is risk of pregnancy, at any time in the cycle.
- Oral EC provides no ongoing contraception and will not protect further episodes of unprotected intercourse in that cycle.
- Ask patients about their history of use of EC and hormonal contraception, when deciding which EC method is suitable.
- *Figure 3.1* provides an algorithm to help decide between use of oral EC and a Cu-IUD, and between both types of oral EC.

3.12.2 Mechanism of action

- Oral emergency hormonal contraception works by delaying ovulation.
- Cu-IUD works by preventing fertilisation and implantation.

3.12.3 Assessing pregnancy risk

To assess pregnancy risk, you need to know:

- Exact date of the first day of the last menstrual period.
- The longest and shortest cycle length in the last 6 months, to help work out the earliest and latest predicted dates of ovulation.
- Exact dates and times of all episodes of unprotected intercourse since the start of the last period.

3.12.4 Copper intrauterine device

- This is the most effective method and should be offered to all women, if suitable.
- If a person opts to have an IUD, oral EC should also be offered, in case they later change their mind, or it is not possible to fit the copper IUD.
- Can be fitted if all episodes of unprotected sexual intercourse since the last menstrual period have occurred either within the last 5 days, or you are fitting the IUD within 5 days after the earliest predicted date of ovulation (see *Section 3.12.5*).
- Can legally be fitted at any time prior to implantation.
- Can be retained until pregnancy is excluded, e.g. onset of period, or at least 3 weeks after the last episode of unprotected sex, or can remain in place for the licensed duration of the IUD.

3.12.5 Assessing the earliest predicted date of ovulation when considering a Cu-IUD for EC

- Ovulation occurs 14 days before the next menstrual period.
- Ask what the longest and shortest cycle length has been in the last 6 months.

- The earliest likely ovulation date is the shortest cycle length minus 14 days. For example, a patient with a shortest cycle length of 26 days in the last 6 months, has an earliest likely ovulation date of day 12 (26 minus 14). Pregnancy risk is highest in the 6 days leading up to and including ovulation, so for a 26-day cycle, the days at highest risk are days 7 to day 12.
- Sperm survive up to 5 days in the genital tract. The ovum survives for 24 hours after ovulation. Once ovulation occurs, if an egg has been fertilised by sperm in the fallopian tubes a zygote forms. It takes time for the zygote to move into the uterus, where it implants and starts to develop into a fetus.
- In the UK, prevention of implantation of a fertilised egg is contraception and not abortion. Pregnancy starts at the point of implantation. This normally occurs 8–10 days after ovulation, and no earlier than 6 days after ovulation, so the Cu-IUD can be fitted within 5 days after the earliest predicted date of ovulation, before implantation could occur.

3.12.6 Oral emergency contraception

- Oral EC delays ovulation by delaying the LH surge, so ovulation will occur about 5 days later than predicted. This means any sperm in the genital tract will no longer be viable when the egg is released.
- For oral EC to have the best chance of delaying ovulation it needs to be taken at the earliest opportunity, before ovulation has occurred.
- Both oral EC preparations are unlikely to have any effect after ovulation has occurred, but should be offered at any time in the cycle.
- Refer to *Section 3.2.11* for details about oral EC use and BMI/weight, and *Section 3.2.20* about drug interactions and oral EC, and about starting contraceptives after the use of oral EC.
- Both types of oral EC can be used more than once in a cycle, but if the patient has taken LNG-EC she should not take UPA-EC in the following 7 days, as levonorgestrel is a progestogen and may affect the effectiveness of UPA-EC. Similarly, if the patient has used UPA-EC, then LNG-EC cannot be used in the following 5 days.

3.12.7 Oral selective progesterone receptor modulator: UPA

- 30mg single oral dose, to be taken within 120 hours of unprotected sex or contraception failure.
- May be able to delay ovulation if the LH surge has started.
- More effective than levonorgestrel.
- Never given as a double dose.
- Absorption may be reduced if the gastric pH is raised, as in patients taking antacids or proton pump inhibitors.
- Check for interacting medications taken in the last 4 weeks (e.g. some anti-epileptics and St John's wort).
- As described in *Section 3.2.7*, no progestogen-containing contraception should be started within 5 days of use of UPA-EC, and if the woman has taken any progestogens in the last 7 days, then UPA may not work as emergency contraception.

3.12.8 Oral progestogen-only EC: LNG-EC

- 1.5mg single oral dose licensed to be used up to 72 hours after unprotected sex, but can be taken up to 96 hours (off-licence).
- Use in preference to UPA-EC if any progestogen has been taken in the last 7 days.
- Will only delay the LH surge if it is taken before the LH surge begins.
- Can be given if there has been an episode of unprotected sex earlier in the same cycle as well as within the last 5 days, as evidence suggests it does not disrupt an existing pregnancy.
- Advise to resume or start contraception with additional barrier cover as necessary. Hormonal contraception can be started immediately and does not need to be delayed as with UPA-EC.

3.12.9 After taking emergency contraception

Advise about STI screening and ongoing contraception. Advise a pregnancy test:

- 3 weeks after the last episode of unprotected sex.
- If the next period is late by 7 days.
- If the period is lighter than usual.
- If the period is associated with atypical abdominal pain.

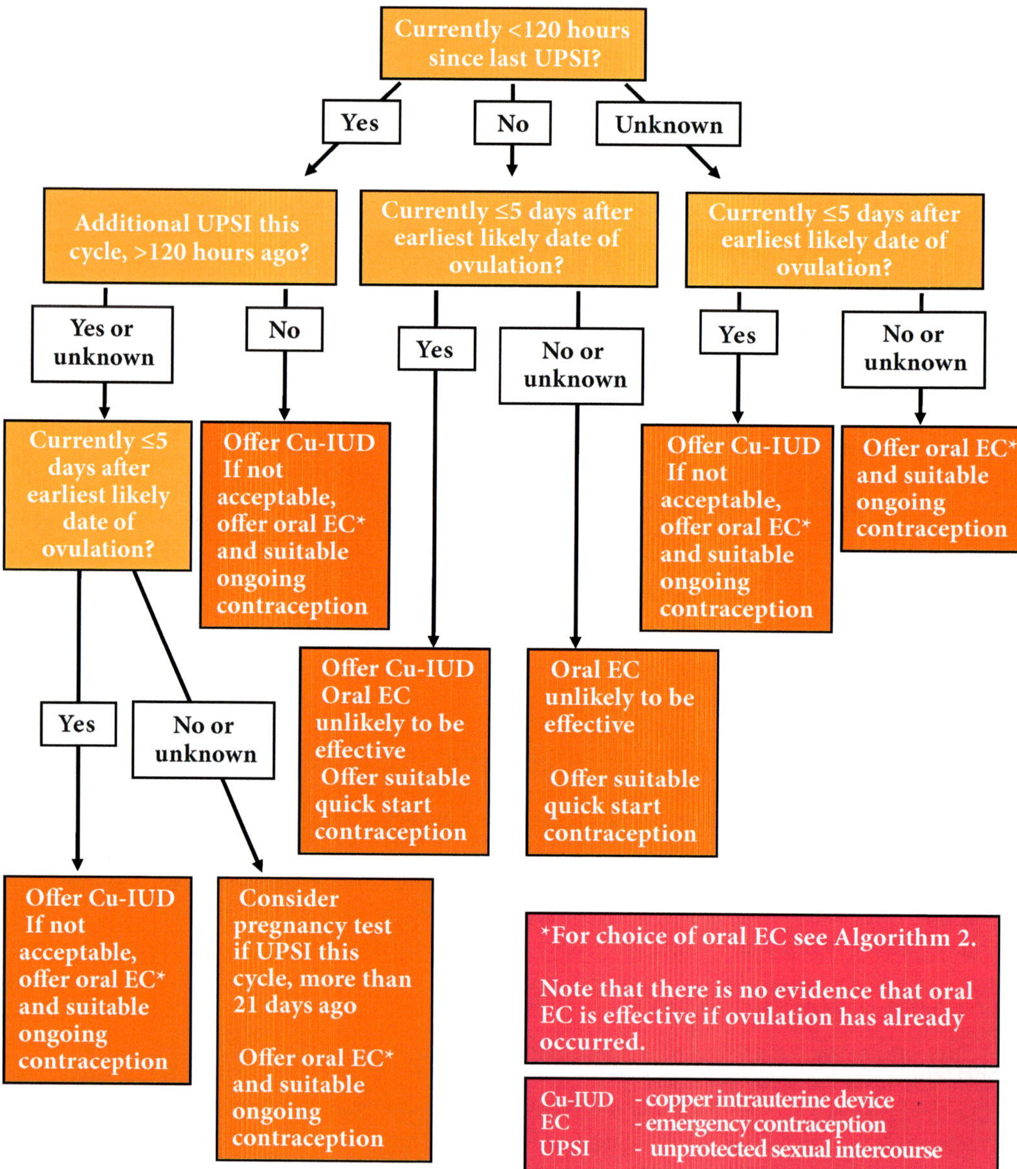

Figure 3.1: CoSRH decision algorithm for emergency contraception: Cu-IUD vs. oral EC. Reproduced with permission from CoSRH 2025.

3.13 Further reading

British Menopause Society (2022) *HRT preparations and equivalent alternatives.* Available at: https://thebms.org.uk/wp-content/uploads/2024/02/15-BMS-TfC-HRT-preparations-and-equivalent-alternatives-JAN2024-B.pdf

Brook; Sexual health and wellbeing website (www.brook.org.uk)

Chakrabarti, R. and Chakrabarti, R. (2021) Prescribing the oral contraceptive pill: key considerations for primary care physicians. *BJGP*, 71(712): 522–4.

CoSRH: Contraception choices (www.contraceptionchoices.org)

CoSRH (undated) *Contraception for specific populations.* Available at: www.cosrh.org/Public/Public/Standards-and-Guidance/Contraception-for-Specific-Populations.aspx

CoSRH (amended 2015) FSRH Clinical Guideline: *Barrier methods for contraception and STI prevention.* Available at: www.cosrh.org/Public/Public/Documents/ceu-guidance-barrier-methods-for-contraception.aspx

CoSRH (2015) FSRH Clinical Guideline: *Fertility awareness methods.* Available at: www.cosrh.org/Public/Documents/ceu-guidance-fertility-awareness-methods.aspx

CoSRH (2015) FSRH Clinical Guideline: *Problematic bleeding with hormonal contraception.* Available at: www.cosrh.org/Public/Public/Documents/ceu-guidance-problematic-bleeding-hormonal-contraception.aspx

CoSRH (2017) FSRH CEU Statement: *Contraceptive choices and sexual health for transgender and non-binary people.* Available at: www.cosrh.org/Public/Public/Documents/fsrh-ceu-statement-contraceptive-choices-and-sexual-health-for-non-binary-people.aspx

CoSRH (2018) FSRH CEU Statement: *Contraception for women using known teratogenic drugs or drugs with potential teratogenic effects.* Available at: www.cosrh.org/Public/Public/Documents/fsrh-ceu-statement-contraception-for-women-using-known-teratogenic-drugs.aspx

CoSRH (amended 2019) FSRH Clinical guideline: *Contraceptive choices for young people.* Available at: www.cosrh.org/Public/Public/Documents/fsrh-ceu-guidance-young-people-mar-2010.aspx

CoSRH (2019) FSRH Guideline: *Combined hormonal contraception.* Available at: www.cosrh.org/Common/Uploaded%20files/documents/fsrh-guideline-combined-hormonal-contraception-october-2023.pdf

CoSRH (2019) FSRH Clinical Guideline: *Overweight, obesity and contraception.* Available at: www.cosrh.org/Public/Public/Documents/fsrh-clinical-guideline-overweight-obesity-and-contraception.aspx

CoSRH (amended 2020) FSRH Guideline: *Contraception after pregnancy.* Available at: www.cosrh.org/Common/Uploaded%20files/documents/contraception-after-pregnancy-guideline-oct2020.pdf

CoSRH (2021) FSRH Statement: *Pain associated with insertion of intrauterine contraception.* Available at: www.cosrh.org/Common/Uploaded%20files/documents/fsrh-clinical-statement-pain-associated-with-insertion-of-iut-jul-2021.pdf

CoSRH (amended 2021) FSRH CEU Guidance: *Recommended actions after incorrect use of combined hormonal contraception (e.g. late or missed pills, ring and patch).* Available at: www.cosrh.org/Public/Public/Documents/fsrh-ceu-guidance-recommended-actions-after-incorrect-use.aspx

CoSRH (2022) FSRH CEU Guidance: *Drug interactions with hormonal contraception.* Available at: www.cosrh.org/Public/Public/Documents/ceu-clinical-guidance-drug-interactions-with-hormonal.aspx

CoSRH (amended 2023) FSRH Guideline: *Emergency contraception.* Available at: www.cosrh.org/Common/Uploaded%20files/documents/fsrh-guideline-emergency-contraception03dec2020-amendedjuly2023-11jul.pdf

CoSRH (amended July 2023) FSRH Clinical Guideline: *Progestogen-only implant.* Available at: www.cosrh.org/Public/Public/Documents/clinical-guidance-progestogen-only-implants.aspx

CoSRH (amended 2023) Clinical Guidance: *Progestogen-only injectable contraception.* Available at: www.cosrh.org/Common/Uploaded%20files/documents/progestogen-only-injectable-december-2014-amended-11july2023.pdf

CoSRH (amended 2023) FSRH Guideline: *Progestogen-only pills.* Available at: www.cosrh.org/Common/Uploaded%20files/documents/fsrh-ceu-clinical-guideline-progestogen-only-pills-aug22-amended-11july-2023-.pdf

CoSRH (2023) FSRH CEU Guidance: *Switching or starting methods of contraception.* Available at: www.cosrh.org/Public/Public/Standards-and-Guidance/Switching-or-Starting-Methods-of-Contraception.aspx

CoSRH (2023) *FSRH Response to new study on use of CHC and POC and breast cancer risk.* Available at: www.cosrh.org/Public/Public/Documents/response-to-study-on-use-of-chc-and-poc-and-breast-cancer.aspx

CoSRH (2023) FSRH CEU Guidance: *Supporting contraceptive choices for individuals who have or have had breast cancer.* Available at: www.cosrh.org/Common/Uploaded%20files/documents/fsrh-cadbc-guidance-document-15-nov-2023.pdf

CoSRH (2025) FSRH patient information leaflet: *GLP-1 agonists and contraception.* Available at: www.cosrh.org/Public/Public/Documents/fsrh-clinical-guideline-overweight-obesity-and-contraception.aspx

CoSRH (amended 2025) FSRH Guideline: *Intrauterine contraception.* Available at: www.cosrh.org/Common/Uploaded%20files/documents/fsrh-clinical-guideline-intrauterine-contraception-mar-23-amended.pdf

GMC (updated 2018) *0–18 years: guidance for all doctors.* Available at: www.gmc-uk.org/-/media/documents/0_18_years_english_0418pdf_48903188.pdf?la=en%26hash=3092448DA3A5249B297C4C5EAEF1AD7549EEB5C7

HerLifeHerHealth magazine (spring 2023), page 4: *Hormonal contraceptives and breast cancer risk.*

NICE (updated 2023) *Familial breast cancer: classification, care and managing breast cancer and related risks in people with a family history of breast cancer* [CG164]. Available at: https://www.nice.org.uk/Guidance/CG164

NICE (revised 2024) CKS: *Combined oral contraceptive.* Available at: https://cks.nice.org.uk/topics/contraception-combined-hormonal-methods/management/combined-oral-contraceptive

NICE (revised 2024) CKS: *Combined transdermal patch.* Available at: https://cks.nice.org.uk/topics/contraception-combined-hormonal-methods/management/combined-contraceptive-patch

NICE (revised 2024) CKS: *Combined vaginal ring.* Available at: https://cks.nice.org.uk/topics/contraception-combined-hormonal-methods/management/combined-contraceptive-vaginal-ring

NICE (revised 2024) CKS: *Contraception – combined hormonal methods*. Available at: https://cks.nice.org.uk/topics/contraception-combined-hormonal-methods

NICE (revised 2024) CKS: *Copper intrauterine device*. Available at: https://cks.nice.org.uk/topics/contraception-iuc/management/copper-intrauterine-device

NICE (revised 2024) CKS: *Emergency hormonal contraception*. Available at: https://cks.nice.org.uk/topics/contraception-emergency/management/management

NICE (revised 2024) CKS: *Levonorgestrel intrauterine device*. Available at: https://cks.nice.org.uk/topics/contraception-iuc/management/levonorgestrel-intrauterine-device

NICE (revised 2024) CKS: *Progestogen-only implant*. Available at: https://cks.nice.org.uk/topics/contraception-progestogen-only-methods/management/progestogen-only-implant

NICE (revised 2024) CKS: *Progestogen-only injectables*. Available at: https://cks.nice.org.uk/topics/contraception-progestogen-only-methods/management/progestogen-only-injectables

NICE (revised 2024) CKS: *Progestogen-only pill*. Available at: https://cks.nice.org.uk/topics/contraception-progestogen-only-methods/management/progestogen-only-pill

NICE (2024) *Ovarian cancer: identifying and managing familial and genetic risk* [NG241]. Available at: www.nice.org.uk/guidance/ng241

NICE (updated 2025) *British National Formulary (BNF)*. Available at: https://bnf.nice.org.uk

RCOG (2016) *Management of premenstrual syndrome*. Available at: www.rcog.org.uk/guidance/browse-all-guidance/green-top-guidelines/premenstrual-syndrome-management-green-top-guideline-no-48

UK teratology information service (UKTIS) website: https://uktis.org

Chapter 4
Sexual health

4.1 Introduction

- Sexual problems are common, but the subject of sex remains largely absent from the medical curriculum.
  - 1 in 6 women admitted to a health problem affecting their sex life in the previous year, but only 1 in 5 of these sought help with it.
  - More than half of all women had sexual difficulties lasting more than 3 months in the last year.
- Sexual difficulties are distressing, and correlate with lower quality of life and relationship satisfaction scores.
- The majority of patients expect their clinician to be the one to raise the subject of sex in a consultation.
- Doctors cite personal and health system limitations, presuppositions and assumptions, and socio-cultural barriers, as well as lack of training, as the reasons these questions are not asked.

4.2 How to talk with patients about sex

There are many ways to open up a conversation about sex with our patients. They will usually follow our lead and find it easier to open up with a practitioner who seems comfortable and at ease with discussing the subject.

- Talking about sex gets easier with practice. With repetition, the language and questions we use become second nature, and approaching the subject will become easier.
- Asking questions about sex does not necessarily have to mean long consultations are needed. Research shows that brief intervention is often important in validating patients' concerns and can improve their sexual wellbeing.
- Direct, clear language usually works best when talking about sex. Ask simple, open questions such as "*Sometimes X can affect sex. Have you noticed any changes you would like to talk about?*".
- The PLISSIT Model (see *Fig. 4.1*) is a validated framework which works well in the healthcare setting and is endorsed by European Society for Sexual Medicine and Institute for Psychosexual Medicine training.

P: Permission – we can seek the patient's permission to discuss sex by mentioning that sexuality can change with illness, medication, relationship and hormonal shifts; this also gives the patient permission to think about the issue and legitimises the subject.

LI: Limited Information – give the patient limited information about the ways in which whatever is happening can impact sex.

SS: Specific Suggestions – make specific suggestions that address the sexual problem. For example, for a menopausal patient to consider the use of vaginal oestrogen or lubricant for vaginal dryness.

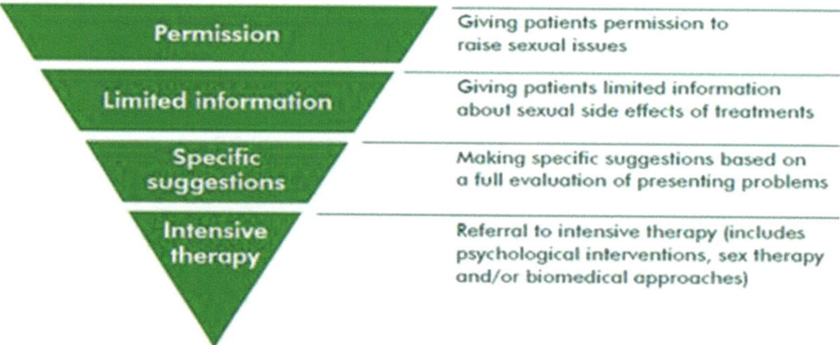

Figure 4.1: The PLISSIT model for addressing sexual functioning. Reproduced from Annon, J.S. (1974) The PLISSIT model: a proposed conceptual scheme for the behavioral treatment of sexual problems. *J. Sex Education Therapy*, 2:1, with permission from Taylor & Francis.

IT: Intensive Therapy – if the patient needs more, then you can signpost for more intensive therapy with an IPM-trained clinician (www.ipm.org.uk/patients/specialists), COSRT-accredited therapist (www.cosrt.org.uk/the-cosrt-registers), or other source of support.

4.2.1 Further training in psychosexual medicine

Further training in psychosexual medicine is available to both doctors and allied health professionals. The Institute of Psychosexual Medicine (IPM) and College of Sexual and Relationship Therapists (COSRT) websites also provide a list of qualified practitioners.

- **The Institute of Psychosexual Medicine** provides introductory courses followed by seminar-based training (www.ipm.org.uk).
- The **College of Sexual and Relationship Therapists** has accredited a number of courses in Clinical Sexology and Psychosexual Therapy (www.cosrt.org.uk).
- **The European Society of Sexual Medicine** has an annual 10-day 'School of Sexual Medicine', available at basic and advanced level. There is the option to sit the Multidisciplinary Joint Committee of Sexual Medicine membership examination for Fellowship of the European Committee of Sexual Medicine – this is the gold standard qualification in sexual medicine (www.essm.org).

4.3 Supporting sexual wellbeing in our patients

Sexual wellbeing goes beyond simply the absence of problems with sexual function. The World Health Organization (WHO) defines sexual health as:

> *"... a state of physical, emotional, mental and social well-being in relation to sexuality; it is not merely the absence of disease, dysfunction or infirmity. Sexual health requires a positive and respectful approach to sexuality and sexual relationships, as well as the possibility of having pleasurable and safe sexual experiences, free of coercion, discrimination and violence."*

Addressing sexual problems holistically requires us to apply a biopsychosocial model (see *Fig. 4.2*) which integrates physical health with other factors that have equal capacity to impact sexual health. The biopsychosocial model takes account of social factors (religious and cultural norms, relationship and roles), and also considers our psychological state (sexual identity, coping skills, previous traumas and experiences, mental health and behaviour) as well as our physical health. This is in contrast to the biomedical model which traditionally separated physical and mental health and did not recognise the complex interaction and interplay of body and mind.

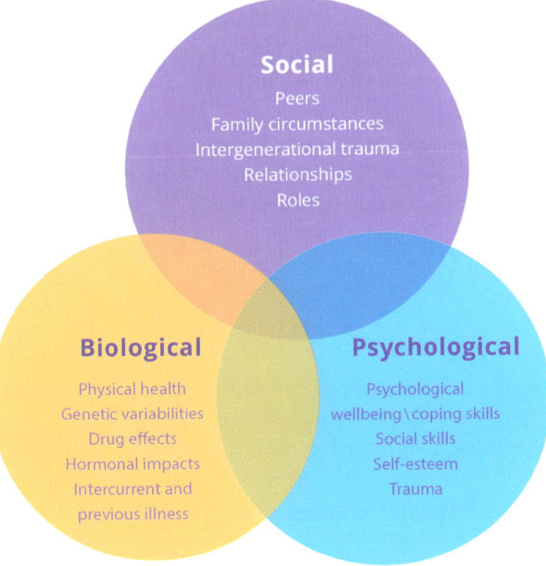

Figure 4.2: The biopsychosocial model.

4.4 What is sexual health?

- The WHO definition of sexual health is shown in *Section 4.3*.
- Achieving sexual health depends upon:
  - access to comprehensive, good-quality information about sex and sexuality
  - knowledge about the risks faced with unprotected sexual activity
  - access to sexual healthcare
  - living in an environment that affirms and promotes sexual health.
- Sexual health issues are wide-ranging. They may encompass sexual orientation and gender identity, sexual expression, relationships and pleasure. They also include negative consequences or conditions such as:
  - infections (i.e. HIV, STIs and reproductive tract infections (RTIs) and their adverse outcomes (such as cancer and infertility))
  - unintended pregnancy and abortion
  - sexual dysfunction
  - sexual violence (thought to impact 1 in 4 women and 1 in 6 men)
  - harmful practices (such as female genital mutilation (FGM)).

4.4.1 Where does pleasure fit in?

- Too often, when we do discuss sex in clinical settings, we focus on 'dysfunction' rather than seeing problems through a pleasure-focused lens. Pleasure is a key aspect of sexual motivation and improves sexual function.
- Sexual desire is known to be experienced in more than one way:
  - spontaneous desire (similar to hunger)
  - responsive desire (where desire is triggered by a sexual cue – similar to feeling hungry only when you smell baking bread when walking past a bakery).
- Rosemary Basson's work on sexuality in women showed that the majority of desire in long-term monogamous relationships is experienced in response to a cue. Where we have an expectation of a rewarding experience (pleasure, orgasm, renewed closeness to a partner, relaxation), we are more likely to respond to a cue with desire and a willingness to have sex.
- Where sex has become associated with negative reward (pain, urine infections, difficulty reaching climax or becoming aroused) then we tend to ignore or block out cues.
- When dealing with sexual problems in practice, it can help to ask questions about what is really going on, and to tackle individual components as they come up: for example, prescribing vaginal oestrogen when women are complaining of low libido at menopause can help them to feel pleasure rather than pain, and prevents urinary tract infection after penetration. This is likely to do more to help libido than prescribing testosterone in the presence of ongoing negative impacts from sex.
- Remember vaginismus and avoidance are logical end points of sexual pain. Trainer therapy alone is unhelpful if we do not focus on supporting patients to explore the cause of pain, to modify this, and to develop a new expectation of a better experience.
- Simple resources in practice can help patients tackle sexual issues:
  - *Mind The Gap* by Karen Gurney – a summary of sexual function and pleasure that provides an excellent self-help guide.
  - *Better Sex Through Mindfulness* by Lori Brotto – a workbook that helps bring focus to the body and away from anxiety or distraction in sex.
  - Post-baby Hanky Panky – a website focused on the impact of childbirth and pregnancy on sexuality (https://postbabyhankypanky.com).
  - The "Oh-Nut" – a series of ring buffers to minimise depth of penetration, helpful in pelvic pain conditions.
  - www.jodivine.com – a website with toys and aids and resources to support patients.

4.5 Barriers to care and intersectionality

4.5.1 What is intersectionality?

- The term 'intersectionality' has its roots in Black feminist activism, and was originally coined by American legal and critical race scholar Kimberlé Williams Crenshaw in 1989.
- Crenshaw used the term intersectionality to refer to the double discrimination of racism and sexism faced by Black women (she called this 'misogynoir').
- She provided the following definition of intersectionality:

  "Intersectionality is a metaphor for understanding the ways that multiple forms of inequality or disadvantage sometimes compound themselves and create obstacles that often are not understood among conventional ways of thinking."

- Research by Stonewall showed that the more layers of intersectionality a person faces, the more barriers to care they face. They are also more likely to have experienced trauma, and to have physical and mental health issues.
- We are often blind to our own privilege and may not consider the problems faced by others with more barriers. Despite the increasing diversity of relationship, gender and sexual expression in our patients, medical training often remains cis, mono and heteronormative.
- Failure to use inclusive language can create further obstacles for those with diverse identities, and may feel shaming or excluding. This may lead to missed opportunities to improve access to care.
- Be curious and respectful: ask your patient how they would prefer you to refer to them and avoid making assumptions about the gender of sexual partners, about relationship structures or about sexual preferences. The patient is always the expert.

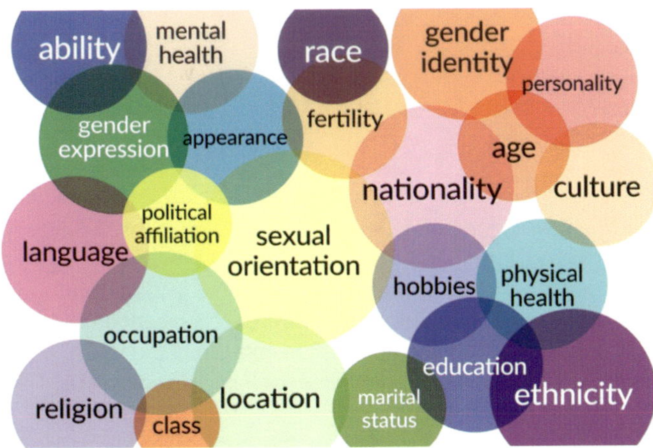

Figure 4.3: Intersectionality. Graphic created by Misty McPhetridge, BSSW.

4.6 Providing trauma-informed care

4.6.1 What do we mean by trauma?

- Trauma can be defined as when we experience very stressful, frightening or distressing events that are difficult to cope with or out of our control.
- This can be one event, a series of events, or an ongoing event that happens over a long period of time (see *Box 4.1*). Trauma may take many forms and can be passed down through families (known as intergenerational trauma).

- Most of us will experience some trauma over the course of our lives, but we do not all respond to it in the same way. Many of our patients will be affected by trauma. They may also be unaware that a historic event is still impacting them.
- The experience of significant trauma correlates with an increased likelihood of physical and psychological/relational health sequelae. For example, women with a history of adverse childhood events are more likely to experience a more symptomatic and distressing menopause and to experience sexual dysfunction as a result, and are less likely to attend routine screening, e.g. smear tests.
- Trauma-informed practice is essential to change these trends and create experiences of safety and bodily autonomy in healthcare environments (see *Box 4.2*).

BOX 4.1: Examples of types of trauma

Sexual assault or abuse (likely to affect 1 in 4 women and 1 in 6 men, though under-reported)

Physical assault or abuse

Emotional abuse

Neglect

Domestic violence

Serious accidents or illness (including childbirth or hospitalisation, or post suicide of a loved one)

War-related trauma

Natural or man-made disasters

School violence

Bullying or workplace mobbing

Historical or intergenerational trauma

4.6.2 How can trauma affect us?

- Trauma is not stored normally in the brain, which means certain cues can trigger the survivor into one of the reflex responses known as the 'four Fs' – fight, flight, freeze or fawn (appeasing others). This may occur immediately after, or many years after the original event.
- MRI studies show that when the trauma response has been triggered, the area coordinating speech in the brain goes 'offline'. **This can mean it is impossible for a patient re-experiencing their trauma, e.g. during an intimate examination, to be able to vocalise their distress or ask us to stop.**
- Common activators of a trauma response can be imagery, lighting, memory, physical space, sensations, smells, thoughts, words or feelings.
- It is easy to see how triggering could occur in a healthcare consultation, especially if the original trauma relates to sexual abuse/assault or medical trauma. The responsibility therefore lies with us as healthcare professionals to be informed as to the types and impacts of trauma, and to adapt our approach to all patients to consider that trauma may be present and patients may not choose to declare it to us.

BOX 4.2: Principles of trauma-informed practice

The four Rs of trauma-informed care

- **R**ealise that trauma can affect individuals, groups and communities and that there is potential for recovery
- **R**ecognise the signs, symptoms and widespread impact of trauma
- **R**espond by integrating knowledge of trauma into policies, procedures and practices
- **R**esist re-traumatisation

Key principles of trauma-informed care

1. Safety
2. Trustworthiness/transparency
3. Peer support
4. Collaboration and mutuality
5. Empowerment, voice and choice
6. Cultural, historical and gender issues must be considered

Adapted from https://library.samhsa.gov.

4.6.3 How to conduct a trauma-informed examination

- We should approach all patients as if they may have experienced trauma: the onus is not on the patient to declare their history to us.
- A trauma-informed approach to examination goes beyond simply asking for consent to proceed. There is often a power dynamic in a clinician–patient relationship and some traumatised individuals may reflexively say "yes" to our request in order to avoid conflict, a form of 'fawn' response. Watch body language, and repeatedly assure the patient they are in control.
- Discuss what any examination may involve, offering time to ask questions. Offer a chaperone.
- Ask the patient if they find examination difficult, and if so, what would help them? (e.g. time to prepare, a friend or relative present, a longer appointment).
- Discuss ahead of time how they will tell you to pause or stop. Verbalising may be impossible when triggered, so agreeing to raise a hand, for example, may help.
- Observe for signs of distress throughout: are they breathing quickly, wringing hands, avoiding eye contact, shaking, tensing? Are they very quiet and seeming to be absent?
- Keep in constant communication and check in with them frequently. Ask permission at every stage of the exam or procedure.
- Stop the exam immediately if the patient is in distress. Help with grounding (offer water, bring their attention to something in the room).
- Allow the patient to dress before continuing the appointment.

The rest of this chapter will focus on diagnosing and managing clinical issues in sexual health.

4.7 Vaginal discharge

4.7.1 Normal physiological discharge

- Normal vaginal discharge is fluid produced by the cervix and vagina to help protect against infections. This physiological discharge is not associated with redness, itching or swelling, and does not have a strong odour.
- Discharge naturally varies in colour, consistency and amount throughout the female life course. Pregnancy, hormonal contraceptives and menopause can all change its characteristics.
- Research indicates that 10% of women presenting with vaginal discharge will be describing normal physiological discharge.

4.7.2 Vaginal discharge during the menstrual cycle

- Vaginal discharge varies during the menstrual cycle, with ovulation leading to clear, stretchy and plentiful discharge (known as 'egg white cervical mucus'). Discharge becomes slightly thicker and more yellow in the luteal phase. These changes are often tracked by women who use natural fertility methods to manage pregnancy.

4.7.3 Vaginal discharge with contraceptives, and during pregnancy and menopause

- Hormonal contraceptives can alter the amount, consistency and type of vaginal discharge.
- Discharge usually becomes heavier during pregnancy, reflecting the increased level of blood flow to the genitals and pelvis and the higher levels of circulating sex hormones.
- Women may experience a reduction in vaginal discharge at menopause and when breastfeeding. The vaginal biome will change in the absence of oestrogen and normal physiological discharge can change in quantity, colour, smell and consistency.
- Women with symptomatic discharge or vulvovaginal itch or discomfort whilst on hormonal contraceptives, when breastfeeding, during perimenopause or post menopause may benefit from vaginal examination and the use of regular vaginal and vulval topical oestrogen. See *Section 6.7* for more detail on genitourinary syndrome of menopause.

4.7.4 When to investigate vaginal discharge and test for STIs

- Where discharge is distressing, or associated with itch, discomfort or other symptoms, further assessment (including examination and/or swabs) may be appropriate.
- Symptomatic vaginal discharge may be associated with a variety of infections, including bacterial vaginosis, candidiasis (thrush) or STIs such as gonorrhoea, chlamydia and trichomoniasis.
- Initial presentations of candidiasis and bacterial vaginosis can usually be reliably identified by history and examination alone. Charcoal swabs for microscopy, culture and sensitivities (MC&S) are expensive and not needed in the first instance. Treat symptomatically and investigate further only if there is failure to improve.
- In contrast, remember that most STIs can be asymptomatic and that assessment of 'risky' sexual behaviours is often flawed and prone to stigmatising patients, and can be misleading clinically. In addition, leading relationship therapist Esther Perel estimates that the rate of non-consensual non-monogamy in relationships (i.e. affairs and infidelity) may be as high as 46%. This suggests many patients are unaware of their own risk of exposure.
- **The bottom line is, if a patient is sexually active, they are at risk of STIs.** Have a low threshold for testing with polymerase chain reaction (PCR) for gonorrhoea, chlamydia and trichomonas, and make few assumptions about who may have it. It is also important to remember blood testing for HIV and syphilis in all patients – particularly those with unexplained symptoms.

- Have a lower threshold for investigation of problematic discharge in pregnancy. Preterm rupture of membranes and preterm birth are associated with vaginal infections during pregnancy, therefore high vaginal swab (HVS) is more often indicated in this group.

4.8 Vulvovaginal candidiasis

4.8.1 What is vulvovaginal candidiasis and who does it affect?

- Genital thrush (or vulvovaginal candidiasis) is a common presentation in primary care. It affects 75% of women at least once in their lifetime, usually causing vulval/vaginal itch or irritation, and non-offensive vaginal discharge.
- 20% of women of reproductive age may be asymptomatically colonised by candida species and do not require treatment.
- Vulvovaginal candidiasis is caused by superficial fungal infection (usually due to overgrowth of commensal yeasts from the *Candida* family). *Candida albicans* is the commonest cause (80–89% of cases). Other species may be implicated in the remaining cases.
- 40–45% women will have two or more episodes of thrush in their lifetime.

4.8.2 How do we diagnose vulvovaginal candidiasis?

- **Most women with an acute presentation of vulvovaginal candidiasis do not need a charcoal HVS.** Treat on the history and symptoms (and examination if necessary) alone. Reserve swabs for treatment failure, recurrence, diagnostic uncertainty, or higher-risk women (e.g. in pregnancy).

4.8.3 Recurrent vulvovaginal candidiasis

- 20% of women will report recurrent vulvovaginal candidiasis in the 12 months after an initial infection. This is distinct from treatment failure, where there is a failure of symptoms to resolve within 7–14 days of treatment.
- Recurrent thrush is defined as four or more symptomatic episodes in one year (in this instance ensure HVS is offered and at least two symptomatic episodes have been confirmed by microscopy or culture).
- Risk factors for recurrent vulvovaginal candidiasis are:
  - non-compliance with treatment
  - recent antibiotic use, changing vaginal flora
  - local irritants (soaps, shampoos, shower gels or douching)
  - uncontrolled diabetes mellitus
  - HIV and long-term corticosteroid use
  - persistent infection with *Candida* or azole-resistant candida species
  - increases in endogenous or exogenous oestrogen (pregnancy, COCP, HRT).

4.8.4 Self-care advice for vulvovaginal candidiasis

- Women with vulvovaginal candidiasis should be advised regarding self-management measures to provide symptomatic relief:
  - Use of simple emollients as a soap substitute to wash and/or moisturise the vulval area.
  - Avoid contact with irritants such as soap / shampoo / bubble bath.
  - Avoid vaginal douching.
  - Avoid tight-fitting / non-absorbent clothing which may irritate the area further.
  - Avoid use of complementary therapies such as applying yoghurt, or tea tree or other essential oils.

4.8.5 Treatment of vulvovaginal candidiasis

- Offer first-line treatment with oral antifungal drugs such as fluconazole 150mg given as a single dose.
- Women who prefer to avoid oral treatment can be offered a 500mg intravaginal clotrimazole pessary as a single dose. Advise that these may damage latex condoms and diaphragms.
- It may take 3–4 days after treatment for symptoms to resolve.
- If symptoms seem severe, advise repeating oral or topical treatment after 72 hours.
- If there are troublesome vulval symptoms, women can also be offered clotrimazole 1–2% cream applied 2–3 times daily.
- These treatments are all available over the counter.
- Antihistamines (e.g. cetirizine 10mg) can help to reduce the severity of itch and irritation in both acute and recurrent infection.
- Advise women to come back for review if things have not settled in 7–14 days. At this stage a HVS and PCR for STIs should be considered.
- It is not necessary to routinely treat a partner unless they have symptomatic infection themselves.
- If the patient is diabetic, take care to ensure glucose control is optimised.

4.8.6 Treatment of recurrent vulvovaginal candidiasis

- Reinforce self-management advice and assess for risk factors for recurrent infection, such as uncontrolled diabetes or immunocompromise, e.g. HIV.
- Arrange examination and HVS as well as considering a PCR screen for STIs.
- Offer induction then maintenance treatment, e.g. fluconazole 150mg every 72 hours for three doses, then weekly for 6 months.
- Concomitant use of topical imidazoles should not be necessary and is not advised.
- If treatment fails, consider patient concordance and the possibility of non-albicans strains of candida or resistance to a particular imidazole. Specialist advice may be required.
- Women starting vaginal oestrogen for genitourinary syndrome of menopause (GSM) sometimes experience recurrent thrush. This usually settles when the vaginal biome improves with re-oestrogenisation. Some will benefit from 3–6 months of weekly fluconazole use when starting treatment.

4.8.7 Treatment of vulvovaginal candidiasis in pregnancy and breastfeeding

- Both asymptomatic colonisation and symptomatic infection are more common in pregnancy. There is no association between infection and low birthweight or preterm birth.
- Prescribe antifungal drug treatments such as clotrimazole pessaries. Some women may require longer-term suppression. Avoid oral antifungals in pregnant and breastfeeding women.
- Where treatment fails, consider patient compliance and risk factors for recurrent infection, and repeat the examination and swabs.

4.9 Bacterial vaginosis

4.9.1 What is bacterial vaginosis and who does it affect?

- Bacterial vaginosis (BV) is a dysbiosis of the vagina, usually as a result of overgrowth of anaerobic organisms, e.g. *Gardnerella vaginalis, Pevotella* species and *Mycoplasma hominis*. There is a loss of lactobacilli leading to a loss of normal acidity, and the vaginal pH rises above 4.5.
- About 50% of women with BV are asymptomatic. When present, symptoms include a fishy-smelling, grey/white homogenous discharge. There is no associated itch or soreness.

- It is the most likely cause of abnormal vaginal discharge, affecting 23–29% of women of childbearing age.
- Recurrent BV is common, affecting up to 80% of women again within 9 months of first infection.
- It has previously not been considered as an STI, but this may be changing. There is higher prevalence amongst sexually active women and recent evidence showed it may be transmitted between partners – including by sharing of sex toys and in women who have sex with other women.
- Factors making BV more likely include:
  - having multiple male sexual partners
  - women having sex with other women
  - changes in partner / multiple partners
  - not using condoms (semen raises vaginal pH)
  - menstruation (menstrual blood also raises vaginal pH)
  - seropositivity for herpes simplex virus 2 (HSV-2)
  - ethnicity (more common in black women).

4.9.2 How do we diagnose bacterial vaginosis?

- **Charcoal swabs for HVS are not needed as a first line for symptomatic women.** Some labs are now stopping routine testing for BV on MC&S. Diagnosis is clinical where symptoms are classical, i.e. fishy, grey/white homogenous discharge. Treatment can be offered on history and symptoms alone.
- Where there is diagnostic uncertainty, take a swab from the lateral wall of the vagina and rub the swab onto litmus paper to test the vaginal pH. If the pH is high, treatment may be offered.
- If there is diagnostic doubt, or litmus paper is not available, then the swab may be sent for MC&S and testing for BV requested. Consider also sending PCR for gonorrhoea, chlamydia and trichomonas in this instance. The presence of BV is associated with an increased likelihood of other STIs – possibly because BV reduces natural defences against infection.

4.9.3 How do we treat bacterial vaginosis?

- Offer non-pregnant women with symptomatic BV one of the following options:
  - oral metronidazole 400mg bd for 5–7 days
  - a single 2g stat dose of oral metronidazole
  - intravaginal metronidazole or clindamycin gel.
- Test of cure is not routinely recommended.
- Women should be advised, where possible, to reduce exposure to contributory factors such as smoking, vaginal douching, and the use of antiseptics, bubble baths and shampoos in the bath.
- If a patient has recurrent symptoms and/or ongoing high pH on litmus testing, consider the possibility of trichomonas. PCR testing is not universally available in primary care: if unavailable locally, refer to specialist sexual health services for further evaluation.
- True recurrent BV may be treated with suppressive 0.75% metronidazole gel twice weekly. There is also some evidence for Balance Activ gel and dequalinium chloride (e.g. used to force the pH back down after unprotected sex where the partner ejaculating seems to be a trigger for BV; condom use can also be helpful where acceptable).

4.9.4 Bacterial vaginosis in pregnancy

- Pregnant women should not routinely be screened for BV.
- Where BV is found but a woman is asymptomatic, discuss with her obstetrician whether treatment is appropriate. Symptomatic BV in pregnancy is associated with adverse pregnancy outcomes (e.g. miscarriage, preterm delivery, low birthweight), postsurgical or postpartum infections and pelvic inflammatory disease (PID).

- Symptomatic BV can be treated with oral metronidazole 400mg bd for 5–7 days. High-dose regimes (2g oral single dose) are not advised during pregnancy.
- Topical treatment with intravaginal metronidazole gel or clindamycin cream is also possible.
- Women should be advised to reduce exposure to contributory factors such as smoking, vaginal douching, and the use of antiseptics, bubble baths and shampoos in the bath.
- Repeat testing can be offered after 1 month (with further treatment) if the woman remains symptomatic or is considered at risk of preterm birth.

4.10 Sexually transmitted infections

4.10.1 Identification – who is at risk of STIs?

- Having sex is the main risk factor for STIs – and if we don't test, we don't find them. Late diagnosis is a significant issue, particularly with HIV and syphilis, and we are well placed in primary care to think more often about testing for these conditions.
- The overall prevalence of newly diagnosed STIs in the UK appears to be fairly stable, but the picture of relative prevalence of each STI is changing (see *Fig. 4.4*).
- Rates of human papillomavirus (HPV) are falling due to the national vaccination programme. Chlamydia diagnoses appear stable, but rates of gonorrhoea are the highest on record as of 2022, and syphilis rates are the highest since 1948.
- The impact of STIs remains greatest in young people aged 15–24, gay and bisexual and men who have sex with men (GBMSM), and some ethnic minority groups – but this needs interpreting with care. Having unprotected sex is the main risk factor for STIs, and traditional assumptions about 'risky populations' and 'risky sexual behaviours' are increasingly outdated, potentially shaming, and may reflect historical prejudice.
- Nearly half of all new HIV diagnoses in England in 2023 were in men and women having heterosexual sex. Late diagnosis is a particular concern with HIV because early treatment can normalise life expectancy. Late diagnosis is particularly common in adults aged over 50.
- We should be regularly testing for, but not treating, gonorrhoea, HIV and syphilis in the community. These conditions should be referred to secondary specialist sexual health services for management.
- Chlamydia can and should be routinely tested for and treated in primary care. Trichomonas testing is not available in primary care in all areas, but where identified can be managed in primary care.

4.10.2 How do we know who needs to be tested and what for?

- Talking to a healthcare professional about your sex life is not easy for many patients. Although it is important to ensure a safe, confidential, non-judgemental environment and attitude, we should also bear in mind that many people will not know the full extent of their risk exposure, and we may be falsely reassured.
- Patients should be offered a clinician of their preferred gender where possible. A trauma-informed approach (as described in *Section 4.6*) is essential.
- Where reasonable, in primary care we can ask about sexual behaviours and habits to help assess risk, but interpret this with caution bearing in mind data on groups most prone to late diagnosis.
- Being sexually active is the main risk factor for STIs, and we should get comfortable with seeing STI screening as routine, rather than unnecessarily stigmatising or shaming certain sexual orientations or practices. The under-25s chlamydia screening programme is a good example of this.

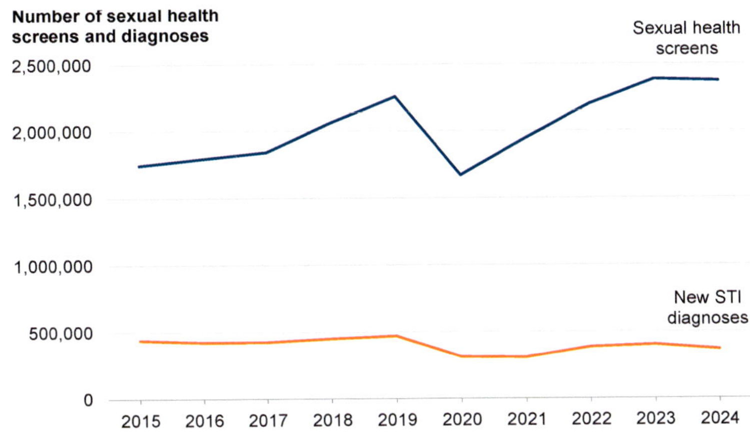

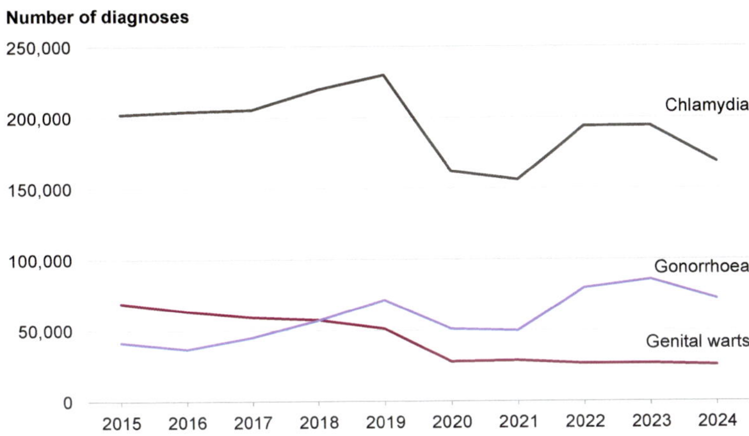

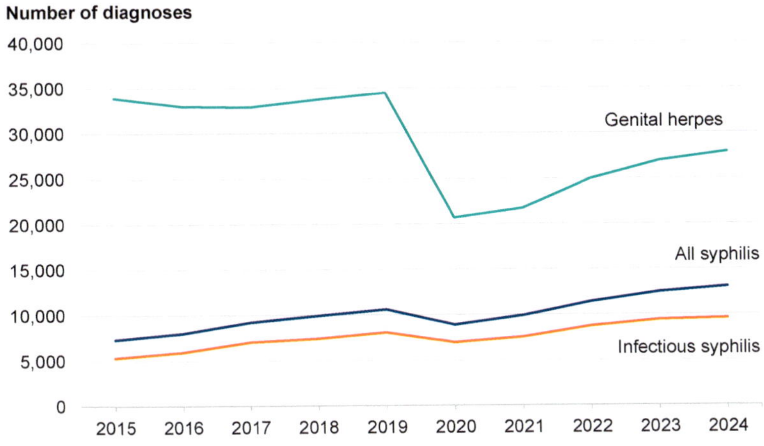

Figure 4.4: Number of new STI diagnoses and sexual health screens among England residents accessing sexual health services, 2015–24. Reproduced from UK Health Security Agency Official Statistics, licensed under the Open Government Licence v3.0.

- Discuss symptoms to guide examination and testing but remember many STIs are asymptomatic. Ask about:
    - dysuria
    - genital skin problems
    - unusual vaginal discharge
    - unusual/changed vaginal bleeding, including postcoital and intermenstrual bleeding
    - urethral discharge
    - abdominal or pelvic pain / dyspareunia
    - perianal/anal symptoms.
- Consider HIV and viral hepatitis risk, i.e. IV drug use, sex with a partner from a country with high prevalence, use of HIV pre-exposure prophylaxis (PrEP) and post-exposure prophylaxis (PEP), sex with cisgender men who have sex with men, and transgender women, hep B risk (men who have sex with men (MSM), sex workers, people injecting steroids or recreational drugs, people from countries where hep B is endemic). Ensure you do not dismiss the possibility of blood-borne viruses in 'lower-risk' groups where late diagnosis is common and confers greater morbidity and mortality.
- Asking more detailed questions about sexual habits, intravenous (IV) drug use, higher-risk practices and previous infection can help us clinically, but we need to approach the issue with care; many patients will not fully disclose all partners and sexual activities, and many are unaware of the extent of the sexual activities of their partners.
- Consider safeguarding concerns, e.g. vulnerability to abuse, evidence of domestic violence, coercion, age, power imbalance within relationships and non-consensual sexual activities, history of FGM.
- Consider whether there is alcohol or recreational drug use (e.g. chemsex), as this may need further referral. Chemsex is a risk factor for enhanced sexual risk-taking. A recent global meta-analysis found a pooled prevalence of 22% for chemsex among MSM.
- The gold standard screening for STIs is now a self- or clinician-performed vulvovaginal swab (PCR test) for chlamydia, trichomonas and gonorrhoea and a blood test for HIV and syphilis (see *Fig. 4.5*). Traditional 'triple swabs' are now considered outdated.
- Charcoal swabs are not routinely needed for BV or candida as these can be treated on the basis of history and examination alone. Charcoal HVS should not routinely be performed when screening for STIs.

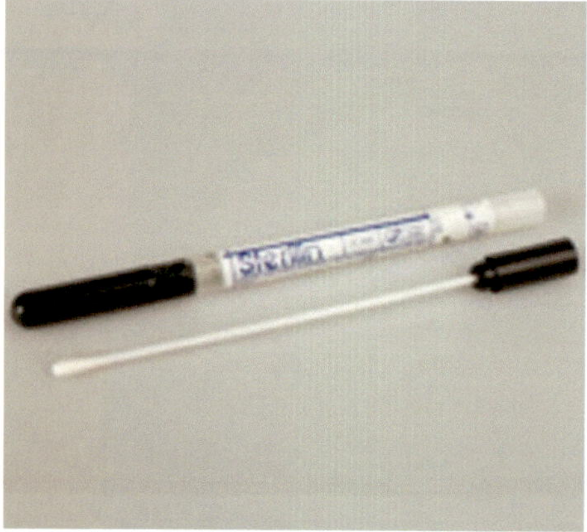

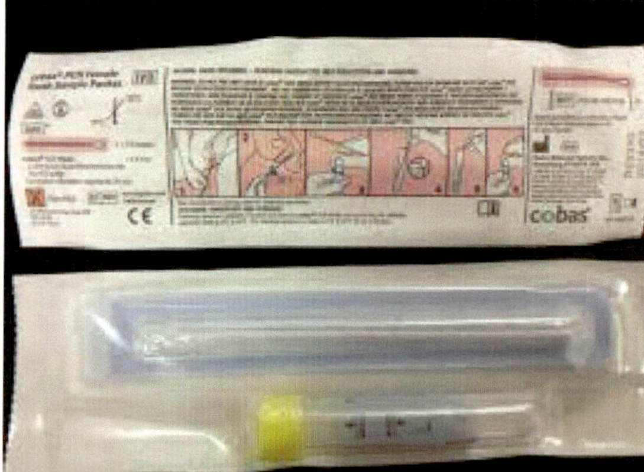

Figure 4.5: A charcoal swab (left) and a PCR swab (right).

4.11 Chlamydia

4.11.1 What is chlamydia and who is at risk?

- Genital chlamydia is caused by *Chlamydia trachomatis*.
- **It is the most commonly reported curable bacterial STI in the UK and should be routinely screened for and treated in primary care.** The highest prevalence is amongst those aged 15–24.
- It has a high frequency of transmission, with concordance rates of up to 75% of partners.
- Infection is primarily through penetrative sexual intercourse, but the bacterium is also found in the conjunctiva and nasopharynx without concomitant genital infection.
- If untreated, studies suggest that up to 50% of infection will resolve spontaneously approximately 12 months from initial diagnosis. The remainder persist.
- Chlamydia may cause significant short- and long-term morbidity, including PID, tubal infertility and ectopic pregnancy.
- In women:
  - **Infection is usually asymptomatic.**
  - If symptomatic, there may be:
    - increased vaginal discharge, postcoital or intermenstrual bleeding, dysuria, abdominal pain or painful sex
    - cervical inflammation with mucopurulent discharge, with or without contact bleeding
    - pelvic tenderness on examination, or pain on movement of the cervix
    - rectal discharge and pain.
  - Pharyngeal infection is usually asymptomatic.

4.11.2 How do we diagnose chlamydia?

- Testing should be with nucleic acid amplification tests (NAATs), usually available as a PCR test. These are considered gold standard. Standard charcoal swabs are not suitable for chlamydia testing.
- **Vulvovaginal swabs are the specimen of choice in women.** Endocervical swabs and first catch urine, although possible, are both much less sensitive than a vulvovaginal swab and should not be used.

4.11.3 How do we treat chlamydia?

- Treatment of uncomplicated infection is appropriate to initiate in primary care.
- Offer doxycycline 100mg bd for 7 days, or azithromycin 1g orally given as a single dose, followed by 500mg once daily for 2 days. Further alternatives can be found in the BASHH 2015 Chlamydia Guidelines.
- Treatment guidelines were updated in 2018 to reflect growing clinical significance of *Mycoplasma genitalium* (Mgen), often present as a co-infection with chlamydia. Single-dose azithromycin was thought to be leading to macrolide resistance in Mgen and is now no longer recommended: the azithromycin dosing schedule above is advised instead.
- Contact tracing may be appropriate and is usually done through referral to the local genitourinary medicine (GUM) clinic who have appropriate training in partner notification.

4.12 Gonorrhoea

4.12.1 What is gonorrhoea and who is at risk?

- Gonorrhoea is caused by the Gram-negative diplococcus *Neisseria gonorrhoeae*. It is the second most common bacterial STI worldwide. Its prevalence has been rising, but may be showing signs of levelling off. It is strongly associated with deprivation, mainly amongst young heterosexuals in urban areas.
- The primary sites of infection are the urethra, endocervix, pharynx and conjunctiva.
- In most women, gonorrhoea infections resolve spontaneously. However, untreated infections can result in complications such as PID, pregnancy complications and perinatal mortality.
- Transmission is by direct inoculation from infected secretions. Secondary infection can also occur to other anatomical sites through systemic or transluminal spread, leading to disseminated gonorrhoea (0.5–3% of cases).
- **Very often women are asymptomatic.** Where symptoms are present, there may be:
  - dysuria or frequency (urethral infection)
  - increased or altered vaginal discharge (endocervical infection)
  - lower abdominal pain
  - intermenstrual bleeding or menorrhagia
  - anal discharge / anal or perianal pain; rectal infection is common in cis-gender women and present in up to one-third of cases of urogenital infection, despite individuals not reporting a history of anal sex
  - pharyngeal infection may be asymptomatic or be associated with a sore throat
  - skin lesions, arthralgia, arthritis and tenosynovitis may result from disseminated gonococcal infection.

4.12.2 How do we diagnose and treat gonorrhoea?

- Diagnosis is through vulvovaginal, pharyngeal or rectal swabs using a PCR swab.
- MC&S with charcoal swab should no longer be done.
- Patients diagnosed with gonorrhoea should be referred to a GUM clinic for partner notification and treatment.
- The 4CMenB vaccine is now being offered as a vaccine against gonorrhoea. The bacteria causing meningococcal disease and gonorrhoea are closely related, so individuals given the 4CMenB vaccine produce antibodies offering some protection against gonorrhoea. This was made available in August 2025 to individuals at highest risk, such as MSM.

4.13 Syphilis

4.13.1 What is syphilis and who is at risk?

- Syphilis is caused by the spirochaete bacterium *Treponema pallidum*.
- Syphilis is frequently diagnosed late. It is known as 'the great mimic' and, due to historic stigma about who may be at risk, is often not considered despite being a possible cause of commonly presenting symptoms in primary care, e.g.:
  - alopecia
  - systemic rash, often affecting palms and soles
  - generalised fever and lymphadenopathy
  - cranial nerve palsies
  - abnormal LFTs.
- Most cases are sexually transmitted during contact with an infectious lesion or infected secretions. It may also be passed from mother to child if she is untreated.

- Data shows syphilis rates are rising, nearly doubling between 2013 and 2018. Although syphilis predominates amongst younger GBMSM, rates are also climbing amongst heterosexual men and women.
- Syphilis is a multisystem, multistage disease. **All stages of syphilis are frequently asymptomatic:** referred to as early or late latent disease.
- Infection may be classified into two types, early and late.

Early stage (0–2 years from infection)

- **Primary syphilis**
  - **When symptomatic** is characterised by an often painless ulcer (known as a chancre) at the site of infection (for example images see https://dermnetnz.org/topics/syphilis). Painful multiple ulcers are also possible. These occur most commonly on the genitals. There is usually local lymphadenopathy.
- **Secondary syphilis**
  - Will develop in about 25% of untreated individuals with primary disease. It describes a system-wide involvement including, when symptomatic, a wide range of clinical signs and symptoms such as:
    - skin and hair changes (maculopapular rash involving palms and soles, condylomata lata – may look like soft genital warts, patchy alopecia)
    - oral lesions (known as snail tract lesions, may be mistaken for aphthous ulcers)
    - generalised lymphadenopathy
    - low-grade fever, headache, or malaise – there may be a neurological component including acute meningitis or cranial nerve palsies (commonly involving the eyes and ears).
- **Early latent syphilis**
  - If untreated, the disease enters an asymptomatic latent stage. It is defined as early latent if <2 years from infection.

Late stage (≥2 years from likely infection)

- **Late latent syphilis**
  - Confirmed infection in the absence of any current clinical features when more than 2 years from infection.
- **Cardiovascular**
  - e.g. aortic aneurysm.
- **Gummatous**
  - Cutaneous disease – may be persistent and often misdiagnosed.
- **Neurological**
  - e.g. tabes dorsalis, general paresis.

4.13.2 How do we diagnose and treat syphilis?

- It is vital to consider the possibility of syphilis and to test for it more often.
- Syphilis can be cured if treated with appropriate antibiotics before complications have developed.
- When untreated, one-third of cases will progress to cause severe, irreversible cardiovascular, neurological and ocular complications.
- Treatment of syphilis should take place in a GUM clinic where a full sexual history, examination and contact tracing can take place.
- Diagnosis is by dark-ground microscopy, molecular diagnostics (e.g. PCR) and/or serological tests (which may not be specific for syphilis and may not become positive until around 6–12 weeks after infection, meaning early tests may need repeating).
- Patients with early, infectious syphilis should be advised to abstain from sexual contact until all lesions have resolved, or until 2 weeks after treatment completion.
- Parenteral treatment with an appropriate penicillin is the treatment of choice.

4.14 Herpes simplex virus

4.14.1 What is herpes simplex virus and who is at risk?

- **Despite ongoing stigma, herpes simplex virus (HSV) infection should be considered a 'state of normality'.**
- **In the UK, about 70% of people will have been infected with either HSV-1 and/or HSV-2 by their 25th birthday.**
- **HSV comes from the same family of viruses as chickenpox and shingles (varicella zoster and herpes zoster).**
- Most people who acquire HSV will be asymptomatic and therefore do not realise they have been infected, but are still able to transmit the virus to others.
- The persistent nature of HSV can lead to anxiety about future attacks and concerns about new partners or impact on relationships. Much of this can be allayed with good psychoeducation on the prevalence of HSV in the population.
- Genital herpes is an infection caused by the HSV; both types of HSV present identically:
  - HSV-1 was traditionally considered to cause oro-labial herpes (cold sores). HSV-1 is the commonest cause of genital herpes in the UK.
  - HSV-2 was associated more with genital herpes and is more likely to be associated with recurrent genital infection.
- **Primary infection** refers to the first time HSV-1 or HSV-2 is acquired. In the vast majority of cases, primary infection is asymptomatic. A proportion of individuals will develop painful herpetic lesions (crops of red lesions which then become vesicular before breaking open then healing over), which are usually bilateral in primary infection. There may be an accompanying flu-like illness.
- Following primary infection, the virus becomes latent and persists lifelong in local sensory ganglia.
- **Recurrent HSV** occurs when clinical symptoms result from re-activation of the existing HSV-1/HSV-2 infection following a latent period. There may be asymptomatic shedding (no visible lesions but the ability to pass on the infection to a partner) or visible herpetic vesicular lesions and associated pain.
- Recurrent HSV may be more likely with local trauma, after exposure to ultraviolet (UV) light, with immunosuppression or hormonal changes. There is some evidence that intense psychological stress can be a factor.
- Herpes spreads by skin-to-skin contact in any type of sex. Transmission occurs at mucosal surfaces or breaks in the skin through contact with infected secretions (which may be present with visible sores, or from asymptomatic shedding from the cervix, anorectum, urethra and external genitalia).
- Most transmission with HSV is from asymptomatic shedding. Transmission is more likely with HSV-2, recent or recurrent infection or in the immunocompromised.
- Lesions can be prone to secondary infection with candida or streptococcal species and may be progressive or coalescing in the immunocompromised. Urinary retention can occur.

4.14.2 How do we diagnose and treat HSV?

- Suspect HSV in patients with multiple crops of painful blisters that quickly burst leaving erosions and ulcers on the external genitalia, perineum and/or perianal region.
- There may be prodromal tingling or burning pain up to 48 hours prior to the appearance of blisters.
- Primary episodes may persist for up to 3 weeks. Recurrences usually heal in 6–12 days.
- There may be accompanying dysuria, vaginal discharge, headache, malaise and/or fever (commonest in first episodes).

- To diagnose in primary care, take a viral swab from the base of an anogenital lesion (pop a fluid-filled blister if needed). Referring to GUM can introduce unnecessary delay in treatment.
- Start treatment as soon as possible (whilst waiting for results) with, for example, aciclovir 400mg tds for 5 days. This can be extended to 10 days if new lesions continue to form.
- Always screen for other STIs with a vulvovaginal PCR for gonorrhoea and chlamydia (delay by a week if patient is too sore to tolerate vulvovaginal swab).
- If HSV swab returns as negative, remember to consider syphilis in the differential diagnoses (see *Section 4.13*).
- Self-care advice is useful:
  - Saline bathing (e.g. one teaspoon of salt in a pint of water) can ease discomfort and promote healing of lesions / prevent secondary infection.
  - OTC analgesia, i.e. ibuprofen or paracetamol as needed.
  - Petroleum jelly can be applied to form a barrier, e.g. before passing urine.
  - Consider increasing fluid intake to dilute urine or pouring water over genitals when passing urine.
  - Dress in loose natural fibres.
- Advise abstaining from sexual activity until lesions have cleared, to prevent transmission.
- Reassure that a first episode may not necessarily indicate recent infection: transmission can occur from an asymptomatic partner years into a monogamous relationship.
- Patients can be referred to GUM if they wish, but do not delay testing and treatment, as by the time they are seen the lesions may have healed and diagnosis may be difficult.
- www.herpes.org.uk is an excellent resource for patients and doctors alike.

4.14.3 What about HSV infection in pregnancy or immunocompromised individuals?

- A first episode of HSV in pregnancy creates risk of neonatal transmission, particularly if it occurs in the third trimester. Refer all to specialist sexual health services for treatment and a midwife / obstetric care plan.
- Individuals who are immunocompromised (e.g. untreated HIV-positive) are more at risk of severe infection and require more intensive antiviral treatment, e.g. aciclovir 400mg 5 times a day for 7–10 days.

4.14.4 What about recurrent HSV infection?

- If recurrent episodes do not resolve with self-care measures alone, and are distressing, patients may be offered:
  - episodic oral antiviral treatment, e.g. aciclovir 800mg tds for 2 days / aciclovir 400mg tds for 5 days
  - suppressive treatment if >6 episodes/year, e.g. aciclovir 400mg bd. This should be continued for a maximum of 1 year then a break taken to assess for further recurrences. If >2 occur, suppressive treatment may be restarted.

4.15 Anogenital warts

4.15.1 What are anogenital warts and who is at risk?

- Genital warts (see *Fig. 4.6*) are very common benign growths occurring in the genital, perineal, anal and perianal areas.
- Lesions may also occur in the urethral meatus, vagina, cervical canal and anal canal.
- They are usually asymptomatic but may be painful, friable or itchy and lead to bleeding, painful sex or local irritation.

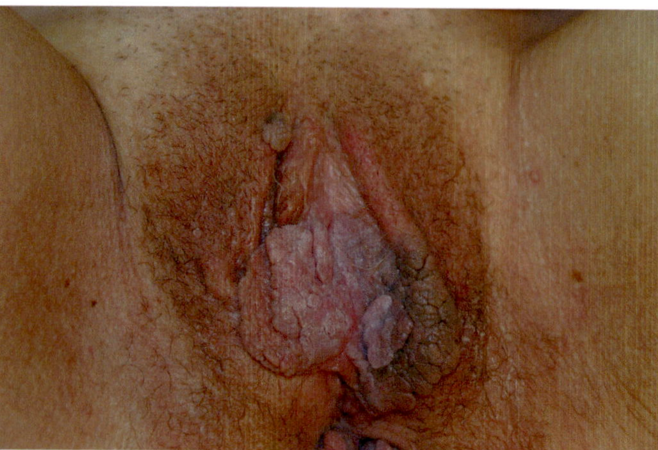

Figure 4.6: Genital warts. Reproduced with permission from ©DermNet dermnetnz.org 2026.

- They may vary in size from a few millimetres to several centimetres and tend to occur most commonly at the vaginal introitus.
- Anogenital warts are caused by human papillomavirus (HPV), usually due to the non-oncogenic types 6 and 11.
- There are at least 150 different types of HPV and around 40 that can infect the genitals.
- Infection with HPV occurs due to direct skin-to-skin contact with an infected individual. They may not have visible lesions but can shed the virus in genital secretions. Virus transmission usually occurs with sexual contact but can also occur perinatally and from hand warts, orogenitally or from contaminated surfaces or objects.
- Lifetime risk in sexually active people is about 10%. Nine out of ten new diagnoses are in heterosexual men and women.
- Rates are falling as a result of quadrivalent HPV vaccination.
- Although warts are caused by low-risk genotypes of HPV, co-infection with oncogenic strains may occur, leaving individuals at higher risk of anogenital cancer.

4.15.2 How do we diagnose and treat anogenital warts?

- **Diagnosis is usually clinical**, and does not generally require biopsy or GUM referral unless lesions are atypical, e.g. significant bleeding, pigmented, ulcerated or seem affixed to underlying tissue. Carcinoma *in situ* often has a lichenoid or pigmented appearance and the surface is usually smooth and velvety. Condylomata lata are often softer.
- Warts usually look like soft, cauliflower-like lesions of varying sizes. Less commonly they may be pigmented, whitish or erythematous.
- On hairless skin, the lesions are usually soft and non-keratinised.
- On hairy skin, they are usually harder and keratinised.
- Left untreated, 10–30% of anogenital warts will resolve spontaneously within 3–6 months.
- 95% of infected individuals will clear the HPV virus within 2 years.
- Offer a speculum examination and ask about the presence of intermenstrual or postcoital bleeding.
- Offer referral to specialist sexual health services if you are unsure of the diagnosis. If you are confident in the diagnosis, consider the following treatment:
    - Self-applied treatment (unsuitable in pregnancy) can be offered for non-keratinised, soft lesions, e.g. podophyllotoxin (0.5% solution or 0.15% cream). Cream is usually slightly easier to apply. Monitor any patients covering an area >4cm^2 for itch/pain and irritation).
    - Imiquimod 5% cream can be used for both keratinised and non-keratinised lesions.
    - Sinecatechin 10% is licensed for external genital warts in over-18s.

  - Patients should ideally be screened for co-existing STIs.
  - Specialist sexual health services can apply cryotherapy/electrocautery or excise warts and apply more abrasive solutions, e.g. trichloroacetic acid.

4.15.3 What about HPV in pregnancy / immunocompromised individuals?

- In both pregnancy and immunocompromise warts may enlarge, multiply and be more easily irritated.
- Wart removal may be considered in pregnancy, but warts do not generally impact pregnancy outcomes. Removal is usually delayed until after delivery.
- Spontaneous resolution often occurs within 6 weeks postpartum.
- Topical treatment is avoided in pregnancy, with cryotherapy, trichloroacetic acid or surgical excision preferred if needed.
- There is a low risk of vertical transmission of HPV to the baby or recurrent respiratory papillomatosis in the child.

4.16 Human immunodeficiency virus

4.16.1 What is HIV and who is at risk?

- Human immunodeficiency virus (HIV) is a form of retrovirus. It causes immunodeficiency by targeting and destroying cells in the immune system, in particular CD4 cells.
- There is often a long latent phase between infection and development of symptoms.
- Alarming public health campaigns in the past have resulted in significant outdated stigma and stereotype remaining regarding HIV.
- False assumptions about who is at risk from HIV lead to failure to consider the diagnosis and test for the condition. **This contributed to a 43% late presentation rate in 2018.**
- When HIV viral load is unrecordable, as is usually the case with antiretroviral treatment (ART), the virus is untransmissable. This is the premise of the U=U campaign. The UK government recently committed to the elimination of HIV by 2030 – through testing and early use of ART.
- **Individuals with HIV, when treated early, have a normal life expectancy.**
- At the end of 2018 it was estimated that 103 800 individuals in the UK had HIV and 7500 were unaware they had the condition. Approximately 50% of these individuals were gay or bisexual men, and **50% were heterosexual** (19 000 men and 29 600 women). **Only 2300 were IV drug users.**
- **Primary HIV** (or HIV seroconversion illness)
  - In the first few weeks after infection a flu-like illness may occur.
  - Viral load at this stage is very high, and the individual is very infectious.
- **Asymptomatic phase**
  - Once initial symptoms settle, there is an asymptomatic period of infection. The length of this period varies between individuals.
- **Advanced HIV disease** (formerly known as AIDS or acquired immune deficiency syndrome).
  - Advanced HIV disease is defined as when the number of CD4 cells is very low (<200 cells/ml), or if 'AIDS-defining' conditions (opportunistic infections such as pneumocystis pneumonia, or malignancies such as Kaposi's sarcoma) develop.
  - The term AIDS is less commonly used now.

4.16.2 How do we diagnose and treat HIV?

- Testing for HIV should be considered routinely in certain higher-risk groups (i.e. paid sex workers, men who have unprotected sex with men, people from high-prevalence areas) but **we should also bear in mind that anyone can have undiagnosed HIV and our patients may not divulge their risk factors.**

- All women are offered screening as part of antenatal care and in termination of pregnancy (TOP) services.
- Consider testing people who have unexplained symptoms consistent with HIV infection, e.g.:
  - Unusually severe, prolonged, recurrent or unexplained infections.
  - Conditions related to immunosuppression, such as oral candidiasis or shingles.
  - Glandular fever-like illness, pyrexia or lymphadenopathy of unknown origin.
  - Unexplained weight loss of >10kg.
  - The full list of symptoms is available at https://bhiva.org/file/5f68c0dd7aefb/HIV-testing-guidelines-2020.pdf.
- Patients should be counselled about HIV testing prior to the test being done.
- Testing may need to be repeated if performed too early, because it may take up to 12 weeks for antibodies to appear.
- Patients newly diagnosed with HIV should be referred to the nearest specialist clinic for follow-up – usually patients will be seen between 2 days and 2 weeks after a positive result. Unwell patients may need admission.
- Emphasise safer sexual practices until treatment is started and viral load is adequately suppressed with ART.

4.16.3 HIV prophylaxis options

- Pre-exposure prophylaxis (PrEP)
  - Prevention of HIV in high-risk groups may be achieved through the use of PrEP, usually prescribed by GUM services.
  - This can be offered to high-risk groups, e.g. MSM, partners of HIV-positive individuals who have not yet achieved unrecordable plasma viral load.
- Post-exposure prophylaxis (PEP)
  - PEP is also available from the Emergency Department when an individual thinks they have been exposed to HIV. This is best taken within 24 hours of the exposure but is available up to 72 hours post-exposure.
- Useful resources for clinicians include:
  - Aidsmap – www.aidsmap.com.
  - British Association for Sexual Health and HIV (BASHH) – www.bashh.org.
  - British HIV Association (BHIVA) – www.bhiva.org.
- Useful resources for patients include:
  - Terrence Higgins Trust – www.tht.org.uk.
  - Avert – www.avert.org.

4.17 Trichomoniasis

4.17.1 What is trichomoniasis and who is at risk?

- Trichomonas vaginalis (TV) is a sexually transmitted infection caused by the flagellate protozoan *Trichomonas vaginalis*.
- Transmission is almost always through sexual contact, although vertical infection is possible.
- It is the most common STI worldwide, but relatively rare in the UK. Around 6000 cases are reported annually (prevalence around 0.3%) compared to 200 000 chlamydia cases.
- 90% of trichomoniasis is diagnosed in women. Men clear the protozoa more rapidly.
- 10–50% of infections are asymptomatic. Where symptoms are present, women most commonly report discharge, vulval itch, dysuria or odour.
- 20–25% of infections will clear spontaneously.
- Recurrence is common, likely due to reinfection, and affects 5–37% of cases.

- There may be complications in pregnancy (preterm delivery, low birthweight and increased likelihood of maternal sepsis). PID can also result.
- TV alters the vaginal biome and can increase susceptibility to BV.
- Women with TV may be at increased risk of cervical cancer.

4.17.2 How do we diagnose and treat trichomoniasis?

- **Up to 50% of women with TV are asymptomatic.**
- PCR testing is not universally available routinely – you may need to specify that you wish samples to be tested for TV or if this option is not available, refer suspected cases to local secondary sexual health services for diagnosis. When running a PCR, the lab should also routinely check for the presence of gonorrhoea and chlamydia. Consider also testing for HIV and syphilis.
- Classically, TV-related discharge is frothy, offensive-smelling and may be yellow–green.
- Suspect TV where BV does not respond to treatment or seems recurrent.
- Litmus testing vaginal discharge will show high pH.
- Speculum examination may rarely show a strawberry appearance of the cervix.
- TV is usually managed by GUM but can be managed in primary care. BASHH has a useful patient information leaflet on TV (www.bashh.org/resources/66/trichomonas_vaginalis_tv).
- Offer treatment with oral metronidazole 4–500mg tds for 7 days. A 2g stat dose is an alternative if preferred.
- When pregnant or breastfeeding, offer 400mg metronidazole bd instead. Inform the midwife or obstetrician involved in care about the diagnosis and treatment.
- Abstain from sex for at least one week until treatment is completed. Partners will also need treatment.

4.18 Mpox

- Mpox (formerly known as monkeypox) is caused by the **mpox virus**, a zoonotic orthopoxvirus related to smallpox.
- The UK experienced a sizable mpox outbreak in **2022**, with **3732 confirmed and highly probable cases** of the Clade IIb (less severe) virus by the end of that year.
- From **2023 to mid-2025** there have been **around 556 additional cases** reported, substantially **lower** than in the 2022 peak.
- Most UK cases have been among **MSM**, although anyone can be infected.
- A **very small number of Clade I (more severe) cases** linked to travel have also been reported.
- Spread requires **close physical contact** with a person who has mpox, especially contact with their **rash, blisters or scabs**. It can spread through sexual contact but also via **respiratory secretions** and by touching **contaminated materials** such as bedding or clothing.
- Symptoms can resemble other conditions (e.g. chickenpox), so professional evaluation is needed.
- Refer suspected cases to local secondary sexual health services for testing and management. **PCR swabs are taken** from samples of lesions.
- Most people with mpox experience **mild illness** and **recover within weeks** with **supportive care** (managing symptoms such as pain, fever and skin lesions).
- An **mpox/smallpox vaccine** (e.g. Imvanex) is used in the UK for **pre- and post-exposure prophylaxis** and is offered to people at higher risk (e.g. MSM with multiple partners or close contacts of confirmed cases).
- The vaccine can help **prevent infection** or **reduce severity** if given early.

4.19 Urogenital commensals

- The commercialisation of home STI and biome testing kits means that patients may present with concerns about urogenital commensals (e.g. *Ureaplasma urealyticum, U. parvum, Mycoplasma genitalium* and *M. hominis*).
- The British Association of Sexual Health and HIV (BASHH) has issued a position statement warning against the use of such kits. Some online providers are offering treatment regimens which do not comply with national recommendations for first-line therapy.

4.19.1 *Ureaplasma urealyticum* and *U. parvum*

- **BASHH guidelines do not recommend routine testing for the presence of ureaplasma, as it is considered an 'organism of dubious significance'.**
- They are part of the Mycoplasma genus and are considered normal commensal organisms in the urogenital, oral and anal areas. They are amongst the normal vaginal flora of 60% of healthy sexually active women. They are typically a benign finding on a swab and do not require routine treatment.
- In certain situations, when a patient is symptomatic and other pathogens have been excluded, ureaplasma presence may be related to PID, cervicitis and genital discomfort.
- Pregnancy complications can rarely be associated with ureaplasma, including preterm birth and neonatal infections including meningitis. If ureaplasma is identified in a symptomatic patient, or during pregnancy, advice should be sought from specialist sexual health services regarding the need for treatment.

4.19.2 Mycoplasma bacteria

Mycoplasma genitalium

- *M. genitalium* is an emergent STI. It has been more extensively researched in men with non-gonococcal urethritis than in women.
- Women with *M. genitalium* may have a two-fold increased risk of cervicitis, endometritis, PID, preterm delivery, spontaneous abortion and infertility.
- The majority of women with *M. genitalium* infection are asymptomatic. Infection may be associated with:
  - dysuria
  - postcoital bleeding
  - painful intermenstrual bleeding
  - cervicitis
  - lower abdominal pain.
- Infection testing and management should be done by secondary sexual health services.

Mycoplasma hominis

- In contrast to *M. genitalium*, ***M. hominis*** **is considered a normal commensal of the urogenital tract and an 'organism of dubious clinical significance'. Up to 50% of women may carry it.**
- Detection is via PCR or culture from high vaginal swabs. **Routine screening is not advised.**
- Its presence may be more clinically relevant when it is associated with BV.
- There is possible association with PID and with postpartum/post-TOP infection. Evidence linking the presence of *M. hominis* to tubal infertility remains inconclusive. Where the organism is found in pregnant women or in symptomatic individuals where other pathogens have been excluded, advice should be sought from secondary sexual health services regarding the need for treatment.

4.20 Further reading

Barrett, G., Pendry, E., Peacock, J. *et al.* (2000) Women's sexual health after childbirth. *Br J Obstet Gynaecol*, **107(2)**: 186–95.

Bartellas, E., Crane, J.M., Daley, M., Bennett, K.A. and Hutchens, D. (2000) Sexuality and sexual activity in pregnancy. *Br J Obstet Gynaecol*, **107(8):** 964–8.

BASHH (updated 2018) *Chlamydia 2015*. Available at: www.bashh.org/resources/15/chlamydia_2015

BASHH (updated 2020) *Gonorrhoea 2018*. Available at: www.bashh.org/resources/14/gonorrhoea_2018

BASHH (updated 2021) *Position statement on the inappropriate use of multiplex testing platforms, and suboptimal antibiotic treatment regimens for bacterial sexually transmitted infections*. Available at: www.bashh.org/resources/72/bashh_position_statement_on_the_inappropriate_use_of_multiplex_testing_platforms_and_suboptimal_antibiotic_treatment_regimens_for_bacterial_sexually_transmitted_infections

BASHH (2023) *Summary guidance on testing for sexually transmitted infections*. Available at: www.bashh.org/_userfiles/pages/files/resources/bashh_summary_guidance_on_stis_testing_2023.pdf

BASHH (updated 2025) Mycoplasma genitalium 2025. Available at: www.bashh.org/resources/19/mycoplasma_genitalium_2018

BHIV/BASHH (2018) Guidelines on the use of HIV pre-exposure prophylaxis (PrEP). Available at: https://bhiva.org/wp-content/uploads/2024/10/2018-PrEP-Guidelines.pdf

Brook, G., Church, H., Evans, C. *et al.* (2020) 2019 UK National Guideline for consultations requiring sexual history taking: Clinical Effectiveness Group British Association for Sexual Health and HIV. *Int J STD AIDS*, **31(10):** 920–38.

Cadman, L., Waller, J., Ashdown-Barr, L. and Szarewski, A. (2012) Barriers to cervical screening in women who have experienced sexual abuse: an exploratory study. *J Fam Plann Reprod Health Care*, **38(4):** 214–20.

Crenshaw, K.W. (1989) Demarginalizing the intersection of race and sex: a black feminist critique of antidiscrimination doctrine, feminist theory and antiracist politics. *University of Chicago Legal Forum*, **1989:** 139–67.

Georgiadis, N., Katsimpris, A., Vatmanidou, M.A. *et al.* (2025) Prevalence of chemsex and sexualized drug use among men who have sex with men: a systematic review and meta-analysis. *Drug Alcohol Depend*, **275:** 112800.

Kingston, M., Apea, V., Evans, C. *et al.* (2024) BASHH UK guidelines for the management of syphilis 2024. *Int J STD AIDS*, **0(0):** 1–19. Available at: www.bashh.org/_userfiles/pages/files/syphilis_2024.pdf

Kletzel, H.H., Rotem, R., Barg, M., Michaeli, J. and Reichman, O. (2018) Ureaplasma urealyticum: the role as a pathogen in women's health, a systematic review. *Curr Infect Dis Rep*, **20(9)**: 33.

Mind (undated) *Trauma?* Available at: www.mind.org.uk/information-support/types-of-mental-health-problems/trauma/about-trauma

National Guideline Alliance (UK) (2021) Management of symptomatic vaginal discharge in pregnancy: antenatal care. NICE.

Natsal-3 (undated) *Sexual attitudes and lifestyles in Britain: highlights from Natsal-3*. Available at: www.natsal.ac.uk/natsal/wp-content/uploads/2023/03/Natsal-3-infographics.pdf

NICE (revised 2023) CKS: *Bacterial vaginosis in women who are pregnant*. Available at: https://cks.nice.org.uk/topics/bacterial-vaginosis/management/women-who-are-pregnant

NICE (revised 2023) CKS: *Candida – female genital: management*. Available at: https://cks.nice.org.uk/topics/candida-female-genital/management/during-pregnancy

NICE (revised 2024) CKS: *Herpes simplex*. Available at: https://cks.nice.org.uk/topics/herpes-simplex-genital/background-information/definition

NICE (revised 2024) CKS: *Warts – anogenital*. Available at: https://cks.nice.org.uk/topics/warts-anogenital/management/management

NICE (revised 2025) CKS: *Gonorrhoea: how common is it?* Available at: https://cks.nice.org.uk/topics/gonorrhoea/background-information/prevalence

One in Four (charity supporting those who have survived child sexual abuse): https://oneinfour.org.uk

Palfreeman, A., Sullivan, A., Rayment, M. *et al.* (2020) British HIV Association / British Association for Sexual Health and HIV / British Infection Association adult HIV testing guidelines 2020. *HIV Medicine*, **21(6):** 1–26.

Pretorius, D., Mlambo, M.G. and Couper, I.D. (2022) "We are not truly friendly faces": primary health care doctors' reflections on sexual history taking in North West Province. *Sex Med*, **10(6):** 100565.

Quan, M. (2010) Vaginitis: diagnosis and management. *Postgrad Med*, **122(6):** *117–27.*

Saadedine, M., Faubion, S., Kingsberg, S. *et al.* (2023) Adverse childhood experiences and sexual dysfunction in midlife women: is there a link? *J Sex Med*, **20(6):** 792–9.

Serati, M., Salvatore, S., Siesto, G. *et al.* (2010) Female sexual function during pregnancy and after childbirth. *J Sex Med*, **7(8):** 2782–90.

SAMHSA's Trauma and Justice Strategic Initiative (2014) *SAMHSA's concept of trauma and guidance for a trauma-informed approach*. Available at: www.health.ny.gov/health_care/medicaid/program/medicaid_health_homes/docs/samhsa_trauma_concept_paper.pdf

Stonewall (undated) *Resources*. Available at: www.stonewall.org.uk/resources

Terrence Higgins Trust (undated) *HIV diagnoses in England in 2023*. Available at: www.tht.org.uk/hiv/about-hiv/hiv-statistics#:~:text=Nearly%20half%20(49%25)%20of,were%20of%20Black%20African%20ethnicity

UK Health Security Agency (updated 2025) Official Statistics, *Sexually transmitted infections and screening for chlamydia in England: 2024 report*. Available at: www.gov.uk/government/statistics/sexually-transmitted-infections-stis-annual-data-tables/sexually-transmitted-infections-and-screening-for-chlamydia-in-england-2024-report

WHO (undated) *Sexual health*. Available at: www.who.int/health-topics/sexual-health

Wiesenfeld, H.C. and Manhart, L.E. (2017) Mycoplasma genitalium in women: current knowledge and research priorities for this recently emerged pathogen. *J Infect Dis*, **216(suppl 2):** S389–S395.

Chapter 5
Pregnancy and fertility

5.1 Introduction

- Healthcare professionals in primary care are often the first to be involved in supporting women through pre-conception advice, pregnancy and the postnatal period, as well as dealing with problems along the way such as miscarriages and fertility issues.
- Comprehensive, patient-centred care during this journey can have a significant positive impact on outcomes for both parents and the child.
- This chapter outlines key areas of reproductive and antenatal/postnatal care relevant to primary care.

5.2 Antenatal checks

- Around 660 000 women give birth in England and Wales each year.
- Antenatal care gives women (and their partners) support and information about pregnancy, birth and the postnatal period. It assesses and manages pregnancy complications and identifies safeguarding issues.
- Good-quality antenatal care can enable women to identify and manage potential problems, which can reduce the chance of poor outcomes for both the woman and the baby. It can enhance the experience of pregnancy and childbirth for both the woman and her partner.
- Antenatal consultations are usually provided under a shared care agreement between primary care and the maternity team at a local NHS hospital. Appointments are divided between primary care and the maternity team. In some areas where shared care is not available, care may be provided entirely by a community midwifery team. Some women may also choose private care or an independent midwife in addition to NHS care, or may opt for private care only.
- The maternity team / obstetrician will provide advice about the frequency of antenatal visits required, at certain agreed stages of gestation for crucial checks.
- In an uncomplicated first pregnancy a woman will have all the antenatal visits as listed in *Table 5.1*. Some of these recommended appointments may not be required in subsequent uncomplicated pregnancies.

Table 5.1: Planned prenatal appointments

Appointment	Timing
First antenatal appointment in primary care	
First antenatal booking visit in hospital or with community midwife	before 10 weeks
First ultrasound scan	between 11+2 and 14+1 weeks
16 week antenatal appointment	between 14 and 18 weeks
Second ultrasound scan appointment	between 18+0 and 20+6 weeks
25 weeks antenatal appointment (*for nulliparous women only*)	
28 weeks antenatal appointment	
31 weeks antenatal appointment (*for nulliparous women only*)	
34 weeks antenatal appointment	
36 weeks antenatal appointment	
38 weeks antenatal appointment	
40 weeks antenatal appointment (*for nulliparous women only*)	
41 weeks antenatal appointment (*for women who have not given birth yet*)	

- If complications arise, women are usually cared for by the hospital maternity team, and primary care reviews may not be required. However, a woman may approach the primary care team at any time during the pregnancy, so it is important to have a consistent approach during consultations with pregnant women.
- Closer monitoring may be needed for women and their babies from Black, Asian and other ethnic minorities, and those who live in deprived areas, because they are at an increased risk of adverse outcomes. This is due to several factors such as poorer social conditions, higher burden of health problems, and barriers to getting high-quality, timely maternity care.

5.2.1 Pre-conception care

- Pre-conception care is important for women, to improve their short- and long-term health outcomes and those of their children. It should be offered to all women of child-bearing age before they become pregnant, whenever the opportunity arises.
- This is a chance to optimise medical, psychological and social issues prior to a pregnancy, to inform women of any risks if they become pregnant, and to provide advice about how to manage risk. This helps women make an informed decision about becoming pregnant.
- A history should consist of plans for timing of future pregnancies, previous obstetric history, medical history, drug history (including recreational drugs), family history especially of genetic conditions, any workplace hazards, future travel plans, smear status and weight, BP and BMI (see also *Section 5.13* on how to take a fertility history).
- Advise women that fertility starts to decline, and the risk of certain pregnancy complications increases, after the age of 35 so, if possible, they should consider planning for a pregnancy before this.
- To improve the chances of conceiving, the couple should be encouraged to have sex every two or three days. It is best to avoid timing having sex around the date of expected ovulation, as this can cause stress for the couple, and does not improve the chance of getting pregnant.
- They should be advised that there is an 85% chance of becoming pregnant within the first year of actively trying to conceive. 50% of women that do not become pregnant within the first year are likely to conceive in the second year of trying.
- If a woman has not become pregnant after one year of trying to conceive and she is below the age of 35, or after six months if she is over the age of 35 or has any risk factors that may impact fertility such as PCOS, she should seek medical advice.
- All women should be advised to take folic acid whilst trying to conceive (400mcg daily until they are 12 weeks pregnant) to reduce the risk of neural tube defects. If they have any of the risk factors listed below, they should be offered 5mg of folic acid daily until they are 12 weeks pregnant:
  - Diabetes.
  - Family history or previous history of neural tube defects or congenital malformation in either side of family.
  - Sickle-cell anaemia or thalassaemia (they should take folic acid throughout their pregnancy).
  - Medications that reduce the absorption or metabolism of folic acid, e.g. epilepsy or HIV medications.
  - Note: women with a BMI >30kg/m^2 were previously advised to have high-dose folic acid, but a recent NICE review of the evidence has suggested that there is no clear evidence of benefit and they do not need high-dose folic acid unless there are other risk factors also present.

- Teratogenic drugs can cause developmental abnormalities in a fetus when taken by the pregnant mother. Examples include ACE inhibitors, angiotensin II receptor blockers (ARBs) and some anticonvulsants. Review teratogenic medications in women at risk of pregnancy, and offer effective contraception, or, if the woman would like to become pregnant, stop the teratogenic medication and find an alternative medication. The UK Teratology Information Service provides detailed information on the safety of medicines in pregnancy, available at www.uktis.org. Herbal remedies should be avoided if trying to get pregnant.
- Women with a history of mental health illness should be referred to their psychiatrist or a perinatal mental health team (see *Section 8.2* for more information) to assess the impact of a pregnancy on their mental health and any medications they may be taking. NICE CKS: *Depression – antenatal and postnatal* has helpful information about management of women with a history of, or a newly-diagnosed mental health problem in pregnancy. It contains guidance about use of antidepressants in the antenatal and postnatal period.
- Women with chronic disease such as asthma, diabetes, cardiac or thyroid problems should optimise management of these conditions before getting pregnant. They should discuss this with their usual healthcare professional in primary care, who may seek specialist advice about how their condition will be managed during pregnancy and what impact it might have.
- Encourage women who are due for their cervical screening test to have this taken before they plan to become pregnant. In most cases, it is recommended to postpone routine cervical screening until at least 12 weeks after delivery. Some women, for example those requiring a repeat smear after a previous abnormality, should have their smear during pregnancy.
- Smoking cessation: refer to smoking cessation services if needed. Avoid using bupropion or varenicline in women who are trying to conceive.
- Encourage women to stop drinking alcohol, or reduce consumption, and refer to alcohol services if needed.
- Offer dietary advice and weight management advice if required. Direct towards the Eatwell guide to healthy eating (see *Further reading*):
  - Women with a BMI >30kg/m^2 should be supported and encouraged to lose weight. A weight loss of 5–10% has been shown to have significant health benefits and can increase their chances of conceiving.
  - Women with a BMI <18.5kg/m^2 are at risk of fertility problems, miscarriage, preterm birth, low birthweight and gastroschisis.
  - Consider eating disorders and offer support and refer to specialist services if required.
  - Remember that people with obesity can have disordered eating patterns and may need support to manage this.
- Immunity: check rubella and varicella immunity or offer serological testing if unsure. Vaccinate if not immune and advise to avoid getting pregnant for one month after the vaccines. Hepatitis B vaccine should be considered for those at high risk, e.g. healthcare workers, IV drug users, frequent sexual partners and chronic kidney or liver disease. Further information about vaccines can be found in the Green Book.
- Workplace hazards should be assessed. If women are at risk of being exposed to any toxic substances, they should inform their employer who can refer them to occupational health for a health and safety risk assessment. If they do not wish to inform their employer, they can contact a health and safety expert for advice via www.hse.gov.uk.
- Future travel plans should be discussed. Women should be advised to avoid getting pregnant if travelling to a country with active Zika virus transmission (a useful website to check is https://travelhealthpro.org.uk/countries).
  - If a woman travels to an affected country, and her partner does not accompany her, she should avoid becoming pregnant for 2 months after leaving the affected country.
  - If her partner does accompany her, she should avoid becoming pregnant for 3 months after leaving the affected country, to avoid harm to the developing baby.

- Domestic violence can begin or escalate in pregnancy. It is important to provide support, and effective contraception, if needed, to protect women from unwanted pregnancy.

5.2.2 First antenatal appointment

- *Usually in primary care / with community midwife.*
- Women should have access to timely antenatal care at a local NHS hospital by self-referral or referral via a healthcare professional, school nurse / community centre or refugee hostel.
- Most women will first approach a healthcare professional in primary care if they have a positive pregnancy test, especially during their first pregnancy.
- If there is doubt, you can perform a urine pregnancy test for confirmation.
- Assess the number of weeks of gestation based on the first date of the last menstrual period or, in an *in vitro* fertilisation (IVF) pregnancy, the date of embryo transfer. This can then be used to calculate an expected due date. Most primary care IT clinical systems will have a pregnancy due date calculator.
- Ask about previous obstetric history, any complications and whether the pregnancy was natural or via IVF. Medical history is important, especially a history of chronic disease or mental health problems, along with family history, drug history, occupation and any hazards at work, alcohol, smoking status, relationship status and whether there are any safeguarding issues. Also ask about allergies, blood group / Rhesus status if known, and rubella immunisations.
- Take a baseline weight, BMI and BP. Assess the heart and lungs and perform a urine dipstick. Palpate the abdomen if there is any pain.
- Women should be advised to take folic acid 400mcg daily (5mg for high risk – see *Section 5.2.1*) and vitamin D 400IU/10mcg daily for the duration of the pregnancy.
- Advise women that they are eligible for a flu jab, Covid vaccine (at any time), whooping cough vaccine (between 16 and 32 weeks) and respiratory syncytial virus vaccine (between 28 and 36 weeks) during their pregnancy.
- This appointment is where women may ask lots of questions and information should be provided about the antenatal visits and how to have a healthy pregnancy. They should be directed towards any free pregnancy books such as *The Pregnancy Book* and apps such as Mum and Baby / Emma's diary / Baby buddy. Hospitals may also have their own resources they want pregnant women to be directed to.

5.2.3 First antenatal booking visit

- *With midwife – hospital or community-based.*
- A hospital / community midwife booking appointment should be offered to all women before 10 weeks. If referred later than 9 weeks, then an appointment will be offered within 2 weeks. Reasons for a late presentation in pregnancy should be explored, considering social, psychological or medical issues.
- Women will be given their patient-held antenatal notes to bring to each visit, so that advice and information can be shared between all healthcare professionals involved in their care.
- Some women may not have been seen in primary care and may self-refer directly to the community or hospital midwives, so they will be asked the questions covered in the primary care first antenatal appointment described in *Section 5.2.2*.
- Baseline BP, weight, BMI and urine dipstick will be carried out.
- Women will have screening blood tests: blood group, Rhesus status, FBC, HbA1c (if risk), HIV, hepatitis B/C, syphilis, vitamin D.
- Risk assessments are carried out including VTE, mental health, pre-eclampsia, diabetes, domestic violence and FGM.
- Comorbidities are reviewed and referral to specialist care considered, if required, e.g. diabetes and epilepsy.

- Antenatal screening options will be discussed: combined check of ultrasound scan and blood tests (between 11+2 and 14+1 weeks) to check for fetal anomalies such as Down's syndrome and sickle-cell / thalassaemia screening, as well as blood tests to check for HIV, hepatitis B or syphilis.
- A schedule of antenatal visits will be agreed and information on diet, lifestyle advice and keeping healthy in pregnancy will be offered.
- The woman will be risk-assessed for pre-eclampsia and if high risk they will be advised to take aspirin 75–150mg from week 12 until birth (see *Section 5.7*).

5.2.4 First ultrasound scan

- The first scan is arranged for between 11+2 and 14+1 weeks gestation in the hospital or in a community setting.
- It determines gestational age, and the expected due date.
- It can detect multiple pregnancy.
- It is part of the fetal anomaly screening programme (FASP) in the first trimester (for more information on FASP see *Further reading*).

5.2.5 16 weeks antenatal appointment

- A general health check undertaken between 14 and 18 weeks for BP and urine dipstick for proteinuria and glucose.
- Any concerns about symptoms or mental health will be assessed.
- Whooping cough vaccine will be made available between 16 and 32 weeks.
- Discussion around birth preferences, implications, benefits and risks.

5.2.6 Second ultrasound scan

- This scan is between 18+0 weeks and 20+6 weeks in the hospital or in a community setting.
- It is to screen for fetal abnormalities.
- It checks the growth of all the baby's organs.
- It can determine the sex of the baby for the parents if they wish to know.
- Checks the location of the placenta.

5.2.7 25 weeks antenatal appointment

- *For nulliparous women only – primary care or community midwife.*
- Symphysis fundal height will be measured together with listening to the fetal heart and checking the position of the baby.
- If there are any concerns with the symphysis fundal height at any point in the pregnancy, then a woman should be referred for an ultrasound scan to check the growth of the baby. The only exception may be if the baby has already moved into the pelvis.
- Provide advice on monitoring of baby's movements and when to seek help if concerned.
- Continued discussion about birth preferences, general health and any concerns.
- BP check and urine dipstick for proteinuria and glucose.
- A MATB1 certificate can be issued any time after 20 weeks to officially inform an employer of the pregnancy.

5.2.8 28 weeks antenatal appointment

- *Hospital or community midwife.*
- Blood test for FBC, blood group and antibodies.
- Anti-D prophylaxis for Rhesus-negative women.

- Information and discussion about preparing for birth, labour, vitamin K prophylaxis, feeding / looking after a baby, mental health and pelvic floor health.
- Women should be advised to avoid sleeping on their back after 28 weeks, to reduce risk of late stillbirth.
- Respiratory syncytial virus vaccine will be recommended.
- BP, urine dipstick for proteinuria and glucose, symphysis fundal height, fetal heartbeat and position of baby will all be checked.

5.2.9 31 weeks antenatal appointment

- *For nulliparous women only – primary care or community midwife.*
- Address any concerns and check general health and wellbeing.
- Review any risk factors in pregnancy.
- BP and urine dipstick for proteinuria and glucose, symphysis fundal height, fetal heartbeat and position of baby will all be checked.

5.2.10 34 weeks antenatal appointment

- *Hospital or community midwife.*
- Address any concerns and check general health and wellbeing.
- Review any risk factors in pregnancy.
- BP and urine dipstick for proteinuria and glucose, symphysis fundal height, fetal heartbeat and position of baby will all be checked.
- Discussion around birth plan, preparation for labour, infant feeding choices and newborn screening.

5.2.11 36 weeks antenatal appointment

- *Could be primary care or community / hospital midwife.*
- Address any concerns and check general health and wellbeing.
- Review any risk factors in pregnancy.
- BP and urine dipstick for proteinuria and glucose.
- Assess position of baby, looking for breech positions (external cephalic version will be offered), check fetal heartbeat and symphysis fundal height.
- Discussion around birth plan, place of birth and contraception choice.

5.2.12 38 weeks antenatal appointment

- *Primary care / community midwife / hospital midwife.*
- Address any concerns and check general health and wellbeing.
- Discussion of prolonged pregnancy and how this is to be managed.
- Review any risk factors in pregnancy.
- BP check and urine dipstick for proteinuria and glucose.
- Assess position of baby and fetal heart rate; however, symphysis fundal height may no longer be accurate if baby has started to move into the birth canal. Assess degree of engagement.
- Women should be advised to be aware of their baby's individual pattern of movements. If they are concerned about a reduction in or cessation of fetal movements after 28 weeks of gestation, they should contact their maternity unit.
    - The RCOG Green-top Guideline No. 57 about reduced fetal movements is helpful.
- Offer advice about the postnatal period. This would involve discussion about what happens after discharge from the hospital, when the initial midwife and subsequent health visitor visits are planned, followed by the 6-week check for both mum and baby (including the information in *Section 5.3*).

5.2.13 40 weeks antenatal appointment

- *For nulliparous women only – hospital or community midwife.*
- Address any concerns and check general health and wellbeing.
- Discussion of prolonged pregnancy and how this is to be managed.
- Review any risk factors in pregnancy.
- BP and urine dipstick for proteinuria and glucose.
- Assess position of baby and the fetal heart rate, and be aware that the symphysis fundal height may no longer be accurate if baby has started to move into the birth canal. Assess degree of engagement.
- Monitor baby's movements and if any concerns or reduction in movements, involve the midwife as soon as possible.

5.2.14 41 weeks antenatal appointment

- *For women who have not given birth yet – hospital or community midwife.*
- Address any concerns and check general health and wellbeing.
- Options and choices for induction of labour and a membrane sweep will be discussed.
- Review any risk factors in pregnancy.
- BP and urine dipstick for proteinuria and glucose.
- Assess position of baby and the fetal heart rate, and be aware that symphysis fundal height may no longer be accurate if baby has started to move into the birth canal. Assess degree of engagement.
- Ask women to monitor their baby's movements and if they have any concerns or reduction in movements, they should contact the midwife as soon as possible.

5.3 Birth to the six weeks postnatal appointment

NICE guideline NG194 has helpful recommendations about postnatal care for the woman and the baby. This information should be given to women so they are familiar with what problems may occur in the immediate postnatal period and beyond. The guideline includes advice about the following:

- A general health assessment and assessment of psychological and emotional wellbeing.
- Advice about symptoms and signs of potential postnatal mental health problems, and how to seek help.
- The importance of pelvic floor health, including how to do pelvic floor exercises, and when to seek help. Advice about urinary incontinence and pelvic organ prolapse.
- Signs and symptoms of postnatal physical problems, and how to seek help. These include:
  - symptoms and signs of infection, pain, vaginal discharge and bleeding, bladder and bowel function, nipple and breast discomfort and signs of infection or inflammation, symptoms of signs of thromboembolism, anaemia and pre-eclampsia
  - depending on the type of birth: perineal or wound healing
  - signs of potentially serious conditions such as sudden or heavy vaginal bleeding that could indicate retained placenta or endometritis; abdominal pain, fever, shivering, vaginal discharge that could indicate infection; leg swelling or shortness of breath or chest pain which could indicate thromboembolism; persistent or severe headache, which could indicate hypertension or pre-eclampsia; symptoms or signs of sepsis.
- Lifestyle.
- Contraception.
  - Counselling should ideally be initiated at the booking appointment.
  - Women can be advised that although contraception is not required until day 21 postnatal, most methods (except for combined hormonal contraception) can be safely initiated immediately after birth.
- Sexual intercourse.

- Safeguarding, including domestic violence.
- Planning and supporting the baby's feeding, including general feeding principles and information and support for both breast and formula feeding, and what to do if there are problems.
- Postnatal care of the baby, assessment and care of the baby, advice about bed sharing and emotional attachment.

5.4 Postnatal check

- A postnatal check is usually done between 6 and 8 weeks postpartum.
- It can be done by the community midwife and/or in primary care.
- It is an opportunity for healthcare professionals to assess for domestic violence and safeguarding issues and refer appropriately.
- The different areas to explore are covered below.

5.4.1 Review of pregnancy / birth experience

- Start with a review of any antenatal care issues that may have arisen during the pregnancy.
- Discuss the birth experience, mode of delivery and any concerns about the delivery and postnatal period in the hospital:
  - Some women who may have concerns about their birth experience will need referral to a 'Birth Afterthoughts Clinic' to review with an experienced midwife what happened during labour and the delivery.
  - These clinics provide a space to explore any questions, concerns or emotional reactions to the birth, and they help women understand what happened and potentially plan for future births.
  - They can be accessed soon after birth or even years later.

5.4.2 Check for physical recovery

- Ask about physical recovery in terms of:
  - bleeding post-delivery (lochia)
  - vaginal discharge or pain
  - wounds (C-section scar or any tears / episiotomy scars)
  - pelvic floor and bladder and bowel function; guide women towards useful resources for pelvic floor health such as www.bladderandbowel.org.
- Do a physical examination which should include:
  - temperature if fever/sepsis suspected
  - blood pressure
  - BMI
  - mood and mental state
  - perineal or wound healing (if appropriate)
  - abdominal or pelvic examination if there is abnormal vaginal bleeding and/or pain or suspected vaginal prolapse, depending on clinical judgement
  - assessment for FGM if suspected.
  - assessment of abdomen for abdominal diastasis, by asking women to do a gentle sit-up; you can then feel for a gap between the left and right rectus abdominis muscles, by palpating just above and below the umbilicus – if there is more than a two-finger gap, refer to pelvic health physiotherapy.
  - check for any signs of deep vein thrombosis or pulmonary embolus.
- Arrange additional investigations such as:
  - blood tests, urine tests or vaginal swabs, depending on clinical judgement
  - HbA1c for women who had gestational diabetes during their pregnancy
  - TSH if there is a history of thyroid problems
  - FBC/ferritin if any iron transfusion or previous anaemia in pregnancy.

- Arranging urgent referral to specialist maternity services if there is suspected perineal wound breakdown or healing concerns.
- Arranging emergency hospital admission if there are any clinical features of a potentially serious or life-threatening medical or psychiatric condition, such as postpartum haemorrhage, sepsis, postpartum pre-eclampsia or eclampsia, VTE or postpartum psychosis.

5.4.3 Cervical screening, contraception and sexual health

- If the woman was due for routine cervical screening during pregnancy, it can be postponed and arranged for 12 weeks after birth.
- Discuss contraception (see *Chapter 3* for further details).
- Contraception should be offered to both non-breastfeeding and breastfeeding women as soon as possible, as sexual activity and ovulation may resume very soon after birth.
- Many maternity units are now sending women home with some form of contraception. If they haven't started any contraception this should be discussed at the 6-week check. It may be a sensitive area for some women who may feel pressured to restart their sex life, so it should be explored carefully.
- Women who are breastfeeding should be informed that the available evidence indicates that progestogen-only methods of contraception have no adverse effects on lactation, infant growth or development.
- Women who are breastfeeding should wait until 6 weeks after childbirth before initiating a combined hormonal contraceptive method (CHC). They should be informed that there is currently limited evidence regarding the effect of CHC use on breastfeeding; however, the better-quality studies of early initiation of CHC found no adverse effects on either breastfeeding performance (duration of breastfeeding, exclusivity and timing of initiation of supplemental feeding) or on infant outcomes (growth, health and development). If there are risk factors for VTE then CHC should not be used within 6 weeks of birth. If low risk for VTE and not breastfeeding, then CHC can be commenced after day 21 (UKMEC 2).
- Discuss sexual health sensitively because they may be reluctant to raise this issue themselves (see *Section 5.12*).

5.4.4 Assessment of perinatal mental health

- Timely identification and management of perinatal mental illness is critical (see *Section 8.2*):
  - 67% of maternal deaths occur postnatally, with suicide a leading cause between 6 weeks and 1 year.
  - Assess their mental health with a screening tool such as the Edinburgh Postnatal Depression scale and refer to the mental health team or perinatal mental health if there are any concerns.
  - It is important to be aware that early symptoms of postpartum psychosis may include insomnia, anxiety, irritability or mood fluctuation before abnormal thoughts and/or behaviours may become apparent.

5.4.5 Infant feeding

- Breastfeeding can be an empowering experience for many women, but for some it can also cause significant anxiety and stress, especially if they have been struggling. Discussion and questions about feeding should always be raised with empathy and in a supportive manner.
  - Determine the most appropriate ongoing method of feeding such as breastfeeding, bottle feeding or mixed for mum and baby. Explore any concerns about the method of feeding. Provide information and support if needed.
  - Review any breast problems such as lumps, infections, nipple/breast pains, and latching problems that may indicate tongue tie.

- If there are any concerns then referral to a community lactation consultant should be arranged (see *Section 12.8* for more on breastfeeding).
- The NHS recommends that breastfeeding mothers take a 10mcg (400IU) daily vitamin D supplement. Breastfed infants should receive a daily vitamin supplement of 8.5–10mcg (340–400IU).

5.5 Miscarriage

- Miscarriage is the spontaneous loss of pregnancy before the fetus reaches viability. The term includes all pregnancy losses from the time of conception until 24 weeks of gestation.
- Miscarriages can be termed early miscarriage if before 13 weeks and late miscarriage if between 13 and 24 weeks of gestation.
- Recurrent miscarriage is the loss of three or more pregnancies before 24 weeks of gestation. In 50% of cases no cause is found.
- Miscarriage affects 20% of recognised pregnancies, with recurrent miscarriages affecting approximately 1%.
- Miscarriages are common, and 25% of women will experience a miscarriage in their lifetime.
- It can be a very distressing experience and is often not spoken about. 20% will experience depression and anxiety, and these symptoms may last for up to 3 years.
- 80% of miscarriages will occur in the first trimester and chromosomal abnormalities are the most common cause.
- Risk factors and causes for miscarriage include:
  - maternal age (over 35) and paternal age (over 45) causing chromosomal abnormalities
  - structural issues: congenital uterine abnormalities or incompetent cervix
  - endocrine disorders, e.g. PCOS, luteal phase defect, diabetes, thyroid disorder
  - placental failure
  - multiple pregnancy
  - infections, e.g. rubella
  - immunological causes
  - vitamin D deficiency
  - Black ethnic background
  - lifestyle factors: smoking, drinking, excess caffeine, obesity, environmental toxins.
- Risk factors for recurrent miscarriage include:
  - chromosomal abnormalities
  - parental chromosomal anomaly
  - blood clotting factors, e.g. antiphospholipid syndrome
  - PCOS
  - male factor: increased sperm DNA fragmentation has been linked with recurrent miscarriages
  - thyroid disorders
  - abnormal BMI: <19kg/m^2 or >25kg/m^2 can lead to increased risk of miscarriages.

5.5.1 Types or stages of miscarriage

- **Threatened miscarriage**
  - When vaginal bleeding, with or without lower abdominal pain, occurs in the first 24 weeks of gestation. The bleeding is generally not heavy, and pain is minimal. Pregnancy may continue.
- **Inevitable miscarriage**
  - With heavy bleeding with clots and crampy abdominal pain, and the woman may be at risk of collapse. The pregnancy is being expelled from within the uterine cavity. Pregnancy will not continue and will proceed to incomplete or complete miscarriage.

- **Incomplete miscarriage**
  - When products of conception are partially expelled from the uterus. Many incomplete miscarriages may be missed miscarriages.
- **Complete miscarriage**
  - When all the products of conception have been expelled from the uterus, and the bleeding has stopped.
- **Missed miscarriage**
  - When a non-viable pregnancy is identified on an ultrasound scan without associated pain and bleeding.

5.5.2 Role of the healthcare professional in managing miscarriages

- Miscarriages can be a traumatic experience for women and consultations should be done in a sensitive, empathetic manner.
- Confirm pregnancy with a pregnancy test.
- Take a detailed gynaecological and obstetric history.
- Examination to assess bleeding and pain and exclude other causes such as ectopic pregnancy.
- Assess BP, pulse and temperature to check signs of infection and haemodynamic status.
- Four options for management depending on the findings:
  - Immediate admission to hospital if signs of haemodynamic shock: pale, clammy, hypotension, tachycardia, tachypnoea or collapse, or if there are concerns regarding heaviness of bleeding and pain.
  - Urgent referral to local Early Pregnancy Assessment Unit (EPAU) for pelvic ultrasound scan if pregnant and lower abdominal pain or pelvic or cervical tenderness.
  - Assessment in EPAU if bleeding and pain and around 6 weeks pregnant or unknown gestation. Urgency depending on symptoms.
  - Expectant management: women who are less than 6 weeks pregnant with bleeding but no pain and no risk of ectopic pregnancy. Repeat pregnancy test after 7–10 days and review if positive. If ongoing bleeding and pain refer to EPAU. If negative confirms miscarriage.
- Discuss potential management options that the EPAU may offer:
  - Expectant management monitoring and a further follow-up scan / pregnancy test should be arranged.
  - Medical management:
    - For missed miscarriage: 200mg oral mifepristone and 48hrs later 800mcg of misoprostol (vaginal/oral/sublingual unless the gestation sac has been passed).
    - For incomplete miscarriage: single dose of 600mcg misoprostol (vaginal/oral/sublingual).
  - Surgical management: evacuation of retained products of conception (ERPC). Anti-D should be offered to all Rhesus-negative women after surgical procedures.
- Offer a follow-up appointment after any miscarriage to discuss ongoing emotional support that may be needed and a referral for counselling. Cancel any future antenatal appointments. Discuss avoiding sex until miscarriage symptoms have settled; if they wish to try again their next period may start 4–8 weeks later and they can start as soon after that as they feel physically and emotionally ready.
- For women with recurrent miscarriages check local referral guidelines but refer to a recurrent miscarriage clinic for further investigations into the likely causes.

5.5.3 Ectopic pregnancy

- This occurs when the fertilised egg implants outside of the uterine cavity.
- 97% implant in the fallopian tubes, although rarely there may be implantation in the ovary, abdomen, C-section scar or cervix.
- The prevalence is 11 in 1000 pregnancies.

- It can lead to tubal rupture and maternal death; it may impact future fertility, result in recurrent ectopics, and have psychological impacts.
- Symptoms may be atypical but usually feature lower abdominal pain and a period of amenorrhoea with vaginal bleeding. Other presentations include gastrointestinal problems, symptoms of urinary tract infection (UTI), shoulder tip pain or dizziness. If severe or close to rupture, they may present with signs of shock.
- Urgency of referral depends on the severity of symptoms:
  - women who are in pain and shock should be admitted immediately
  - for others a referral to the EPAU for a pelvic scan is sufficient to confirm the diagnosis.
- Management is either:
  - expectant
  - medical with methotrexate
  - surgical
  - follow-up after a visit to the EPAU is important to offer support, information and advice.

5.6 Nausea and vomiting in pregnancy

5.6.1 Prevalence

- This is a common symptom in early pregnancy and generally starts around 4–7 weeks, peaks at around 9–16 weeks and then ends by 16–20 weeks of gestation.
- It affects around 70% of pregnant women.
- Hyperemesis gravidarum is a very severe form of nausea and vomiting in pregnancy that impacts the ability to eat and limits daily activities. Some women (0.3–3% of pregnancies) with hyperemesis gravidarum will need to be admitted to hospital.
- The psychological impact must not be underestimated: around 10% of women with hyperemesis gravidarum will terminate their pregnancy due to the severity of the symptoms and some women may feel suicidal.
- Complications that can arise include weight loss, dehydration, electrolyte imbalance, nutritional and vitamin deficiencies, abnormal LFTs, Mallory–Weiss tears, acid reflux, retinal haemorrhages, VTE, emotional distress / depression / anxiety.
- If the symptoms start after 11 weeks of pregnancy, then other causes should be explored such as hypertensive disorders of pregnancy, hepatobiliary disease, gastrointestinal infection, urinary infection, and other systemic causes.

5.6.2 Management

- Assess the severity of the symptoms and how it is impacting them psychologically.
- Check for dehydration (temperature/BP/pulse/weight) and rule out a urine infection.
- If dehydration and vomiting is severe then blood tests including FBC, U&Es, LFT, blood glucose may be needed.
- Direct women towards a support service such as Pregnancy Sickness Support: https://pregnancysicknesssupport.org.uk.
- For mild symptoms general dietary advice may be sufficient: small, frequent protein-rich meals low in carbohydrates and fat; ginger; plain crackers / digestives in the morning, avoid triggers. Drinking little but often.
- Acupressure may help over the P6 point on the ventral aspect of the wrist by finger pressure or a wrist band.
- For more severe symptoms start with first-line anti-emetics: cyclizine **or** promethazine **or** prochlorperazine **or** Xonvea (doxylamine/pyridoxine); reassess symptoms 24–72hrs later.
- If first-line drugs have all been tried and they do not work, consider second-line anti-emetics: ondansetron (short-term: 5 days and small risk of cleft palate/lip) **or**

metoclopramide (short-term: 5 days) **or** domperidone (short-term: 7 days); reassess after 24hrs.

- Some women may need different classes of drugs in combination to manage the symptoms.
- Rarely third-line drugs such as oral prednisolone (40–50mg daily) may be needed, then tapering dose to level where symptoms are controlled.
- If not managed with anti-emetics/steroids or dehydrated, then hospitalisation for IV fluids may be needed. Ambulatory daycare may be suitable for some women but consider inpatient management if there is at least one of the following:
  - continued nausea and vomiting and inability to keep down oral anti-emetics
  - continued nausea and vomiting associated with ketonuria and/or weight loss (>5% of body weight), despite oral anti-emetics
  - confirmed or suspected comorbidity (such as UTI and inability to tolerate oral antibiotics).
- Sometimes thiamine may be needed for severely reduced food intake, laxatives for constipation and proton pump inhibitor for reflux symptoms.
- Consider a perinatal mental health referral if there are severe psychological impacts.

5.7 Hypertension in pregnancy and postnatal hypertension

5.7.1 Prevalence

- Hypertensive disorder can occur in 8–10% of pregnancies.
- Hypertension during pregnancy can result in:
  - increased risk of preterm deliveries
  - intrauterine growth restriction and low birthweight babies
  - babies needing neonatal ITU care
  - placental abruption
  - increased risk of fetal death and maternal death
  - an increased risk of hypertension, stroke and cardiovascular disease in the future.
- Different types of hypertension may impact women at different times during their pregnancy:
  - **Hypertension** – women with diastolic BP of 90–109mmHg and/or systolic BP of 140–159mmHg should have increased monitoring of their blood pressure.
  - **Severe hypertension** – women with a diastolic BP of ≥110mmHg and/or systolic BP of ≥160mmHg require treatment if systolic BP >160mmHg on two consecutive readings 4 hours apart.
  - **Chronic hypertension** – hypertension that is present at, or prior to the booking visit, or before 20 weeks of gestation.
  - **Gestational hypertension** – new hypertension presenting after 20 weeks of gestation without significant proteinuria; 10–25% will go on to develop pre-eclampsia.
  - **Pre-eclampsia** – new hypertension presenting after 20 weeks of gestation with significant proteinuria; pre-eclampsia is a multisystem disorder which can affect the placenta, kidney, liver, brain and other maternal organs.
  - **HELLP syndrome** (haemolysis, elevated liver enzymes and low platelets syndrome) – a severe form of pre-eclampsia associated with a high rate of maternal and perinatal morbidity and mortality.
  - **Eclampsia** is the occurrence of one or more seizures in a woman with pre-eclampsia.

5.7.2 Risk factors for hypertension and pre-eclampsia

- Risk factors for gestational hypertension include:
  - nulliparity
  - multiple pregnancy
  - Black ethnicity

- maternal obesity
- maternal type 1 diabetes.

- Women are at high risk of pre-eclampsia if they have one of the following high-risk factors:
  - history of hypertensive disease during a previous pregnancy
  - chronic kidney disease
  - autoimmune disease, such as systemic lupus erythematosus or antiphospholipid syndrome
  - type 1 or type 2 diabetes
  - chronic hypertension.

Or two or more of the following moderate risk factors:
- first pregnancy
- 40 years of age or older
- pregnancy interval of >10 years
- BMI of ≥35kg/m^2 at the first visit
- family history of pre-eclampsia
- multiple pregnancy.

5.7.3 Symptoms

- Some women may have no symptoms, and hypertension may be picked up during routine screening.
- Symptoms of pre-eclampsia:
  - severe headaches (increasing frequency unrelieved by regular analgesics)
  - visual problems, such as blurred vision, flashing lights or photophobia
  - persistent new epigastric pain or pain in the right upper quadrant
  - vomiting
  - breathlessness (due to pulmonary oedema)
  - sudden swelling of the face, hands or feet.

5.7.4 Assessment

- BP and urine dipstick should be checked at every antenatal and postnatal visit.
- If proteinuria (1+ or more) then check albumin:creatinine ratio (≥8mg/mmol is significant) or protein:creatinine ratio (≥30mg/mmol is significant).
- Avoid first morning urine samples. They are not preferred for checking proteinuria because they may underestimate the amount of protein excreted over 24 hours.

5.7.5 Management

- Lifestyle advice for all women: regular rest periods but with gentle exercise, such as walking and yoga, maintain a healthy weight and healthy balanced diet with restriction of dietary salt and excess caffeine.
- **Chronic hypertension and hypertension before 20 weeks**
  - These women will be at risk of pre-eclampsia so will need close monitoring.
  - They will need consultant-led care for specialist management.
  - Start aspirin 75–150mg daily in the evening from 12 weeks gestation until birth. Use the lower dose if there is renal or hepatic impairment.
  - If already on an ACE inhibitor or ARB, these will need to be stopped due to adverse fetal outcomes in the 2nd and 3rd trimester. Consider alternative treatment such as labetolol first line, then nifedipine and then methyldopa.
  - Thiazide and thiazide-like medication will also need to be stopped, and alternative treatment, as mentioned above, should be considered.
  - Target BP is 135/85mmHg.

 - Assess for symptoms of pre-eclampsia at every visit and refer urgently for assessment if suspected.
- **New hypertension after 20 weeks**
  - Women with BP >140mmHg systolic or >90mmHg diastolic will need urgent referral for assessment in hospital within 24hrs.
  - If hypertension is severe (>160/110mmHg) they will need to be admitted on the same day for monitoring and management of blood pressure.
- **Pre-eclampsia**
  - If blood pressure >140/90mmHg and >20 weeks gestation with proteinuria or other maternal organ dysfunction (renal problems, abnormal LFTs, thrombocytopenia, uteroplacental dysfunction, neurological symptoms) then a diagnosis of pre-eclampsia can be made.
  - Refer for secondary care assessment within 24hrs and if >160/110mmHg admit on the same day.
  - Ensure aspirin 75–150mg daily is prescribed from 12 weeks until birth.
- **Proteinuria and normal blood pressure after 20 weeks**
  - These women are at high risk of pre-eclampsia.
  - Admit urgently if symptoms and proteinuria (2+ or more) even if symptoms of UTI.
  - If no symptoms and proteinuria – rule out UTI and monitor BP in 1 week with clear instructions to look for the symptoms of pre-eclampsia and do protein:creatinine or albumin:creatinine ratios. Seek specialist advice if any concerns.

5.7.6 Postnatal hypertension

- If any hypertension problems during their pregnancy, women will only be discharged once stable with a home BP monitor with a clear plan for frequency of monitoring and thresholds for reducing or stopping treatments, when to see their GP about their blood pressure, and advice on self-monitoring.
- They will be advised to monitor their BP daily for the first 2 days, then once between days 3 and 5, and then as clinically advised on discharge.
- Women with pre-eclampsia will need their BP checking every 1–2 days for the first 2 weeks. This can usually be done at home with the midwife or by self-monitoring.
- If not on medication, start treatment if blood pressure >150/90mmHg.
- Consider stopping antihypertensives if normotensive >1 week or reduce dose if below 130/80mmHg. Target BP is <140/90mmHg.
- Check for symptoms of pre-eclampsia.
- Adjust antihypertensives if already on them:
  - avoid ARB/diuretics in breastfeeding, because antihypertensives can pass (in small quantities) into breast milk. Women who are breastfeeding should be advised to monitor their babies for symptoms of hypotension, such as drowsiness, lethargy, pallor, cold peripheries, or poor feeding.
  - stop methyldopa 2 days after delivery and switch to alternatives.
  - enalapril can be used first line (monitor kidney function) or if Black African or Caribbean origin start with nifedipine or amlodipine; if not tolerated or alternative needed then consider atenolol/labetalol.
- Refer to Cardiology if persistent hypertension or treatment needed >6 weeks postpartum.

5.8 Gestational diabetes

5.8.1 Overview

- Gestational diabetes can affect 10–20% of pregnancies in the UK.
- It can cause complications during the pregnancy and birth, and women continue to have a higher risk of developing type 2 diabetes mellitus (T2DM) after the delivery.

- Complications include a larger than average baby, traumatic birth, induction of labour and/or caesarean section, neonatal hypoglycaemia and perinatal death. Good glucose control throughout pregnancy can reduce the risks.

5.8.2 Risk factors for gestational diabetes

- BMI ≥30kg/m^2.
- Previous larger than average baby weighing ≥4.5kg.
- Previous gestational diabetes.
- Family history of diabetes (first-degree relative with diabetes).
- An ethnicity with a high prevalence of diabetes.

5.8.3 Screening

- During routine antenatal urine dipstick testing, women with glucosuria of 2+ on one occasion or 1+ on two occasions should be referred for further testing.
- Offer referral for a 75g 2-hour oral glucose tolerance test (OGTT).
- For women who have previously had gestational diabetes, organise early self- monitoring of blood glucose, or arrange an OGTT at booking and a second OGTT to take place between 24 and 28 weeks, if the first was normal.
- Any woman with risk factors for gestational diabetes should be offered an OGTT between 24 and 28 weeks of gestation.

5.8.4 Diagnosis

- Diagnose gestational diabetes if the woman has either:
  - a fasting plasma glucose level of ≥5.6mmol/L **or**
  - a 2-hour plasma glucose level of ≥7.8mmol/L.
- Women with positive tests should have a specialist review within 1 week.
- They should be taught how to self-monitor their glucose levels with fingerprick testing, aiming to keep levels below (some may use continuous glucose monitors):
  - 5.3mmol/L – fasting
  - 7.8mmol/L – 1hr after eating
  - 6.4mmol/L – 2hrs after eating.

5.8.5 Management

- Dietary advice: all women should be referred to a dietitian.
  - Avoid missing meals and eat three meals a day.
  - Eat starchy and low-GI foods.
  - Five portions of fruit and vegetables daily.
  - Avoid sugary food and drinks.
  - Eat lean sources of protein.
- Exercise advice: 30 minutes 5× per week, e.g. walking briskly for 30 minutes after a meal, cycling, swimming.
- If diet and exercise have not improved blood sugars after 1–2 weeks and fasting glucose at diagnosis is between 5.3 and 7.0mmol/L, then metformin should be started. If blood sugars are still not well controlled, then insulin can be added.
- If metformin is not tolerated or contraindicated, or if fasting glucose at diagnosis is >7.0mmol/L, then insulin should be started.
- Women with gestational diabetes will be offered more ultrasound scans to check fetal growth at 28, 32 and 36 weeks.
- Aim for delivery between 38 and 40+6 weeks.

5.8.6 Managing gestational diabetes postnatally

- Medication can usually be stopped after birth, but blood glucose monitoring will need to be continued for 1–2 days after birth. This helps confirm that blood sugar levels remain stable without treatment.
- Screen at 6–13 weeks postpartum with HbA1c.
- Advise annual diabetes screening thereafter due to increased risk of T2DM.
- Lifestyle advice and weight management.
- Offer a referral into the NHS Diabetes Prevention Programme if eligible based on the results of the fasting plasma glucose test or HbA1c test if abnormal.

5.9 Anaemia in pregnancy

5.9.1 Prevalence

- Iron-deficiency anaemia affects around 23% of pregnant women in the UK. Nearly one-third of women are anaemic postpartum.
- Normal physiological changes in pregnancy result in a rise in plasma volume, and this causes haemodilution which causes a lowering of haemoglobin to 115g/L. Treatment is needed as per *Section 5.9.4*.

5.9.2 Causes

- Iron deficiency (most common), folate or B12 deficiency
- Multiple pregnancy
- Sickle-cell anaemia
- Coeliac disease
- Beta-thalassaemia
- Chronic haemolysis
- Gastrointestinal bleeding
- Leukaemia
- Parasitic disease.

5.9.3 Symptoms

- Some women may be asymptomatic.
- Others may appear pale.
- Fatigue, shortness of breath and dizziness are common.

5.9.4 Screening

- At booking and 28 week appointments (additional if symptomatic).
- Treat if Hb <110g/L (1st trimester), <105g/L (2nd/3rd trimester), <100g/L (postpartum).

5.9.5 Treatment

- Advise that women maintain an adequate balanced intake of iron-rich foods (e.g. dark green leafy vegetables, iron-fortified bread, meat, apricots, prunes and raisins) and consider referral to a dietitian.
- Oral iron: NICE advises that treatment should be one tablet once a day of oral ferrous sulphate, ferrous fumarate, or ferrous gluconate and continued for 3 months after the iron deficiency is corrected. A FBC should be checked in 2–4 weeks to assess the response to iron treatment. If there is lack of response (an increase of <20g/L in the Hb level at this time), then a referral should be made for specialist assessment.

- IV iron for severe cases or if they are unable to tolerate oral preparations, or oral preparations are ineffective.
- Check for haemoglobinopathies if indicated.
- Women with known haemoglobinopathy should have serum ferritin checked and be offered oral supplements if their ferritin level is low (<30μg/L).
- Refer pregnant women to obstetrics if there are significant symptoms and/or severe anaemia (haemoglobin <70g/L), if pregnancy is at advanced gestation (>34 weeks) or if there is failure to respond to a trial of oral iron.

5.10 Perinatal mental health

- Refer to *Section 8.2* for detailed guidance on perinatal mental health.
- Healthcare professionals should screen routinely throughout the perinatal and postnatal period and provide early referral to local perinatal mental health services where needed.

5.11 Abortion care

5.11.1 Legal context

- In the UK a pregnancy can be lawfully terminated by a registered medical practitioner in an NHS hospital, or premises approved for this purpose, if two medical practitioners are of the opinion, formed in good faith, that (from the Abortion Act 1967):
  - *"The pregnancy has not exceeded its 24th week and the continuance of the pregnancy would involve risk, greater than if the pregnancy were terminated, of injury to the physical or mental health of the pregnant person or any existing children of their family.*
  - *The termination is necessary to prevent grave permanent injury to the physical or mental health of the pregnant person.*
  - *Continuing the pregnancy would involve risk to the life of the pregnant person, greater than if the pregnancy were terminated.*
  - *There is a substantial risk that if the child were born, it would suffer from such physical or mental abnormalities as to be seriously handicapped."*

5.11.2 Role of the healthcare professional

- The consultation must be non-judgemental and confidential. Some healthcare providers may refuse to participate in abortion care. They must inform their employer in advance, ensure that patients can be seen without delay by another clinician and maintain non-judgemental communications at all times, but must provide care in an emergency setting regardless of their objections.
- Exclude ectopic pregnancy.
- Discuss all pregnancy options so the woman knows what alternatives are available.
- Refer to abortion service: NHS, British Pregnancy Advisory Service (BPAS) or MSI Reproductive Choices UK or National Unplanned Pregnancy Advisory Service (NUPAS) clinics.
- Abortions are free on the NHS, although some women may opt to go privately.
- Consider safeguarding referral if any concerns.
- Post-procedure care: contraception and emotional support.

5.11.3 Methods

- Medical: mifepristone + misoprostol up to 10 weeks.
- Surgical: manual vacuum aspiration, electric vacuum aspiration or dilatation and evacuation, at 10 to 24 weeks.

5.12 Impact on sexual function

- Sex is a healthy and normal part of pregnancy and the postpartum period.
- Lack of adequate information about sex during pregnancy and concerns about possible adverse obstetric outcomes are the most relevant factors contributing to avoidance of sexual activity in pregnancy.
- Only 31% of pregnant and 15% of postpartum women discuss sexuality with a healthcare provider.
- Healthcare professionals should sensitively initiate conversations about sexual health during and after pregnancy, creating a safe environment for women and couples to discuss their concerns openly.

5.12.1 Common concerns

- Low libido, dyspareunia, vaginal dryness, less clitoral sensitivity causing reduced arousal, and body image issues.
- These concerns can vary with trimester.
- Dyspareunia can get worse in the third trimester and genital sensitivity and arousal improve in the second trimester but reduce in the third as prolactin rises. Sexual activity can be more difficult due to the size of the bump in the third trimester.
- Sexual drive can also fluctuate during pregnancy.
- It may be low during the first trimester due to anxiety, nausea or tiredness but increase in the second trimester due to hormone changes, then taper off in the third trimester as the baby grows causing discomfort and as women get closer to their due date.
- Postnatally the decline in sexual function can continue for 3–6 months or longer. Women may have dyspareunia due to birth trauma, breastfeeding may cause vaginal dryness and nipple sensitivity, and altered body image can also impact sexual function.

5.12.2 Causes

- Hormonal, i.e. breastfeeding.
- Physical trauma, e.g. tears, weak pelvic floor, birth trauma, fatigue.
- Psychological, e.g. postnatal depression, body changes. Distressing feelings including guilt, worry, frustration and embarrassment.

5.12.3 Management

- Try to gently explore the topic during a consultation because the woman/couple may not raise it themselves.
- Reassure them that having sex will not harm the baby and that having orgasms or sex will not increase the risk of going into labour or a miscarriage; however, in later pregnancy they may set off mild Braxton Hicks contractions.
- Whilst sex during pregnancy is generally safe, some women may be advised *not* to have sex if:
  - previous premature labour or at risk of premature birth
  - any heavy bleeding
  - previous cervical problems or surgery
  - low-lying placenta
  - multiple pregnancy
  - their partner has an STD
  - their waters have already broken.
- Consider different positions that may be more comfortable, e.g. woman on top or side by side or on all fours.
- Advise to always use lubricants during sex if there is vaginal dryness.

- If not considering penetrative sex, then it is important to encourage the couple to keep up good communication and to consider other ways they can maintain intimacy, e.g. kissing, hugging, massage, mutual masturbation and oral sex.
- Pelvic floor exercises should be encouraged to strengthen the pelvic floor.
- Some women postnatally may need vaginal oestrogen, especially when breastfeeding, if there is any vaginal dryness. Breastfeeding itself may be sexually arousing for some women, while it may put other women off sex.
- There are no set rules, but it is sensible to avoid sex for 6 weeks postnatally as there is a high risk of infection during this time.
- Discuss contraception at the 6-week postnatal check if they haven't already been offered this at the hospital.
- Most couples will have resumed sexual intercourse within 3 months and the rest between 6 and 12 months postpartum. Reassure them that there is no set time by which they have to start and it can be when they feel ready but if there is a delay that is causing distress, then they should discuss this with a healthcare professional.
- Review any dyspareunia or perineal pain postnatally and refer to gynaecology if it persists. Vaginal oestrogen cream locally for a few weeks may help.
- Referral to psychosexual therapy or pelvic health physiotherapy if needed.
- Good resources to direct patients to are *How not to let having kids ruin your sex life* by Dr Karen Gurney and the website https://postbabyhankypanky.com which has useful short videos that couples can watch.

5.13 How to take a fertility history

5.13.1 Importance of the history

- Infertility can have a devasting impact on a couple trying to conceive.
- A comprehensive history enables early identification of treatable causes or risk factors, such as smoking or obesity.
- It also identifies those couples that need further investigations and prompt referral.

5.13.2 Key components of history-taking

- Age, length of time trying to conceive.
- **Menstrual history:** age at menarche, cycle length, regularity, dysmenorrhoea, amenorrhoea, menorrhagia.
- **Sexual history:** sub-fertility can be a significant cause of psychosexual distress, so it is important to explore this area. Ask about frequency and timing of intercourse, previous STIs or PID, any sexual issues that may arise during intercourse (including partner's issues such as erectile dysfunction) and explore if there is any history of trauma.
- **Obstetric history:** previous pregnancies (gravidity), how many live births (parity), type of births (normal/C-section/instrumental), any miscarriages / ectopic pregnancies, any complications during the pregnancy or deliveries, whether children were with current or previous partners.
- **Medical/surgical history:** ask about PCOS, thyroid disorders, endometriosis, diabetes, inflammatory bowel disease, any previous pelvic or abdominal surgery.
- **Lifestyle factors:** smoking, alcohol, BMI, exercise, occupational exposures, recreational drug use, stress.
- **Contraception:** length of time since stopping contraception, previous use, type and duration. Last smear test.
- **Partner's history:** age, medical and sexual history, any known fertility issues, previous children, lifestyle factors.

5.14 Infertility

- Infertility is defined as failure to conceive after 12 months of regular unprotected intercourse.
- Over 85% of women under the age of 40 will conceive in the first year if having regular (every 2–3 days) unprotected intercourse; 50% of those that do not conceive will do so in the second year.
- Infertility affects 1 in 7 heterosexual couples in the UK. It is classed as primary infertility in couples who have never conceived and secondary infertility in couples who have conceived once before, either with the same or different partners.
- The leading causes of infertility in the UK are:
  - Male factors in 30% of couples (oligozoospermia/azoospermia, testicular damage, varicocele, conditions causing low testosterone, ejaculatory and erectile dysfunction).
  - Ovulatory disorders in 25% of couples (hypothalamic amenorrhoea, hypogonadotropic hypogonadism, PCOS, thyroid problems).
  - Tubal damage in 20% of couples (PID, endometriosis).
  - Uterine or peritoneal disorders in 10% of couples (adhesions, polyps, fibroids/ endometriosis).
  - Combined male and female factors in 40% of couples.
  - Unexplained fertility in 25% of couples – where no clear cause has been found on investigations.

5.14.1 Initial primary care exam and investigations

- Try to investigate both partners at the same time.
- Start investigations after 1 year of trying to conceive, or earlier if above age 35 or if any problems identified that may affect fertility.
- BMI: high BMI >30kg/m^2 is associated with lower fertility.
- Blood pressure.
- Pelvic exam to check for any masses.
- Vaginal exam: bimanual and speculum to check for cysts, fibroids, tenderness, vaginal infections, PID.
- Day 2–5 FSH, LH, prolactin to check for ovulation disorders or pituitary disorders.
- Day 21 progesterone to check ovulation has occurred (level should be >20nmol/L).
- TSH may be tested if any symptoms of thyroid disease.
- STI screen including chlamydia.
- Check smear testing is up to date.
- Chlamydia tests and semen analysis for male partner – inform them they need to abstain from sex/masturbation for 2–7 days prior to collecting the sample. Warn them that they may have to produce the sample in the lab; if not then the sample should be in the lab within 30 minutes and no later than 50 minutes. If it is abnormal it will need to be repeated after 3 months.

5.14.2 What advice to give to couples trying to conceive?

- Involve both partners when discussing management.
- Discuss chances of conception: 80% within 12 months if woman under 40 and having regular intercourse, and 50% of those who did not conceive in the first 12 months will conceive in the second year of trying.
- Have regular intercourse every 2–3 days rather than timing to ovulation because there is no evidence that using ovulation sticks improves fertility rates and instead it can cause a lot of stress for the couple.
- Fertility declines with age.
- Smoking can reduce fertility and harm a developing baby, and may impact semen quality.

- Alcohol is not advised during pregnancy because it can affect the fetus and may affect semen quality if over normal limit of 14 units/week.
- Advise that a raised BMI (>30kg/m^2) in women can reduce fertility and losing weight can increase their chances of getting pregnant. For women with a low BMI (<19kg/m^2) increasing their weight can improve amenorrhoea and improve their chances of conceiving.
- Some medications (including OTC medication such as NSAIDs, decongestants or some herbal products) and illicit drugs can interfere with fertility.
- Stress in either partner can impact libido and reduce the frequency of sex and fertility.
- If there are concerns about any occupational health risks, then a risk assessment should be made at work.
- Women should be up to date with their smears and rubella status and take 400mcg folic acid daily if trying to conceive.
- Direct them to helpful websites for more information:
  - British Infertility Counselling Association (www.bica.net).
  - Fertility Network UK (https://fertilitynetworkuk.org).
  - The Human Fertilisation & Embryology Authority (www.hfea.gov.uk) provides information on IVF clinics, and other fertility treatments from the UK government fertility regulator.

5.14.3 Referral criteria

- Early referral if >35 years old and trying for 6 months, otherwise refer any couple unable to conceive if trying for 12 months under the age of 35 years.
- Refer women early if there are known risk factors, e.g. age, PCOS, or abnormal tests.
- Symptoms that may indicate ovulatory problems that may warrant early referral:
  - menorrhagia (abnormal heavy bleeding)
  - oligomenorrhoea (infrequent or irregular menstrual periods)
  - amenorrhoea (absence of menstruation)
  - dysmenorrhoea (painful periods)
  - galactorrhoea or hirsutism
  - excessive exercise, weight loss or psychological distress.
- Symptoms that may indicate uterine, cervical or peritoneal problems that may require early referral:
  - symptoms of PID or endometriosis, such as dyspareunia (difficult or painful sexual intercourse)
  - dysmenorrhoea
  - intermenstrual or postcoital bleeding.

5.15 Conclusion

Healthcare professionals in primary care provide essential reproductive and pregnancy-related care from preconception to postnatal recovery. Applying evidence-based guidelines and offering compassionate, holistic care ensures optimal outcomes for patients and their families.

5.16 Further reading

Gurney, K. (2024) *How Not to Let Having Kids Ruin Your Sex Life: navigating the parenting years with your relationship intact*. Headline Home.

Human Fertilisation & Embryology Authority: www.hfea.gov.uk

NHS (undated) *Abortion*. Available at: www.nhs.uk/conditions/abortion

NHS England (2023) NHS fetal anomaly screening programme (FASP). Available at: www.gov.uk/government/collections/nhs-fetal-anomaly-screening-programme-fasp

NHS Scotland (2024) *Postpartum hypertension, guideline for management* (322). Available at: https://rightdecisions.scot.nhs.uk/ggc-clinical-guidelines/maternity/common-obstetric-problems-intrapartum-labour-ward/postpartum-hypertension-guideline-for-management-322

NICE (updated 2020) *Diabetes in pregnancy* [NG3]. Available at: www.nice.org.uk/guidance/ng3

NICE (2021) *Antenatal care* [NG201]. Available at: www.nice.org.uk/guidance/ng201/chapter/Recommendations

NICE (2021) *Postnatal care* [NG194]. Available at: www.nice.org.uk/guidance/ng194

NICE (revised 2023) CKS: *Infertility*. Available at: https://cks.nice.org.uk/topics/infertility

NICE (revised 2023) CKS: *Miscarriage*. Available at: https://cks.nice.org.uk/topics/miscarriage

NICE (revised 2024) CKS: *Anaemia – iron deficiency*. Available at: https://cks.nice.org.uk/topics/anaemia-iron-deficiency

NICE (revised 2024) CKS: *Postnatal care*. Available at: https://cks.nice.org.uk/topics/postnatal-care

NICE (revised 2025) CKS: *Depression – antenatal and postnatal*. Available at: https://cks.nice.org.uk/topics/depression-antenatal-postnatal

NICE (revised 2025) CKS: *Hypertension in pregnancy*. Available at: https://cks.nice.org.uk/topics/hypertension-in-pregnancy

NICE (revised 2025) CKS: *Pre-conception*. Available at: https://cks.nice.org.uk/topics/pre-conception-advice-management

Public Health England (2016) *Eatwell Guide*. Available at : https://assets.publishing.service.gov.uk/media/5bbb790de5274a22415d7fee/Eatwell_guide_colour_edition.pdf

RCOG (2011) *Reduced fetal movements*. Green-top Guideline No. 57. Available at: www.rcog.org.uk/media/2gxndsd3/gtg_57.pdf

RCOG Green-top Guidelines. Available at: www.rcog.org.uk

Tommy's: the pregnancy and baby charity: www.tommys.org

UK Health Security Agency (updated 2025) *The Green Book*. Available at: www.gov.uk/government/collections/immunisation-against-infectious-disease-the-green-book

Chapter 6
Menopause

6.1 Menopause definitions

Menopause

- Natural menopause is a biological stage in a woman's life when menstruation stops permanently because the number of oocytes in the ovaries declines, there is loss of ovarian follicular activity and consequently a fall in the levels of oestrogen and progesterone.
- It is diagnosed 12 months after the last natural period, if there is no other cause for periods to have stopped.
- In the UK, menopause usually occurs between 45 and 55 years of age; the average age is 51 years.
- The age of menopause can be affected by factors such as diet, exercise, smoking status, socioeconomic background, ethnicity and BMI.

Perimenopause (the menopause transition)

- This is the time leading up to a natural menopause, when many women start to experience a change in their menstrual cycle and menstruation. Cycles may shorten or lengthen. Periods can become heavier or lighter.
- Women may start to notice menopausal symptoms including vasomotor symptoms, cognitive problems, mood disorders, urogenital symptoms, sleep disturbance, altered sexual function, joint and muscle pains, headaches and fatigue.
- Perimenopause can last between 2 and 10 years, and ends 12 months after the last menstrual period.
- During perimenopause, hormone levels fluctuate significantly.

Early menopause

- Menopause which occurs between the ages of 40 and 45. This affects 12.2% of women.

Premature ovarian insufficiency (POI)

- A clinical condition when there is loss of ovarian activity, either transiently or permanently, before the age of 40 (see *Section 6.8* for more details). This affects 3.7% of women.
- It is characterised by menstrual disturbance (amenorrhoea or oligomenorrhoea) and raised gonadotrophins (FSH and LH), and low estradiol.
- The British Menopause Society (BMS) advises that in clinical practice, the advice and management of the diagnoses of early menopause and POI should be similar.

Surgical menopause

- Occurs following removal of the ovaries (bilateral oophorectomy) before a woman goes through her natural menopause.
- For more details about surgical menopause see *Section 6.10.*

Induced or iatrogenic menopause

- Occurs when a treatment (e.g. chemotherapy or radiotherapy, or gonadotrophin-releasing hormone agonists) causes the ovaries to stop functioning normally.
- This may be temporary or permanent.
- For more details about induced menopause see *Section 6.9.*

6.2 Symptoms of perimenopause and menopause

- By the age of 54, 80% of women will be menopausal.
- Menopausal symptoms will affect about 80% of women, and around 25% of women say their symptoms affect them severely, impacting on their work, relationships and quality of life.

- Symptoms can vary between women, both in how they present and in severity. Some women experience vasomotor symptoms, others may present with depression and sore joints. Symptoms usually last about 5–7 years but can continue for longer, and some women continue to experience symptoms for years after their menopause.

6.2.1 Main symptoms

- Women may experience any combination of the following symptoms.
- During perimenopause, periods can become erratic. They can be lighter, heavier, closer together, further apart and more painful.
  - Women over 40 with a significant change in their bleeding pattern, for example heavier and longer periods, should have a gynaecological assessment and investigations, whether or not they are using a contraceptive method.
- Vasomotor symptoms (VMS): hot flushes, night sweats and chills. These are experienced by more than 80% of women during the menopause transition and show pronounced racial and ethnic differences, with prevalence being highest in Black women and lowest in East Asian women.
  - They are described as a sudden feeling of heat in the upper body which spreads upwards and downwards, or a feeling of being generally hot. They can last from as little as 30 seconds to as long as an hour, but typically last around 3–4 minutes. They are often accompanied by sweating, reddening of the skin and palpitations.
  - They often start for no reason but may be provoked by embarrassment, stress, alcohol, caffeine or temperature change.
  - Consider other causes for VMS, such as hyperthyroidism, anxiety and panic disorder, phaeochromocytoma, malignancy, drugs such as selective serotonin reuptake inhibitors (SSRIs).
- Mood changes.
  - These include low mood, mood swings, anxiety, worry, panic attacks, tearfulness, irritability, anger outbursts, loss of confidence, low self-esteem, loss of joy, worsening of PMS and premenstrual dysphoric disorder (PMDD).
  - Estradiol helps to modulate neurotransmitters including serotonin, dopamine and glutamine, so lack of oestrogen, or fluctuating changing levels seen in perimenopause, can have an impact upon mood and cognition.
  - Underlying mental health disorders can be triggered or can worsen. Some women may be at higher risk of mood changes, including those with a history of depression, premenstrual syndromes or postnatal depression.
  - Mental health and cognitive symptoms can affect quality of life and ability to function in relationships, family and work. It is important to recognise, diagnose and appropriately treat perimenopausal/menopausal anxiety and depression.
- Impaired memory and concentration (known as 'brain fog').
  - These symptoms may be linked to changes in oestrogen, VMS, sleep and mood.
  - They can include difficulty recalling words and numbers, misplacing items (such as keys), trouble concentrating, absent-mindedness, losing a train of thought, being easily distracted and forgetting to attend appointments.
- Sleep difficulties and insomnia can affect 40–60% of women.
  - Take a detailed daytime and nighttime history.
  - Consider causes for waking such as VMS, mood changes, restless legs syndrome, sleep disordered breathing, snoring or obstructive sleep apnoea (OSA), and the need to pass urine at night.
- Fatigue.
- Joint and muscle aches.
  - Oestrogen can affect connective tissue metabolism in places such as joints, bone, skin and intervertebral discs. Pain and swelling most often affects the small joints of the hands and feet, but can also affect the cervical spine, knees and elbows.

  - Consider other musculoskeletal causes such as osteoarthritis and rheumatoid arthritis.
  - During the menopausal transition, and with aging, women tend to gain fat mass and lose lean muscle mass (sarcopenia), which can affect their physical functioning.
- Low libido / loss of interest in sex.
  - Sexual desire is complex and can be influenced by many things including life stressors, relationship problems, depression, vaginal dryness, joint pain, bladder problems and tiredness.
  - There may be a change in spontaneous and/or responsive desire. Sensation in the genital tissues can reduce, affecting pleasure and climax.
  - Sexual problems can have a significant effect upon the woman and her relationships, and it is important to approach this sensitively.
- Genitourinary symptoms (see *Section 6.7*).
  - Vulval and vaginal symptoms including dryness or wetness, soreness, burning, itching and dyspareunia.
  - Bladder symptoms including urinary frequency, urgency, stress incontinence and recurrent UTI.
  - These symptoms can present during perimenopause, are more common in postmenopausal women, and tend to progressively worsen over time without appropriate treatment.

6.2.2 Other symptoms reported by women

- Headaches (new-onset or worsening migraine), digestive changes, changes to skin, hair and nails; palpitations; feeling dizzy and faint; increasing allergies; tinnitus; restless legs; oral health changes; weight gain (particularly around the abdomen) and changes in body shape.
- Evidence is increasing that women who are neurodivergent, with attention deficit hyperactivity disorder (ADHD) or autism, may find their symptoms worsen or present for the first time.
- Hormonal fluctuations leading up to and during menopause can have a marked impact on ADHD. Research is limited, but it is thought that the declining oestrogen level can affect levels of neurotransmitters in the brain, including dopamine and serotonin. This can cause worsening of ADHD symptoms such as difficulty with concentration, regulating emotions, organisational skills and memory. Management includes pharmacological treatment for ADHD and/or HRT, psychological therapies and lifestyle advice.

6.2.3 Menopause in ethnic minority women

- Women from different ethnicities and races experience the menopause differently.
- There may be barriers to them seeking help due to different attitudes or beliefs.
- In many minority communities, menopause is not openly discussed, making it harder for women to talk about their symptoms or seek help.
- Women can experience differences in menstrual changes, the age at which menopause occurs, and the type and severity of symptoms. Examples include the following:
  - In South Asian women, the average age of menopause can be up to 4 years earlier than in Western countries, and they may experience more genitourinary symptoms.
  - South-east Asian women may experience more memory problems, joint and muscle pains.
  - Women of African and Caribbean descent may be more likely to experience significant weight gain and mental health problems. Vasomotor symptoms are often more common, longer-lasting, and potentially more severe.
- For further information see the BMS fact sheet *Menopause in ethnic minority women:* https://thebms.org.uk/wp-content/uploads/2023/07/20-BMS-TfC-Menopause-in-ethnic-minority-women-JULY2023-B.pdf

6.3 Diagnosis of perimenopause and menopause

- Diagnosis of perimenopause and menopause involves taking a detailed history (see *Section 6.4*).
- Consider that the use of hormonal therapy (including oral, injectable, or long-acting contraceptives) may conceal or cause amenorrhoea or irregular menstrual cycles.

6.3.1 Women over the age of 45

- The menopause and perimenopause are clinical diagnoses, based on symptoms and changes in bleeding pattern.
- There is no need to do hormonal blood tests in otherwise healthy women who are ≥45 years old if they have menopause-related symptoms to diagnose perimenopause or menopause, unless they present with atypical symptoms. Menopause management in this age group is not altered by an FSH test.
- It may be appropriate to carry out other blood tests relevant to the woman's age; for example, she may be eligible for an NHS health check, including lipids and HbA1c.
- It may also be appropriate to carry out other blood tests if the diagnosis is uncertain; for example, thyroid function tests.

Diagnosis of menopause

- Menopause can be diagnosed in one of the following two categories:
  - Women who have not had a period for at least 1 year and are not using hormonal contraception.
  - Women who are experiencing menopause symptoms and have had a hysterectomy.

Diagnosis of perimenopause (menopause transition)

- As a woman approaches menopause, ovarian function declines and FSH and oestrogen levels can fluctuate wildly, so it is not helpful to test them. Progesterone levels also fluctuate and decline due to less frequent and eventually absent ovulation. The diagnosis of perimenopause is based on menstrual cycle changes ± menopausal symptoms.

CASE: Sonja is 48

Sonja is fit and well but for the last 2 years her periods have changed and become lighter. She has a period every 6–8 weeks now, instead of every 4 weeks, and she has the occasional heavy period. She tells you she has no symptoms of menopause but tells you she doesn't really know much about what the symptoms of menopause are. She is asking for time off work as she feels overwhelmed, anxious and she is finding it hard to concentrate. Her sleep is disturbed, she wakes in the night two or three times feeling anxious. Her joints are starting to become painful. She is struggling with her relationship and is thinking of leaving her husband.

What is the likely reason for these symptoms?

Sonja is in perimenopause; she has changing periods and symptoms (see *Section 6.6*). It is important to remember that many women do not know the symptoms of perimenopause or menopause. They may tell you they have no symptoms, but when you explain the symptoms to them, they may tell you that they are experiencing lots of them. She does not need an FSH test. She is over the age of 45 and due to the fluctuating levels of FSH in perimenopause, it is not a helpful indicator to her menopause status. Sonja can consider lifestyle changes and HRT, and you can discuss all treatment options with her, offering her choice in how her symptoms are managed.

- Symptoms:
  - Hormonal changes during this transition can cause widespread symptoms which can come and go; see *Section 6.2.1*.
- Menstrual cycle changes:
  - Be aware that marked differences occur in the way women's menstrual cycles change during this transition. For most women, menstrual cycles become increasingly variable in length. Short cycles may occur in the early perimenopause, while long cycles are most frequent in the late perimenopause; see *Section 1.6.3*. Around 15–25% of women experience little or no change in menstrual regularity before their final menstrual period, but they may still experience menopausal symptoms.
  - The duration and volume of blood loss can vary. Some women experience heavy, prolonged bleeding, often linked to anovulatory cycles.

6.3.2 Women under the age of 45

- Consider the diagnoses:
  - Perimenopause, as discussed above: this can last for several years before periods finally stop and symptoms are commonly found in women under the age of 45.
    - FSH is not helpful in making the diagnosis, as it can fluctuate wildly.
  - Early menopause:
    - In women aged 40–45 if you are considering a diagnosis of early menopause, measure serum FSH.
    - The BMS advises that early menopause should be diagnosed on the basis of **menopausal symptoms and menstrual disturbance** (oligomenorrhoea or amenorrhoea for more than three months), together with **elevated gonadotropins** (FSH >30IU/L) on **at least two occasions**, measured **4–6 weeks apart**, in women aged **40–45 years**. If the diagnosis remains uncertain, **seek advice from a specialist menopause service**. This condition should be managed in a similar way to POI.
  - Premature ovarian insufficiency (POI):
    - In women <40, if you are considering a diagnosis of POI, measure serum FSH and estradiol.
    - Symptoms of menopause may or may not be present.
    - FSH >25IU/L and oligo-/amenorrhoea for at least 4 months is sufficient to make the diagnosis (FSH concentration >25IU/L represents a value greater than the physiological peak observed in premenopausal women). If there is diagnostic uncertainty the FSH can be repeated after 4–6 weeks. If the diagnosis is inconclusive, seek advice from a specialist menopause service.

CASE: Carolyn is 36

Carolyn has just had a total abdominal hysterectomy and bilateral salpingo-oophorectomy to manage her heavy painful periods and endometriosis. She was not given any treatment after her operation. She is visiting you in general practice to discuss her hot flushes, anxiety and difficulty sleeping.

What is the likely reason for her symptoms?

She has had a surgical menopause (as her ovaries have been removed before she went through menopause.) She has POI, as her ovaries were removed before the age of 40. She should be managed with continuous combined HRT, due to the possibility of remaining endometriosis lesions, unless there are contraindications. This should be continued until at least the average age of menopause, 51 years. HRT will relieve her symptoms and protect her from future health conditions. HRT is recommended to protect her future health, even if she is asymptomatic (see *Section 6.8*).

  - For more details see *Section 6.8*.
- It is important to consider all causes if a woman presents with amenorrhoea or oligomenorrhoea (see *Section 2.6*).

6.3.3 Follicle-stimulating hormone testing

- Testing FSH in perimenopause is not helpful, as FSH levels fluctuate significantly during this time. A normal FSH does not rule out the perimenopause as a cause for symptoms.
- Testing estradiol levels in perimenopause is not helpful or diagnostic of perimenopause. Estradiol levels change throughout the menstrual cycle and fluctuate wildly in perimenopause.
- If testing FSH is required, aim to test day 2–5 of the cycle, if possible. FSH testing for the diagnosis of POI or early menopause does not have to be timed to a specific day in the cycle, as this may lead to a significant delay in diagnosis.
- FSH should not be tested in women >45 years or in women using CHC methods or HRT, because the exogenous hormone suppresses serum FSH and estradiol. The CHC can be stopped for 2–6 weeks and then an FSH can be tested.

6.3.4 Use of serum FSH measurement in assessing requirement for hormonal contraception

- In general all women can stop using contraception at age 55.
- The CoSRH recommends measuring serum FSH only when advising women over the age of 50 who are using progestogen-only contraception and are amenorrhoeic about their menopausal status and when they can stop using contraception.
- A serum FSH >30U/L does not confirm that contraception can be stopped immediately.
  - A woman aged >50 with single serum FSH of >30U/L (even if using progestogen-only contraception) can stop using contraception after 1 more year. If the FSH result is <30U/L she can continue suitable progestogen-only or non-hormonal contraception until age 55. Alternatively, the serum FSH can be repeated after 1 year.

6.3.5 Contraception in perimenopause

- A copper IUD inserted after the age of 40 can be used for contraception until age 55, when contraception is no longer needed. If a woman becomes amenorrhoeic for a year after turning 50 or two years under the age of 50, the Cu-IUD can be removed.
- Women using the POP, IMP or any LNG-IUD can continue using this method until age 55 and then stop. Women using DMPA can continue to use this method until the age of 50 and then usually would swap to another progestogen-only method, and continue this until the age of 55. These progestogen-only contraceptives can be used alongside HRT, but only the 52mg LNG-IUD can be used for endometrial protection as part of HRT (for 5 years after insertion).
- A 52mg LNG-IUD inserted after age 45 can be used solely for contraception until age 55. Ensure that if HRT is started during this time (and the 52mg LNG-IUD is being used for endometrial protection), it is replaced within 5 years of insertion.
- CHC is not generally recommended after age 50 because of the associated risk of VTE. Women aged ≥50 who use the CHC and who wish to continue contraception can switch to the POP, IMP or LNG-IUD or a non-hormonal contraceptive method and continue contraception until age 55 or follow the advice above.
- Eligible women aged <50 could consider using CHC instead of HRT for menopause symptom management as well as contraception. HRT is generally more effective for symptom control and bone protection and has a smaller effect on thrombotic risk (especially if the HRT contains transdermal estradiol). CHC cannot be used alongside HRT.

CASE: Hanna is 43

Hanna has a 52mg LNG-IUD in place, and due to this has had amenorrhoea since it was inserted 3 years ago. Prior to this her periods were regular. She has started to wake at night with drenching night sweats and has hot flushes in the day which cause her great embarrassment at work. She has started to feel low and cannot concentrate on anything. She has lost confidence and has stopped going out with her friends. She is irritable and bursts into tears telling you she cannot stop shouting at her children. She is tired, is gaining weight and has muscle aches and weakness.

What is the likely reason for her symptoms and what can you do to help her?

There are several things to consider. Hanna could be in perimenopause (when hormones are fluctuating wildly) or she could have an early menopause (menopause between 40 and 45 years). She could have another diagnosis alongside this, such as hypothyroidism. She is amenorrhoeic with her 52mg LNG-IUD, and she has developed new symptoms. Performing blood tests would be recommended, including FSH and thyroid function. An FSH can fluctuate in perimenopause, so could be high or normal. A raised FSH could suggest a diagnosis of early menopause.

Whatever the result of her FSH, if she is in perimenopause or early menopause, she can consider a trial of HRT for 3 months to see if it relieves her symptoms, if there are no contraindications. A shared decision-making discussion should take place, including a risk assessment (see *Chapter 7*). Oestrogen, as an oral tablet, patch, gel or spray, can be taken alongside her 52mg LNG-IUD (which must have been fitted within the last 5 years to provide endometrial protection). She should monitor her symptoms and a review should take place after 3 months to see how she is.

6.4 Patient assessment

Tailor your approach to the person and offer individualised care. Ask about her symptoms and their severity and impact on her life at home and at work. An examination is not routinely needed, but you may wish to do this if the history shows any concerning symptoms.

6.4.1 Patient assessment

Symptom history

- Use a validated symptom questionnaire such as the Greene Climacteric Scale, which is a tool used in the UK to assess the severity of menopause symptoms by measuring various aspects such as psychological, physical and vasomotor symptoms (see *Table 6.1*).

Gynaecological / menstrual history

- Bleeding pattern and last menstrual period (LMP) if she has not had a hysterectomy.
- Include genitourinary and sexual symptoms (see *Section 6.4.3*).
- Exclude suspected pathology, such as abnormal uterine bleeding.
- Irregular bleeding during the perimenopause can be caused by endometrial polyps, fibroids, adenomyosis, endometriosis, endometrial hyperplasia or cancer, or vulval, vaginal or cervical lesions.

Past medical history

- This should include: cancer, CVD or risk factors for this, VTE, migraine, epilepsy, thyroid disorder, diabetes, malabsorption problems.
- Include:
  - History of mental health problems including postnatal depression (PND), PMS and PMDD
  - History of trauma.
  - History of ADHD or autism.

Family history

- This should include: cancer, VTE, CVD, dementia.
- Take a family history from both sides of the family. Refer for family history screening, according to guidelines for breast and ovarian cancer.
- Family history of breast cancer: NICE CG 164: *Familial breast cancer: classification, care and managing breast cancer and related risks in people with a family history of breast cancer* advises which women can be managed in primary care and which need referral to secondary care or genetics services.
- 1 in 450 people in the UK carry a *BRCA* gene mutation. This rate is higher in people with Jewish ancestry, particularly those of Ashkenazi Jewish descent. Free *BRCA* gene testing is available for anyone living in England, aged ≥18 with one or more Jewish grandparent.
- Family history of ovarian cancer: NICE NG241: *Ovarian cancer: identifying and managing familial and genetic risk* advises who to refer. Anyone with a first- or second-degree relative with ovarian cancer qualifies for referral to genetics services.
- Lynch syndrome: an inherited condition which causes an increased risk of certain cancers. It is caused by a mutation in one of five different genes. Cancers include colorectal, endometrial, ovarian, upper gastrointestinal, renal, bladder and brain. If this pattern of cancers is present in the patient's relatives, when you take a family history, consider this diagnosis and refer for genetic testing (https://patientinfolibrary.royalmarsden.nhs.uk/lynchsyndrome).

Medication

- Ask about OTC therapies including injectable weight loss drugs, dietary supplements or herbal medicines. Ask patients to take care with supplements and ensure they understand the ingredients.

Complementary and alternative therapies

- Patients may have tried, or are trying therapies including CBT, hypnosis and acupuncture.

Observations

- BP.
- BMI – consider obesity as a risk factor and ask if it is possible to discuss her weight.
- If possible: waist/hip ratio.

Screening

- Discuss importance of attending national screening programmes including breast, cervical and bowel screening.

Contraception

- Does she need/use contraception? (see *Section 6.3.5*)
- History of side-effects with contraceptive hormones in the past.
- Offer advice about this and about sexual health if appropriate.

Lifestyle and social history

- Taking a detailed lifestyle history and giving advice about this is important to help with symptom control.
- Symptoms can be worse in those who suffer obesity or who smoke, for example.
- Working pattern, living arrangements, smoking, alcohol, exercise, diet and stress levels.
- Offer support as needed.

Manage risk factors for long-term health

- Hypertension, lipids, diabetes.
- Long-term implications of menopause include the risk of cardiovascular disease (CVD) and osteoporosis.

Assessment for fragility fracture risk

- See *Section 6.5.4.*

Consider other causes for symptoms

- Investigate as necessary.

Screen for domestic abuse

- Symptoms of menopause can impact on partner relationships, and may lead to changes or escalation in domestic abuse. More information can be found in this article: *Menopause and Domestic Abuse: brief guidance for staff and clinicians in general practice* (https://irisi.org/wp-content/uploads/2022/02/Menopause-and-Domestic-Abuse-Brief-Guidance-for-Staff-and-Clinicians-in-General-Practice.pdf).

6.4.2 Example of a symptom questionnaire chart

Table 6.1 provides an example of a chart you can give to patients to assess their symptoms.

Table 6.1: Patient menopause symptom chart

Symptom	Yes	No	Details
Changes to periods (heavier, lighter, closer together or further apart, bleeding in between periods)			
Hot flushes			
Night sweats			
Anxiety			
Low mood			
Irritability			
More emotional / mood swings			
Lack of motivation			
Loss of feeling of joy			
Reduced confidence			
Brain fog			
Poor memory			
Difficulty concentrating			
Fatigue/tiredness			
Difficulty sleeping – either getting to sleep or waking in the night. Do you snore or have restless legs?			
Headaches / migraine attacks			
Heart palpitations			
Joint or muscle pain			
Vulval and vaginal symptoms (e.g. soreness, dryness, pain, burning, skin thinning or splitting, labia shrinking, clitoral shrinking, watery discharge, pain during sex, bleeding after sex) *The vulva is not the same as the vagina. The vulva is what you see on the outside of the female genitalia between the legs. It includes the labia (lips), clitoris and the area which can grow pubic hair. The vagina is on the inside, the tube leading from the genitals on the outside to the cervix of the uterus (womb) in women.*			

Table 6.1 *cont'd*

Symptom	Yes	No	Details
Bladder symptoms (increased frequency of passing urine, urine infections, urge to pass urine, leaking urine on the way to the loo (urge incontinence) or when coughing, sneezing or jumping (stress incontinence))			
Loss of sex drive			
Skin, hair and nail changes (dry itchy skin, dry eyes, brittle nails, dry thinning hair)			
Worsening PMS			
Oral health changes, e.g. dry mouth and burning tongue			
Weight gain and change in body shape			
Tinnitus (ringing in the ears)			
Increasing or new-onset allergies			
Digestive issues, e.g. bloating, wind, constipation or indigestion *Seek medical advice if you have changing bowel habit, bleeding from the bottom, abdominal pain, bloating, weight loss and tiredness*			

6.4.3 Assessment of symptoms of genitourinary syndrome of the menopause

- Up to 80% of women suffer with some genitourinary symptoms. Some women feel uncomfortable discussing these symptoms. To help facilitate a conversation, *Box 6.1* provides example questions.
- Consider an examination if there are any concerns in the history, or if the condition is not responding to treatment.
- When examining, ensure you look carefully at the vulva, including the mons pubis, the labia, the entrance to the vagina, the perineum, the anus and back to the natal cleft. This may be best done with the patient in the left lateral position.
- Consider other causes for symptoms, such as lichen sclerosis and lichen planus or a serious cause like a malignancy.
- See *Section 6.7* for guidance about managing GSM.

BOX 6.1: Questions to ask in assessment of symptoms of genitourinary syndrome of the menopause (GSM)

"Does it feel different around your vulva or vaginal area?"

"Have you noticed vaginal dryness or a change in vaginal discharge?"

"Have you experienced any vulval or vaginal itching, soreness, burning or irritation?"

"Is sexual intercourse painful or uncomfortable? Do you bleed after intercourse?"

"Have you lost pleasure, or the ability to orgasm as easily as before?"

"Have you noticed any symptoms such as increased urinary frequency, needing to pass urine at night, or suddenly feeling a need to pass urine?"

"Do you have any discomfort on passing urine?"

"Do you have a history of urine infections?"

6.5 Future health discussion

The menopause is an opportunity to consider conditions which can affect women as they age, and conditions which may affect their future health. Discussions can include metabolic health and risk of cardiovascular disease.

6.5.1 Metabolic health

- Metabolic syndrome is a cluster of common abnormalities, including:
  - Insulin resistance and impaired glucose tolerance.
  - Central obesity.
  - Reduced high-density lipoprotein (HDL) cholesterol levels.
  - Elevated triglycerides.
  - Hypertension.
- According to the new International Diabetes Federation (IDF) definition, for a person to be defined as having the metabolic syndrome, they must have:
  - Central obesity (waist circumference in females ≥80cm) plus any two of the following four factors:
    - Fasting glucose >5.6mmol/L (or previously diagnosed with type 2 diabetes).
    - Reduced HDL <1.29mmol/L (or on a specific treatment for this abnormality).
    - Raised triglycerides >1.7mmol/L (or on a specific treatment for this abnormality).
    - Raised blood pressure BP ≥130/85mmHg (or previously diagnosed hypertension).
  - Note that if BMI is >30kg/m^2, central obesity can be assumed, and waist circumference does not need to be measured.
- Having metabolic syndrome increases the risk of developing cardiovascular disease and diabetes.
- The menopause induces adverse changes in many metabolic factors and is associated with:
  - Vascular changes include increased arterial stiffness, endothelial dysfunction and progression of subclinical atherosclerosis.
  - Weight gain, a change in body composition, increasing fat mass and loss of lean mass. Through midlife, women tend to gain on average around 0.5kg per year, but evidence shows that going through the menopause does not cause women to gain weight. The way fat is deposited in the body changes at the menopause. Oestrogen levels fall, there is a less pronounced decrease in androgen levels (an increase in androgen-to-oestrogen ratio), and simultaneous age-related fall in SHBG, which results in an increase in available androgens. Whether women gain weight or not, they experience a shift in their fat stores to their abdomen. Postmenopausal women have an increase in fat mass, a reduction in lean mass (including muscle) and an increase in visceral and subcutaneous abdominal fat mass. Central obesity is linked with chronic tissue inflammation, which results in oxidative stress and insulin resistance.
  - Increased insulin resistance.
  - The development of a pro-atherogenic lipid profile (increase in total cholesterol, LDL-C, triglycerides and apolipoprotein B levels; a decrease in the quality and anti-atherogenic function of HDL).
- These metabolic changes can increase the risk of cardiovascular disease and diabetes.

6.5.2 Coronary heart disease

- Cardiovascular disease is the leading cause of death and accounts for almost 50% of all deaths in women worldwide.
- In people with metabolic syndrome, prevention of coronary heart disease (CHD) is based on management of established cardiovascular risk factors through:
  - Lifestyle measures (stopping smoking, reducing obesity, eating a healthy diet and doing regular exercise).

CASE: Jill is 53

Jill has come to see you to talk about symptoms of menopause. Her last period was 18 months ago, and she has recently been experiencing vasomotor symptoms, emotional and cognitive symptoms which are affecting her quality of life, ability to sleep and work. She has always been fit and well. She has a family history of cardiovascular disease. She has gained 6kg in the last 2 years, her BMI is now 35, and her body shape is changing, with an increasing waist circumference of 104cm. You arrange some blood tests and her HbA1c is 43mmol/L, she is prediabetic; her lipid profile shows a triglyceride level of 2.8mmol/L and an HDL of 0.9mmol/L. Her home average BP is raised at 141/91mmHg.You discuss the options for managing her menopause symptoms and consider her metabolic health.

Jill fits the criteria to diagnose metabolic syndrome. You can discuss her menopause symptoms and options for managing these. It is also important to discuss her metabolic health and assess her risk of cardiovascular disease. Offer advice about weight management, healthy lifestyle choices and pharmacotherapy (including antihypertensives and, if appropriate, lipid-lowering therapy). If she takes HRT, this can be individualised to her. Oestrogen taken transdermally and a non-androgenic progestogen would be preferred, as they will not have an adverse effect on her metabolic health. For more information about this see *Chapter 7.*

   - Managing lipids, BP, diabetic control and obesity, which also contribute to increasing cardiovascular risk.
- Certain HRT regimes can positively influence metabolic health, improving lipid profiles and insulin sensitivity, depending on the route of oestrogen administration and the type of progestogen prescribed (see *Chapter 7*).

6.5.3 Osteoporosis

- Osteoporosis is a disease which occurs because there is an imbalance in the normal process of bone remodelling by osteoclasts (break down old or damaged bone tissue, also called bone resorption) and osteoblasts (create new bone tissue).
- With aging and particularly after menopause, bone breakdown by osteoclasts increases and is not balanced by new bone formation by osteoblasts. This results in a fall in bone mineral density (BMD) and a change in the composition, architecture and size of the bone.
- Osteoporosis is characterised by low bone mass and a structural deterioration of the bone tissue. Because of this, bones become fragile and are at risk of fracture.
- The prevalence of osteoporosis increases with age, from 21.9% of women aged 50 or over to nearly 50% at 80 years of age.
- Women are at greater risk of osteoporosis, due to the loss of oestrogen at menopause, which accelerates bone loss. Oestrogens are important for maintaining BMD. Oestrogen has an effect on osteocytes, osteoclasts and osteoblasts, leading to inhibition of bone remodelling, decreased bone resorption and maintenance of bone formation. A major consequence of loss of oestrogen at menopause is an increase in bone resorption and a fall in bone density.
- Bone loss leading to osteoporosis begins before the menopause. A period of accelerated bone loss starts 1–3 years before the final menstrual period. This fast bone loss continues for 5–10 years and then the rate of bone loss slows to 0.5% per year. By age 80 women have lost 30% of peak bone mass; this loss is accompanied by a reduction in bone quality and strength.
- Compared with people with normal bone density, those with osteoporosis and osteopenia are at increased risk of fragility fractures, which result from a fall from standing height, or a spontaneous vertebral fracture. Most commonly, they occur at the spine, hip, distal radius and proximal humerus. 50% of women over the age of 50 will suffer from at least one osteoporotic fracture during their lifetime.

- Women who experience menopause at an earlier age have a longer duration of oestrogen deficiency, resulting in lower bone density after menopause, which can increase their risk of fracture.

6.5.4 Assessment of fragility fracture risk

When to assess risk of fragility fracture?

There is no screening programme in the UK for osteoporosis. Targeted case finding is used, assessing people with clinical risk factors. In April 2025, NICE CKS revised its guidelines on osteoporosis; it now advises to consider assessing risk of fragility fracture in all women aged ≥65, and in all women aged under 65 who have these risk factors:

- A previous osteoporotic fragility fracture.
- Smoking.
- Drinking alcohol >14 units per week.
- Family history of hip fracture.
- Low BMI <18.5kg/m^2 (low body weight is a significant risk factor).
- History of falls.
- Current or frequent use of oral corticosteroids.
- A secondary cause of osteoporosis, including:
  - Untreated POI; treatment with aromatase inhibitors or GnRH agonists.
  - Endocrine disorders including diabetes mellitus, Cushing's disease, hyperthyroidism, hyperparathyroidism and hyperprolactinaemia.
  - Conditions associated with malabsorption such as inflammatory bowel disorder, coeliac disease and chronic pancreatitis.
  - Inflammatory arthropathies such as rheumatoid arthritis.
  - Haematological conditions such as multiple myeloma.
  - Chronic obstructive pulmonary disease; chronic liver failure; chronic kidney disease and immobility.
- Consider assessing fracture risk in those using medication such as SSRIs, proton pump inhibitors, anti-epileptic medication, particularly enzyme-inducing drugs such as carbamazepine, thiazolidinediones such as pioglitazone, especially if there are other risk factors as stated above.

There is no need to assess fracture risk in women aged <50 unless they have these major risk factors:

- Current or frequent use of oral corticosteroids.
- Untreated premature menopause.
- A previous fragility fracture.

How to calculate fragility fracture risk

- 10-year fragility fracture risk can be calculated by using an online risk calculator such as the fracture risk assessment tool (FRAX) algorithm. The output is a 10-year probability of hip fracture and the 10-year probability of a major osteoporotic fracture (spine, forearm, hip or shoulder fracture).
- FRAX integrates clinical risk factors for fracture with or without BMD scores at the femoral neck to calculate a 10-year fracture probability.
  - It can be used to help assess the need for BMD testing or pharmacological treatment.
  - The limitations of FRAX include the inability to input information such as specific amounts, duration of use, or dosage of alcohol, smoking or corticosteroids, fall history, number of prior fractures or spinal BMD, which may lead to an underestimation in these patients. FRAXplus is an optional extension of the FRAX tool, used to refine fracture risk assessments by incorporating extra factors such as number of prior fractures and number of falls in the previous year.

  - The FRAX tool links the individual result to the UK National Osteoporosis Guidelines Group (NOGG), which shows a coloured chart explaining recommended intervention thresholds. These are:
    - very high risk: consider specialist referral and treat
    - high risk: treat
    - intermediate risk: measure BMD
    - low risk: give lifestyle advice.
- Women at intermediate risk, near the threshold level (but who have an extra risk that may be underestimated by FRAX, such as high alcohol intake) – consider offering a bone density scan.
- Women with low risk should not be offered a DEXA scan but should be offered lifestyle advice.
- BMD is measured using a dual-energy X-ray absorptiometry (DEXA) scan. It compares the result to that of a young healthy adult of the same sex. The difference is calculated as acstandard deviation (SD) and is called a T-score. A T-score of:
  - above –1 SD is normal
  - between –1 and –2.5 SD shows bone loss and is defined as osteopenia
  - below –2.5 SD shows bone loss and is defined as osteoporosis.
- BMD measurement reflects bone mineral content but does not capture changes in bone microarchitecture or structural integrity that contribute to fracture risk.
- Osteopenia is common (global prevalence is 40.4% compared with osteoporosis at 19.7%). Although the relative risk of fracture is lower in those with osteopenia compared with osteoporosis, the absolute number of fractures is higher among those with osteopenia, due to its greater prevalence. Risk of fracture is determined by a combination of BMD and relevant risk factors. Relying only on BMD might underestimate risk of fracture, especially in those with a T score of above –2.5, and may result in under-treatment of high-risk individuals.

For more detailed advice refer to the NICE guidance: https://cks.nice.org.uk/topics/osteoporosis-prevention-of-fragility-fractures/management/assessment/#interpretation-of-fracture-risk-scores

When to offer a DEXA scan without calculating fracture risk

Offer a DEXA scan to measure BMD, without calculating the fragility fracture risk in women:

- Over 50 years with a history of fragility fracture.
- Younger than 40 who have a major risk factor for fragility fracture, depending upon their BMD T-score (and refer to osteoporosis specialist). BMD alone is a weak predictor of fracture risk if other clinical risk factors are not taken into account.

Advice and treatment options

- The Royal Osteoporosis Society (www.theros.org.uk) is a good source of information for patients, including information about bone health, osteopenia and osteoporosis. It provides information for patients on assessing their dietary calcium intake and vitamin D, and it provides examples of weight-bearing exercises to support bone health.
  - The NOGG recommends intake of ≥700mg/day of calcium for all adults – preferably from dietary sources such as low-fat dairy products, green vegetables, nuts and fortified foods, and ≥800IU/day of vitamin D in those who are at risk of vitamin D insufficiency.
  - If there are no contraindications (such as hypercalcaemia, metastatic calcification, end-stage chronic kidney disease or severe liver disease) an appropriate product of vitamin D can be taken. NICE CKS: *Vitamin D supplements* discusses available preparations, particularly for those with specific dietary requirements (such as those who are vegetarian, vegan or have a peanut allergy), contraindications, cautions and possible drug interactions with vitamin D.

  - Lifestyle advice should include a tailored exercise programme with a combination of exercises, for example balance, flexibility, stretching, endurance and progressive strength exercises; a healthy balanced diet, stopping smoking and drinking alcohol within recommended limits.
- HRT has been shown to prevent bone loss and fragility fractures in postmenopausal women, irrespective of their BMD and their other risk factors. BMD loss is rapid after discontinuation of HRT, and within 2 years reduces to the level of not having taken oestrogen. Changing to other treatments such as bisphosphonates is an option.
- The BMS states that: *"HRT should be considered the first-line therapeutic intervention for the prevention and treatment of osteoporosis in women with premature ovarian insufficiency (POI) and menopausal women below 60 years of age, particularly those with menopausal symptoms."*
- NICE guidance advises to consider prescribing HRT to younger postmenopausal women at high risk of osteoporotic fracture, to reduce the risk of fragility fracture and for relief of menopause symptoms.
- Other treatments are available, including anti-remodelling and antiresorptive drugs, and osteoanabolic agents.

CASE: Emma is 52

Emma is coming to see you to as she has heard about bone health on a podcast and wonders if she might have osteoporosis. Her periods stopped when she was 43; she had no symptoms of menopause, so she didn't see a doctor and did not take HRT. She tells you she is smoking 15 cigarettes a day. She has not had a fragility fracture and there are no other risk factors in her history for osteoporosis.

How should you manage her?

She is 52 and has two risk factors for osteoporosis. She had an untreated early menopause (did not have HRT or CHC), and she smokes. You should assess her fracture risk using an online risk calculator and act on the result of this, according to the NOGG advice linked to her FRAX assessment score. Advise her about lifestyle risk factors, to stop smoking and guide her to the Royal Osteoporosis Society (https://theros.org.uk) for advice about dietary calcium, vitamin D and exercise for bones.

6.5.5 Dementia

- Dementia is a term used to describe a range of cognitive and behavioural symptoms including memory loss, problems with reasoning and communication, a change in personality and a reduction in the ability to carry out daily activities. It is a progressive condition and symptoms gradually worsen over time.
- Cognitive symptoms commonly start in the perimenopause and are often described as brain fog, word-finding difficulty or reduce concentration. They should not be confused with dementia. Young-onset dementia (dementia before age 65) is rare, affecting about 2 per 1000 people.
- Conditions which can present with cognitive impairment include:
  - Normal age-related memory changes.
  - Mild cognitive impairment (MCI).
  - Depression.
  - Delirium (sometimes called an acute confusional state).
  - Vitamin deficiency (thiamine and vitamin B12).
  - Hypothyroidism.
  - Adverse drug effects such as opiates, benzodiazepines, NSAIDs; corticosteroids, drugs with anticholinergic adverse effects such as those used to treat overactive bladder, tricyclic antidepressants, antipsychotics and antiepileptics.
- Refer to the NICE guidance: https://cks.nice.org.uk/topics/dementia.

Cognitive symptoms in perimenopause and menopause

- Cognitive difficulties at menopause are often called 'brain fog' and may include difficulty recalling words or numbers, everyday memory lapses such as misplacing items, reduced concentration with increased distractibility or losing a train of thought, and forgetting appointments or events. They can significantly affect quality of life for some women, and 11–13% of women show a clinically significant impairment.
- These difficulties with learning and verbal memory are linked to changes in estradiol, vasomotor symptoms, sleep and mood. Treating these may improve cognition, although more research is needed to confirm this.
- The memory difficulties resolve for many women, but for some they persist post menopause.
- Address modifiable risk factors which are linked to better cognitive health: obesity, hypertension, diabetes, exercise, smoking, alcohol, sleep, cognitive activity, social interaction, hearing impairment and depression.

Women may ask questions about the use of HRT:

- *"Will taking HRT improve my brain fog and memory?"*
  - The impact of HRT on cognitive abilities is uncertain. There is lack of evidence about the effect of HRT on cognition in women with bothersome VMS and in women in perimenopause. HRT is not prescribed for brain fog alone but can be effective (in some women) for improving this symptom alongside their other menopause symptoms.
- *"Will taking HRT change my risk of developing dementia?"*
  - The BMS states that "*Women should be reassured that HRT is unlikely to increase the risk of dementia or to have a detrimental effect on cognitive function in women initiating HRT before the age of 60.*"
  - Currently HRT is not recommended at any age to treat cognitive symptoms at menopause or to prevent cognitive decline or dementia.
  - More research is needed about the effects of HRT on dementia risk.
- For more information refer to the discussion aid on HRT:
  - www.nice.org.uk/guidance/ng23/resources/incidence-of-medical-conditions-with-and-without-hrt-a-discussion-aid-pdf-13553199901
  - www.imsociety.org/wp-content/uploads/2022/10/IMS-White-Paper-2022-Brain-fog-in-menopause.pdf

CASE: Zara is 49

Zara is perimenopausal and is really struggling at work. She has started to have difficulty recalling words and maintaining concentration, and has developed brain fog. She is woken every 2–3 hours by night sweats and has been drinking alcohol every night to help her get off to sleep. She has no family history of dementia; she is otherwise in good health and takes no medications or supplements. Her vitamin B12, folate and thyroid function are normal.

She wonders if she has early dementia and asks if taking HRT will improve her brain fog.

You can advise Zara that it is common for women to experience cognitive symptoms as they transition through menopause. As the cognitive difficulties at midlife are linked to changes in oestrogen, vasomotor symptoms, sleep and mood, treating these symptoms may improve her cognition.

To answer her question if HRT will improve her brain fog, you can advise her that there is currently no evidence to support this directly in women in perimenopause. Taking HRT may improve vasomotor symptoms and sleep and mood. This could mean she reduces her alcohol intake. The overall result could be an improvement in her cognition. You can reassure her that her cognition is likely to improve over time, and give her advice about the importance of healthy lifestyle choices.

6.6 Management options for perimenopause and menopause

Explain about the stages and consequences of the menopause, including symptoms such as flushes and sweats, psychological symptoms, musculoskeletal, vaginal, bladder and sexual effects, as well as long-term effects on bone and cardiovascular health.

NICE guidance and the BMS consensus statements offer detailed guidance, and this is a summary of some of the points to consider:

- Discuss the benefits and risks associated with each of the options for managing the patient's symptoms.
- Offer appropriate written advice to the person, their family and carers.
- Discuss the need for effective contraception during the perimenopause.
- Give advice on protecting bone health.
- Explain the importance of maintaining muscle mass and strength using physical activity.
- Offer information and support to women who are about to undergo a treatment (medical or surgical) which may lead to menopause, so they understand what to expect and what treatment options are possible for them.
- Offer psychological support, including referral to psychology services, to women who are experiencing menopause under the age of 45 and are distressed by their diagnosis or its consequences.

6.6.1 Lifestyle

- A healthy lifestyle – including taking regular exercise, eating a balanced healthy diet, managing stress, reducing alcohol intake and stopping smoking – can improve menopausal symptoms as well as improving bone and heart health.
- Take a holistic approach, educating women during the menopause transition, discussing modifiable lifestyle factors for symptom improvement and healthy aging.
- Give advice about how lifestyle choices can affect future health conditions including bone health, cardiovascular and metabolic health.
- Advice can include:
  - There is not one diet or way of eating that is right for everyone, but it is important to educate women about core nutrition principles, including the roles of macronutrients (carbohydrate, fat and protein), fibre, vitamins, minerals, and adequate hydration for optimal health and symptom management.
  - The Mediterranean diet offers numerous health benefits.
  - A 'food first' approach focuses on meeting nutritional needs through diet rather than supplements, except when supplementation is required to treat a deficiency.
  - Dietary calcium: advise 700–1000mg daily (calcium calculator: https://theros.org.uk/information-and-support/bone-health/nutrition-for-bones/calcium/calcium-rich-food-chooser).
  - Vitamin D: adequate vitamin D is important so advise about safe sunlight exposure and consider taking a daily supplement (see *Section 6.5.3*).
  - Give advice about gut health.
  - Exercise is the single greatest health intervention.
    - As well as the recommended minimum of 150 minutes of moderate-intensity activity per week, a combination of exercises such as balance, flexibility, stretching, endurance and progressive strengthening is important.
    - Exercise improves insulin resistance, by increasing glucose uptake in skeletal muscles.
    - From the age of 30 women start to lose skeletal muscle mass. This accelerates during perimenopause, leading to sarcopenia.
    - Encourage women to practise exercises to improve balance, to reduce risk of falls.

        - Recommend daily pelvic floor exercises, to protect from prolapse.
            - Squeezy app
            - https://thepogp.co.uk
    - Smoking carries significant health risks and has been shown to trigger vasomotor symptoms and increase risk of osteoporosis, cancer and CVD.
    - Alcohol can increase vasomotor symptoms and affect sleep and mood, and is associated with an increased risk of breast cancer. To minimise health risks, alcohol intake should not exceed 14 units per week. It is safest to spread this evenly and to have several alcohol-free days per week.
    - Stress can worsen menopause symptoms such as vasomotor symptoms and anxiety. Time in nature, and relaxation techniques such as meditation and yoga can reduce stress levels.
    - Try to limit caffeine to 1–2 cups of tea/coffee per day, ideally before midday as it can be associated with anxiety and can affect ability to sleep.
    - Sleep is critical for good health.
        - Sleep deprivation can contribute to brain fog, weight gain and depression. It can have an impact on mental health, cardiovascular health, metabolic health, immune function and bone health.
        - 40–60% of women report midlife sleep disturbance.
        - Advice can include recommending a consistent time of rising 7 days a week, seeing sunlight as soon as possible in the morning, reducing stress and avoiding alcohol.
        - Diagnose insomnia if (even with adequate opportunity to sleep) there is difficulty initiating or maintaining sleep, or early morning awakening, dissatisfaction with sleep resulting in impairment in functioning or wellbeing, or significant distress, which occurs for at least 3 nights a week and for at least 3 months.
        - Consider restless legs syndrome and sleep-disordered breathing, including OSA, as a cause for poor sleep.
        - Treatments are summarised in the BMS Tool for Clinicians: *Managing sleep disturbance during the menopause transition*, and include CBT for insomnia; HRT; non-hormonal treatments; management of restless legs syndrome and sleep-disordered breathing; use of daridorexant and modified-release melatonin. Refer to: https://thebms.org.uk/wp-content/uploads/2025/08/25-NEW-BMS-ToolsforClinicians-Managing-sleep-disturbance-AUGUST2025-A.pdf.
    - For some women the hormonal changes can affect their mental health and close relationships with family and friends, and leave them feeing isolated. Offer advice about supportive relationships and ways to support mental health.
    - Refer women to the Women's Health Concern Menopause Wellness hub (www.womens-health-concern.org/help-and-advice/menopause-wellness-hub).

6.6.2 Hormone replacement therapy

- HRT, also known as menopause hormone therapy (MHT), is the replacement of one or more of the female sex hormones oestrogen, progesterone and testosterone, and it is given to relieve the symptoms of perimenopause and menopause (it is covered in detail in *Chapter* 7).
- As well as being the most effective treatment for managing symptoms of perimenopause and menopause, HRT has some other benefits. It lowers fracture risk and improves bone density, with evidence suggesting cardiovascular benefit when started in healthy women in early or midlife.
- For most healthy women below the age of 60, the benefits of HRT to improve their menopausal symptoms outweigh any risks to them.
- Advise women in England about the HRT prescription prepayment certificate (HRT PPC). It covers all eligible HRT prescriptions, for a set fee each year, no matter how many different medicines they need: www.gov.uk/get-a-ppc/hrt-ppc.

6.6.3 Combined hormonal contraception

- In perimenopause, the goals of treatment are symptom control, cycle control and contraception (if required).
- CHC can be considered in eligible women under 50 years as an alternative to HRT for relief of menopausal symptoms.
- CHC can help manage PMS (which can worsen in perimenopause as hormones fluctuate wildly – ovarian suppression can be helpful), relieve vasomotor symptoms, provide contraception, and regulate menstrual cycles, and may be considered for eligible women in line with UKMEC guidance. It can be tailored, by omitting the HFI, off-licence.
- A low-dose ethinylestradiol pill (20mcg) is preferred, although a 30mcg pill may be used if necessary. Newer combined contraceptive pills containing estradiol or estetrol instead of ethinylestradiol can also be considered and may be preferable. Estradiol has a neutral effect on BP, while estetrol offers a more favourable lipid profile. Refer to UKMEC for guidance.
- CHC methods cannot be used alongside HRT.

6.6.4 Progestogen-only contraception

- All progestogen-only methods of contraception are safe to use alongside HRT.
  - POP, IMP, DMPA and 13.5mg/19.5mg LNG-IUDs are not licensed for endometrial protection as the progestogen part of HRT, but can be used alongside HRT to provide contraception; refer to *Section 3.2.18*.
- Any 52mg LNG-IUD provides effective contraception, suppresses the endometrium, and is a good option for managing heavy bleeding. It offers endometrial protection for up to 5 years and can be combined with oral or transdermal oestrogen as part of a systemic HRT regime.
- With use of a POP, it is important to note that:
  - There is lack of evidence for the use of desogestrel 75mcg as the progestogen part of HRT. If desogestrel 75mcg is used as a contraceptive in women who take HRT, a progestogen such as micronised progesterone 100mg daily, or 200mg for 12–14 days a month should be taken alongside it, to provide endometrial protection.
  - The BMS practical guide *HRT preparations and equivalent alternatives* states use of 150mcg desogestrel (two 75mcg tablets daily), off-licence, is effective as the progestogen component of HRT, with no increase in risk of endometrial hyperplasia.
  - This guide also states that drospirenone 4mg (Slynd) can be used, off-licence, daily as an alternative for women who have side-effects with other HRT preparations. One active hormonal tablet can be taken daily and the four hormone-free (placebo) pills in each pack can be discarded.
  - Refer to https://thebms.org.uk/wp-content/uploads/2024/02/15-BMS-TfC-HRT-preparations-and-equivalent-alternatives-JAN2024-B.pdf (page 3).

6.6.5 Unregulated hormonal preparations

The efficacy and safety of unregulated hormone preparations such as 'compounded bioidentical hormone replacement therapy' is unknown, so it is not recommended by NICE or the BMS (see *Section 7.3*).

6.6.6 Cognitive behavioural therapy

- There is evidence supporting CBT for improving hot flushes, night sweats, low mood, anxiety and sleep.
- CBT for insomnia (CBTi) is a well-researched and effective treatment for insomnia. CBT can take place in groups, individually, online or using self-help books or guides, or apps.

- The Women's Health Concern fact sheet, prepared by Professor Myra Hunter, provides guidance on CBT in a self-help format for women to access directly: www.womens-health-concern.org/wp-content/uploads/2023/02/02-WHC-FACTSHEET-CBT-WOMEN-FEB-2023-A.pdf
- Other resources include:
  - Sleep station: www.sleepstation.org.uk
  - Sleepful: https://sleepful.org.uk
  - The Sleepio app.

6.6.7 Non-hormonal prescribable medications for the relief of vasomotor symptoms

- Some women choose not to take HRT, or are not able to. They can consider some non-hormonal prescribable medications which can help to manage vasomotor symptoms.
- These types of medication offer women choice of different ways to manage their symptoms and significantly improve quality of life.
- Prescribable non-hormonal therapies at specific doses which have been shown to be effective to relieve vasomotor symptoms include some antidepressants, clonidine, oxybutynin, gabapentin and pregabalin (off-licence). For further information about how to prescribe and doses required, refer to: https://thebms.org.uk/wp-content/uploads/2022/12/02-BMS-TfC-Prescribable-alternatives-to-HRT-NOV2022-A.pdf.
- Care is needed when prescribing in women who take tamoxifen, as sertraline and duloxetine (at moderate–high doses), paroxetine and fluoxetine can reduce tamoxifen efficacy.
- *Table 6.2* shows some examples of alternative medications which can be used to relieve vasomotor symptoms, and which may have an impact on mood and wellbeing. Always counsel about possible side-effects.
- SSRIs/SNRIs can cause nausea, dizziness and insomnia, and worsen anxiety/mood in the short term (6 weeks). It can take 8 weeks for side-effects to settle and to see improvement. Reduced libido and sexual response can be a long-term side-effect for some people.

Table 6.2: *Some examples of prescribable alternatives to HRT*

Venlafaxine	Dosage 37.5–150mg/day; start with the lowest dose and titrate upwards Effective at reducing hot flush frequency by up to 65%; beneficial for VMS, low mood and anxiety No interaction with cytochrome P450, so may be safest choice for patients on tamoxifen Counsel for SSRI/SNRI side-effects To improve tolerability, slowly titrate the dose and take in the morning with food
Citalopram	Start at 5mg and slowly increase the dose every 2–4 weeks, if needed, up to 20mg; a dose of 20mg can reduce flushes by 40% Beneficial for VSM, low mood and anxiety Much less effect on cytochrome P450 so can be used in patients on tamoxifen Counsel for SSRI/SNRI side-effects; this drug has the lowest reported impact on sexual dysfunction of this class of drug
Oxybutynin	Dose: 2.5–5mg at night Can be used in women taking tamoxifen or an aromatase inhibitor Beneficial for VSM and bladder symptoms, and can reduce hot flush frequency by 60–77% Side-effects can include dry mouth, difficulty urinating and abdominal pain Care is needed in older women, increased risk of falls and can be associated with cognitive impairment; review to check for side-effects

Adapted from BMS (2022) *Prescribable alternatives to HRT* and Mullin, S. and Manley, K. (2025) Menopause care: alternatives to hormone replacement therapy. *TOG*, 27(4): 308–20.

- Advise about licensing, drug interactions and possible side-effects when prescribing these medications. With all antidepressants, advise that one of the potential side-effects is an effect on libido and ability to climax, which may not improve after the drug is stopped.
- Neurokinin antagonist medication influences changes in brain neurotransmitters which regulate the underlying process of vasomotor symptoms. These treatments are effective and work within days of initiation, reducing hot flush frequency by 70% at 12 weeks. Examples include:
  - Fezolinetant is a neurokinin-3 (NK-3) receptor antagonist. It was approved by the MHRA to manage vasomotor symptoms in December 2023, and it is currently available on private prescription.
    - Fezolinetant has been linked to a risk of drug-induced liver injury. To reduce this risk, new guidelines recommend monitoring liver function both before starting treatment and throughout its duration. The medication should be avoided in individuals with known liver disease or at high risk of liver disease.
    - These are the recommendations for monitoring LFTs if this medication is used: https://thebms.org.uk/wp-content/uploads/_pda/2025/01/Letter-from-Astellas-re-Veoza-fezolinetant-January-2025.pdf.
  - Elinzanetant is a dual neurokinin-1,3 (NK-1,3) receptor antagonist. It was approved by the MHRA in July 2025 to treat moderate–severe vasomotor symptoms caused by menopause and is currently available on private prescription.
  - Trials are currently ongoing looking at safety of these medications in women with a history of breast cancer.

6.6.8 Complementary and alternative therapies

- Complementary and alternative medicine (CAM) and practices (CAP) refer to a range of preparations and practices that are not considered part of conventional medicine but may be used alongside it or as an alternative.
- CAM includes mainly products derived from plants, such as phytoestrogens (including isoflavones and lignans), herbs or minerals. Examples include black cohosh, St John's wort, Chinese herbal medicine and evening primrose oil). Evidence has shown that about 50% of women use CAM to relieve menopause symptoms. CAPs include CBT, clinical hypnosis, mindfulness-based stress reduction, yoga, acupuncture and homeopathy.
- Most studies on complementary medicines and practices are limited by small sample sizes and study design, making their findings inconclusive. There is evidence of benefit for VMS for isoflavones, red clover, CBT and clinical hypnosis.
- Evidence for practices such as yoga is limited, with possibly mild effects on VMS; however, this activity is safe and is likely to contribute positively to a woman's overall wellbeing.
- Refer women to the Women's Health Concern fact sheets on complementary and alternative therapies: www.womens-health-concern.org/wp-content/uploads/2024/11/03-WHC-FACTSHEET-Complementary-And-Alternative-Therapies-NOV2024-B.pdf.

Herbal medicine

- It is important to be aware of herbal treatments, and ask about them, as patients may be taking them.
- Herbal medicines are those with active ingredients made from plant parts.
- Evidence from clinical trials of benefit on menopausal symptoms is limited and conflicting. Different products are not chemically consistent, so comparison between studies is difficult. Herbs may contain many different chemical compounds whose individual and combined effects are unclear.
- If women are buying a herbal medicine they should look for a traditional herbal registration (THR) on the product packaging. This means the medicine complies with the quality standards

relating to safety and manufacturing, and provides information about how and when to use it. However, this doesn't mean the product is completely safe for everyone to use.

- Advise women who wish to have an individualised approach, to consult a qualified medical herbalist, who can provide professional advice about use of herbal medicine.
  - Treatments they provide can include liquid extracts and tinctures, requiring small, individualised doses.
  - Examples of herbs used by medical herbalists include sage, black cohosh and wild yam for night sweats; chaste tree berry for PMS symptoms; shatavari for hot flushes and vaginal dryness; blue skull cap for anxiety, valerian and passionflower for insomnia, St John's wort and rose for anxiety, rage and mood swings.
  - Examples of adaptogens used by medical herbalists (help the body adapt to stress) they may consider include ashwagandha to calm and promote healthy sleep, and rhodiola to improve energy, mood and cognitive function.
- Advise that some herbs may interact with medications and need to be taken with guidance if you have medical conditions such as high BP, diabetes, a thyroid condition or a history of hormone-sensitive cancer, for example.
- Black cohosh may relieve vasomotor symptoms associated with menopause, but advise that it can interact with medications, multiple preparations are available, and safety is uncertain. There is an association with use of black cohosh and liver toxicity.
- St John's wort can relieve anxiety and low mood associated with menopause, but advise that there is uncertainty about variation in nature and potency of preparations, and it can interact with other drugs such as anticonvulsants, anticoagulants and tamoxifen. Do not take St John's wort alongside HRT as they interact.
- Refer to the article (*Menopause care: alternatives to hormone replacement therapy* which looks at the evidence base for common and emerging alternatives to HRT, including lifestyle options, complementary therapies, herbal remedies and prescribable medications, and is useful to discuss with patients) at https://obgyn.onlinelibrary.wiley.com/doi/10.1111/tog.70010.

6.6.9 Menopause and work

- 45% of women say they feel that their menopause symptoms have had a negative impact on their work. Women may take time off work, change their role at work or even leave the workplace due to their menopausal symptoms.
- They may require information about how an employer can support them in the workplace. Guidance for women and employers can be found at: www.womens-health-concern.org/wp-content/uploads/2025/07/07-NEW-BMS-ToolsforClinicians-Menopause-and-the-workplace-JULY2025-A.pdf.

6.6.10 Support for specific symptoms

Support for vasomotor symptoms

- Offer HRT as a first-line treatment to women who suffer with VMS associated with menopause, if there are no contraindications.
- Menopause-specific CBT can be used alongside HRT, or as an alternative option, for women who cannot take or choose not to take HRT.
- Do not routinely offer non-hormonal treatments such as SSRIs or serotonin–noradrenaline reuptake inhibitors (SNRIs) as first-line treatment for women who suffer with VMS alone.

Support for depressive symptoms

- Changes in hormones during the menopause can affect mental health. Low mood in menopause is different from clinical depression.
- NICE guidelines are clear that antidepressants are not the first-line choice of treatment for low mood in menopause, and that women should instead be offered HRT.

- CBT can be used alongside HRT alone, or as an alternative option, in women who cannot take, or choose not to take HRT.
- For those women experiencing menopause who are diagnosed with depression, follow NICE guidance recommendations for treating and managing depression in adults, considering the use of talking therapies and antidepressants. These could be given alongside HRT if clinically indicated: https://cks.nice.org.uk/topics/depression.
- Diagnosing depression can be done using the International Classification of Diseases 11th revision (ICD-11). Depression is defined as *"the presence of depressed mood or diminished interest in activities occurring most of the day, nearly every day, for at least 2 weeks, accompanied by other symptoms such as: reduced ability to concentrate and sustain attention or marked indecisiveness; beliefs of low self-worth or excessive or inappropriate guilt; hopelessness about the future; recurrent thoughts of death or suicidal ideation or evidence of attempted suicide; significantly disrupted sleep or excessive sleep; significant changes in appetite or weight; psychomotor agitation or retardation; reduced energy or fatigue."*

Support for sleep

- Menopause-specific CBT for insomnia can be beneficial for women who have sleep problems (such as difficulty getting to sleep or waking at night) in association with VMS, and can be used alongside HRT, or as an alternative option, in those who cannot take or choose not to take HRT.
- Refer to https://thebms.org.uk/wp-content/uploads/2025/08/25-NEW-BMS-ToolsforClinicians-Managing-sleep-disturbance-AUGUST2025-A.pdf.

Support for low sexual desire

- Use a biopsychosocial approach and consider adding testosterone to HRT in women with a low sexual desire associated with menopause, if HRT alone is not effective (see *Section 7.18*).

6.7 Genitourinary syndrome of the menopause

Genitourinary syndrome of the menopause (GSM) is a term for conditions previously known as vulvovaginal atrophy, atrophic vaginitis and urogenital atrophy. GSM is a chronic, progressive, vulvovaginal, sexual and lower urinary tract condition characterised by a broad range of signs and symptoms. Although it most commonly affects postmenopausal women due to reduced oestrogen levels, symptoms may also occur in premenopausal women, such as during breastfeeding.

This affects about 80% of women. Symptoms typically only improve with appropriate treatment, and can significantly affect sexual health and overall quality of life, yet many women feel too embarrassed to seek help. It is therefore important to ask about them directly and begin treatment promptly.

Symptoms

- These include vaginal dryness, soreness, burning, itching, dyspareunia, postcoital bleeding, decreased arousal and orgasm, urinary frequency, nocturia and urgency.

Signs on examination

- These include dryness, decreased elasticity, pallor, erythema, loss of vaginal rugae, resorption of the labia minora, friable tissues, fissures and petechiae.

Examination and investigations may be necessary

- An examination is recommended if symptoms are not improving using treatment (see *Section 6.7.1*), are worsening, or if there is uncertainty about the diagnosis, to exclude other conditions such as lichen sclerosus. However, women may still experience symptoms even when the examination appears normal.
- Consider urine dipstick, microscopy and genital swabs.
- New-onset irregular bleeding in perimenopausal women, or any bleeding after menopause, should be investigated.

Table 6.3: Localised vaginal oestrogen products

Estriol products	**Products available: gel, cream and pessary**
	Estriol 0.03mg pessary (Imvaggis) Use one pessary daily (inserted into the vagina with a finger) for 3 weeks and then at least twice weekly May damage latex condoms **Estriol 50mcg/g gel** (Blissel) – one applicator contains 50mcg or 0.05mg (in 1ml of gel); 30g tube Use one applicatorful daily for 3 weeks and then at least twice weekly; can be applied to the vulva with a finger Clear, water-based gel, mucoadhesive, hydrating, non-greasy **Estriol 0.1% (1mg/g) cream** – one applicator contains 0.5mg (in 0.5ml of cream); 15g tube Use one 0.5ml applicatorful daily for 2–4 weeks, then reduce to at least twice weekly; can be applied to the vulva with a finger Postmenopausal women can access Ovesse (estriol 1mg/g) in pharmacies without a prescription, but they have to pay for the cost of the drug **Estriol 0.01% (100mcg/g) cream** – one applicator contains 0.5mg (in 5ml of cream); 80g tube Use one 5ml applicatorful daily for 3–4 weeks, then at least twice weekly; can be applied to the vulva with a finger Oily, so may damage latex condoms Not for use if peanut allergy – contains arachis oil
Estradiol products	**Products available: intravaginal pessary and a silicone vaginal ring**
	10mcg intravaginal pessary Inserted with a reusable plastic applicator (Vagirux) or daily single-use plastic applicator (Vagifem); prefer reusable applicator as more environmentally friendly Use daily for 2 weeks then reduce to at least twice weekly ongoing Postmenopausal women in the UK can access Gina 10mcg estradiol vaginal tablets in pharmacies without a prescription, but they have to pay for the cost of the drug **Estring silicone vaginal ring** – 7.5mcg/24hrs Inserted into the vagina and stays in place, being replaced every 90 days Women can self-fit or by fitted by a clinician Can fit inside supportive pessaries for prolapse
Intrarosa prasterone 6.5mg DHEA pessary	Converted in the vaginal mucosa into oestrogen and androgens NICE NG23 recommends considering this if vaginal oestrogen or non-hormonal moisturisers or lubricants have been ineffective, or they are not tolerated; it is not a first-line treatment Pessaries inserted into the vagina once daily May damage latex condoms, diaphragm and cap Assess treatment every 6 months
Ospemiphene 60mg oral tablets (Senshio)	Not a first-line treatment; consider for postmenopausal women who cannot use the above locally-applied products, for example if dexterity is compromised Selective oestrogen receptor modulator (SERM), licensed for use in postmenopausal women, which acts as an oestrogen agonist in the vaginal mucosa, but as an antagonist in breast and endometrial tissue One tablet taken orally daily Cannot be taken with systemic HRT Side-effects include VMS which affect about 10% of women Can be considered in women with a history of breast or endometrial cancer, if they have completed their treatment; there is no data for women with current breast cancer
Laser therapy	Do not offer this unless part of a randomised controlled trial (RCT)

Management

- Give advice about vulval health care:
    - Avoid douching and using soap or shower gel. Recommend a soap substitute and a barrier ointment, such as emulsifying ointment.
    - Wear cotton underwear and opt for unbleached sanitary products.
    - Gently massage the tissues using fingers or a vibrator on a low setting, or engage in solo or partnered sex, to promote healthy blood flow to the genital area.
- Recommend pH-matched non-hormonal moisturisers and lubricants, either alone or alongside low-dose localised vaginal oestrogen. Both oil- and water-based products are available, but advise that oil-based options can damage condoms, as can some local oestrogen preparations such as estriol cream, estriol pessaries and prasterone pessaries.
- Offer localised low-dose vaginal oestrogen (see *Table 6.3*), which is available as a cream, gel, tablet, pessary or ring, and can be used alone or alongside non-hormonal moisturisers or lubricants to improve symptoms of GSM. Other options are vaginal DHEA or ospemifene.
- Offer localised vaginal oestrogen, or vaginal DHEA, to women with GSM who are on systemic HRT.
- Offer localised low-dose vaginal oestrogen to women with GSM and genitourinary conditions (such as overactive bladder or recurrent UTI) to improve symptoms and reduce risk of future UTI.
- Refer the patient to the British Association of Dermatologists vulval skincare: www.bad.org.uk/pils/vulval-skincare.

CASE: Yasmin is 54

Yasmin went through the menopause when she was 50 and did not take HRT because she had a diagnosis of oestrogen receptor-positive breast cancer in her late 40s and is still taking tamoxifen. Recently she has been having discomfort and itching around the vulva, it is burning and is irritated by wearing underwear. She has an increase in frequency of passing urine, she is up at night to pass urine and has developed urge incontinence, so doesn't want to go shopping with her friends in case she can't find a loo in time. She has been living with these symptoms for a few years, but they are progressively getting worse. In addition, Yasmin has rheumatoid arthritis.

She wants to know if this might be a UTI, or if it is just part of getting older?

All urine investigations are normal. You examine Yasmin to exclude other causes for itching, including lichen sclerosus, and you diagnose GSM and advise that she can use localised vaginal oestrogen. Recommend a good vulval care regime and use of non-hormonal moisturisers. You can offer a low-dose localised vaginal oestrogen product with appropriate counselling, as in *Section 6.7.2*. Ask her to choose a product that suits her dexterity. An estriol 0.03mg pessary (Imvaggis) is a good choice to start with, if she can manage this.

6.7.1 Localised vaginal oestrogen products

- When prescribing localised vaginal oestrogen explain that:
    - There may be initial irritation when treatment is started, which usually settles in 2–3 weeks.
    - Symptoms often return when localised vaginal oestrogen is stopped, so there is usually no need to stop it.
    - Creams and gels can be applied to both the vulva and the vagina.
    - Treatment can take 2–4 months to become effective.
    - After treatment is started, reassess women with GSM after 3 months, to monitor the response.
    - If symptoms do not improve with vaginal oestrogen, consider increasing the dose, changing the preparation (consider DHEA) or using an additional treatment such as

systemic HRT or two local treatments (off-licence). You can increase the frequency of using these preparations in women who have persistent symptoms, as the doses of oestrogen in these preparations are very low. Using 10mcg oestrogen pessaries regularly for one year is an equivalent dose to just one 1mg of estradiol HRT tablet.
  - Women using vaginal oestrogen (even long term) do not need to take a progestogen or have their endometrial thickness measured.
  - Localised vaginal oestrogen should be stopped 48 hours ahead of taking a cervical screening sample.
- The BMS states that "*Vaginal estrogen is not associated with an increased risk in breast cancer*".

6.7.2 Use of vaginal oestrogen in women with a personal history of breast cancer

- GSM symptoms can significantly affect the quality of life of women after breast cancer. They experience pain, painful sex (affecting their relationship), increased risk of UTI and urosepsis, and these symptoms can significantly affect quality of life and compliance with endocrine treatment.
- Offer non-hormonal moisturisers or lubricants to people with a personal history of breast cancer and GSM.
- If symptoms persist despite use of non-hormonal moisturisers, then after review of the NICE guidance [NG23] and the British Society for Sexual Medicine Position statement for management for GSM, discuss with the patient the use of low-dose localised vaginal oestrogen.
- NICE guidance NG23 states:
  - If the breast cancer was oestrogen receptor negative, vaginal oestrogen is unlikely to increase the risk of recurrence and is likely to be safe.
  - If the cancer was oestrogen receptor positive, it is not known whether vaginal oestrogen increases breast cancer recurrence risk. Vaginal oestrogen can be used, alongside adjuvants if these are being taken (including tamoxifen), which would reduce such impact.
- The use of vaginal oestrogens for women taking aromatase inhibitors is not absolutely contraindicated. Currently guidelines differ about the use of aromatase inhibitors and localised oestrogen. There is concern that women are experiencing significant symptoms of GSM without receiving treatment. If a woman is taking an aromatase inhibitor it is important to seek the advice of a breast cancer specialist and a menopause specialist with expertise in breast cancer. Joint decision-making between the patient and the breast team, using the latest evidence, can help to find the best treatment option (which may include localised vaginal oestrogen) for that woman, as these symptoms can significantly affect the quality of her life.

CASE: Jenny is 57

Jenny started having menopausal symptoms when she was 49 and started to take systemic HRT. She is happy taking HRT, but recently she has had vulval discomfort, dryness and a burning sensation. Sex is uncomfortable and she is upset as she has just met a new partner and wants to enjoy an intimate relationship.

She wonders if there are any adjustments you can make to her HRT to help with this? You take a full history and examine her to rule out other causes.

You diagnose GSM and advise her that she can add localised low-dose vaginal oestrogen to her systemic HRT. About 25% of women who take systemic HRT still need to take vaginal oestrogen to relieve the GSM. You can advise her about vulval care and use of non-hormonal moisturisers and lubricants. You can ask her which localised oestrogen product she prefers to use, and advise her about the loading dose, how to take it and how long it will take to work. It is a long-term treatment, and if it is stopped the symptoms will recur.

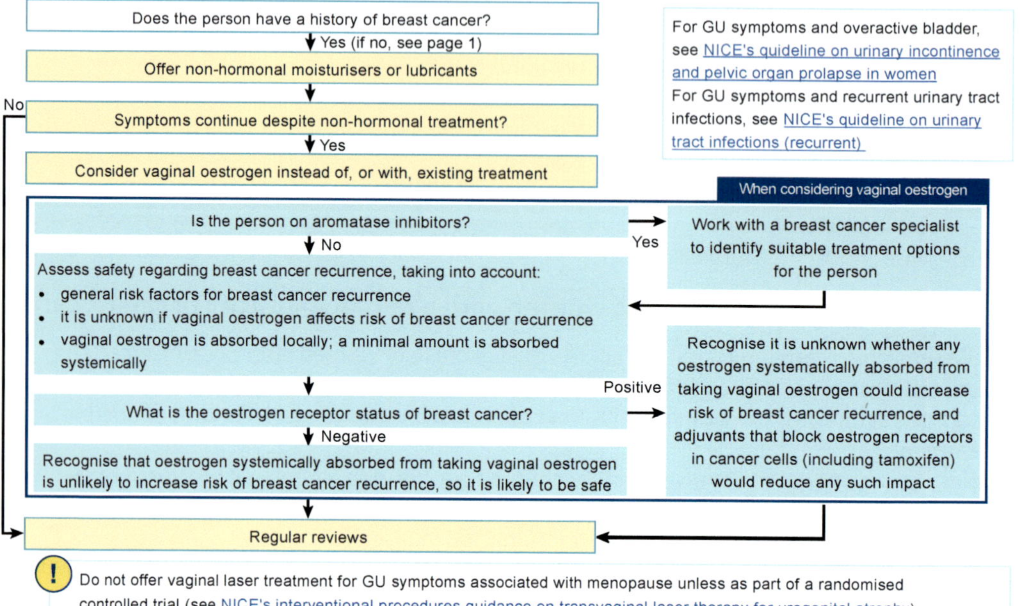

Figure 6.1: Management of genitourinary symptoms associated with menopause in women with a history of breast cancer.

- NICE guidance has useful information to advise about this for women with a history of breast cancer, as shown in *Fig. 6.1*.
- For more information refer to NICE guidance NG23: www.nice.org.uk/guidance/ng23/resources/visual-summary-on-genitourinary-gu-symptoms-associated-with-menopause-pdf-13553202493.

Resources for clinicians

- Primary Care Women's Health Society: *Genitourinary syndrome of the menopause.*
  - www.pcwhs.co.uk/_userfiles/pages/files/resources/pchws_gsm_final_3_5_25.pdf
- British Society for Sexual Medicine: *Position statement for the management of genitourinary syndrome of the menopause.*
  - https://bssm.org.uk/wp-content/uploads/2023/02/GSM-BSSM.pdf

Resources for women

- Menopause Research and Education Fund: *The genitourinary syndrome of the menopause* (https://mref.uk/wp-content/uploads/2024/10/fast-facts-4-GSM.pdf)

6.8 Premature ovarian insufficiency

Premature ovarian insufficiency (POI) affects 3.7% of women and is defined as the temporary or permanent loss of ovarian function below the age of 40. It is characterised by irregular menstrual cycles or amenorrhoea with elevated FSH and LH and low estradiol. Fluctuating ovarian activity may occur, resulting in variable FSH concentrations, including into the normal range.

Comprehensive new guidelines were released in 2024; refer to the healthcare professional toolkit:

- www.eshre.eu/Guidelines-and-Legal/Guidelines/Premature-ovarian-insufficiency
- https://thebms.org.uk/wp-content/uploads/2024/04/05-BMS-ConsensusStatement-Premature-ovarian-insufficiency-POI-APRIL2024-C.pdf

Having untreated POI has a significant impact on future health outcomes, fertility, cardiovascular health, bone health, sexual function, neurological function and psychological health.

Advice and management of POI (and early menopause) differs from the advice given to women who have their menopause aged ≥45.

6.8.1 Causes of POI

- These include chromosomal disorders (e.g. Turner's syndrome), autoimmune disease (e.g. thyroid, adrenal, rheumatoid arthritis), infections (e.g. mumps), metabolic and toxins. Iatrogenic causes include bilateral oophorectomy, chemotherapy, pelvic radiotherapy or pelvic/ovarian surgery.
- Surgery: women who are planning bilateral oophorectomy under the age of 45 should be made aware of the possible detrimental effects of POI or early menopause.

6.8.2 When to suspect POI

- If there has been oligo-/amenorrhoea for at least 4 months in women not using hormones under the age of 40.
- In women experiencing menopausal symptoms under the age of 40, although not all women with POI experience symptoms.
- Family history of POI / early menopause or other risk factors.
- Consider other causes of secondary amenorrhoea (*Section 2.6*).

6.8.3 Criteria for diagnosis

- Diagnose POI in people who are under 40 years based on:
    - Bilateral oophorectomy, in which case no further testing is needed.
    - Menstrual disturbance (amenorrhoea or oligomenorrhoea) for at least 4 months, *and* an elevated FSH level >25IU/L. Repeat FSH in 4–6 weeks if the diagnosis is uncertain.
- Be aware that some hormonal therapy (including hormonal contraceptives) or other medications such as chemotherapy can conceal or cause amenorrhoea or irregular menstrual cycles. Hormonal therapy (CHC and HRT) can potentially lower FSH levels, and may need to be stopped before a diagnosis of POI can be confirmed. Stop CHC for at least 2–6 weeks before measuring FSH and consider use of non-hormonal contraception.
- Do not test for anti-Müllerian hormone in primary care.

6.8.4 Risks of POI

If POI is not treated with hormonal therapy, it is associated with a reduced life expectancy, mainly due to cardiovascular disease.

- POI is associated with an increased risk of:
    - CVD, including hypertension, coronary artery disease, heart failure and stroke.
    - Metabolic problems including T2DM, dyslipidaemia and metabolic syndrome.
    - Depression, which can affect mental and emotional health and quality of life.
    - Musculoskeletal problems, including decreased bone density and osteoporosis, decreased muscle mass and strength.
    - Psychological problems, including anxiety, depression, poor self-esteem and body image.

  - Increased risk of cognitive impairment, dementia and Parkinson's disease.
  - Infertility.

6.8.5 Management and monitoring of POI

- History and examination:
  - Consider the cause for POI, symptoms, sexual function, osteoporosis risk factors, cardiovascular risk factors, psychological risk factors, fertility, pre-existing medical conditions, BP / weight and height.
- After diagnosis investigations include:
  - Thyroid function (including thyroid antibodies), renal function, liver function, fasting lipid profile, HbA1c, vitamin D and fasting glucose.
- If a diagnosis is confirmed or you strongly suspect POI, refer to gynaecology / menopause / fertility services as gold standard for a multidisciplinary approach. They will consider tests such as chromosomal analysis, autoimmune screening including 21-OH adrenal-antibodies depending on the history and examination.
- Encourage healthy lifestyle habits, including a balanced diet, regular physical activity (with weight-bearing exercises), and maintaining a healthy weight (see *Section 6.6.1*).
- It is important to consider assessing BMD at diagnosis. Further BMD assessments should be guided by the initial results, HRT use, and the patient's risk factors for osteoporosis.
- Offer holistic care with sensitivity and empathy. POI can be distressing, particularly for those who feel their family is not yet complete and due to worry about possible future health risks. Refer for psychological support if needed.
- Signpost patients to the POI peer support group, the Daisy Network (www.daisynetwork.org).

6.8.6 Hormone therapy in women with POI

- Women with POI and early menopause should be encouraged to use hormone replacement (unless there are contraindications) until at least the usual age of menopause. This is to replace the hormones they are missing. It acts as primary prevention to reduce risk of morbidity and mortality and should be offered even if there are no menopausal symptoms.
- Either HRT or a CHC method would be suitable options for hormone replacement, but HRT may be more beneficial than CHC in improving bone and cardiovascular health. If CHC is used, then a continuous or extended regimen is recommended to provide continuous oestrogen therapy and avoid bone loss.
- The BMS advises that there is no evidence that HRT use in women with POI until the age of 50 increases risk of breast cancer compared to women of the same age without POI.
- When considering the dose of oestrogen in HRT, usually higher doses of oestrogen are required for women with POI. The dose of progestogen, if required, must balance the dose of oestrogen (see *Section 7.10*).
  - Oestrogen doses recommended in the ESHRE 2024 guidelines are: transdermal patch 75–100mcg; transdermal gel sachet 1.5–2mg daily; transdermal gel pump 3–4 pumps daily; transdermal spray 3–4 sprays daily or oral tablet 2–4mg daily.
- Testosterone therapy can be considered to improve hypoactive sexual desire disorder and sexual function, particularly in those with a surgical menopause.
- Proactively ask about GSM and treat as in *Section 6.7*.
- If hormonal treatment is contraindicated consider non-hormonal treatments, if necessary (*see Section 6.6.7*).
- Patients should have an annual review.
  - It can be helpful to set up reminders to proactively follow women up to improve compliance.

  - The review should include adherence to therapy, review of cardiovascular risk factors (BP, weight, smoking), bone health risk factors, mental health review, symptoms review including GSM, sexual health review.
  - Levels of thyroid-stimulating hormone (TSH) should be checked every 5 years, or if symptoms.

6.8.7 Fertility and contraception

- Some women with POI continue to have ovarian activity, with an estimated 5–10% pregnancy rate, so it is important to advise about use of effective contraception in those women who do not wish to become pregnant. Ovarian activity is likely to reduce with age and longer duration of amenorrhoea.
- Contraception can be continued until the age of 55, when all women can stop using contraception.
- HRT is not a contraceptive unless oestrogen is combined with a 52mg LNG-IUD, so combined hormonal contraception (if there are no contraindications) can be considered following diagnosis of POI in those who wish to avoid pregnancy. This could provide menopause symptom control if taken in a tailored way and may be more acceptable to some women than HRT (but consider benefits and risks of both treatments).
- For women with POI who wish to become pregnant, but are not able to achieve a pregnancy naturally, oocyte donation is the treatment of choice. Taking HRT does not impact upon the chance of conceiving naturally and in women who wish to conceive, the use of sequential HRT is recommended.

CASE: Ana is 35

Ana had regular periods until 6 months ago and then her periods suddenly stopped. She is not using hormonal contraception, has not been under stress or experienced weight change. She is not exercising often and has not been sexually active for over a year. She has no symptoms of menopause and feels well. Her mum had her menopause at age 37. There is nothing in the history to suggest an alternative cause for secondary amenorrhoea. All her investigations to consider causes for secondary amenorrhoea are normal except her FSH which is 47IU/L. The result confirms that she has POI, but she is concerned when you suggest that she considers hormonal therapy such as HRT or CHC.

How do you advise her that this is the best approach? She is concerned as she has heard HRT causes breast cancer. Is this the case for her?

Unless there are contraindications, Ana should be advised to take HRT or CHC until the average age of menopause (51), even though she has no symptoms, for primary prevention to reduce the risk of morbidity and mortality. You can reassure her that HRT taken until she is 51 years old will not cause an increase in breast cancer above her normal baseline risk, as it is replacing her hormones that she has lost. At the age of 51, you can discuss with her whether she wants to continue taking HRT, and discuss the risks and benefits of doing so. If the combined oral contraceptive is used, then a continuous or extended regimen is recommended to provide continuous oestrogen therapy and avoid bone loss.

6.9 Induced menopause

- Induced menopause is also known as a medical or surgical menopause.
- It occurs when a medical intervention, such as surgery or use of a medication, affects ovarian function before a woman goes through her natural menopause. Examples include a bilateral

oophorectomy (surgical removal of both ovaries) or use of GnRH analogues, chemotherapy or radiotherapy.

- *Section 6.10* explains more about surgical menopause.

6.9.1 Reasons for a medically-induced menopause

- This section will discuss use of GnRH analogues, chemotherapy and radiotherapy.

Gonadotrophin-releasing hormone analogues

- GnRH is normally secreted in a pulsatile manner, and its activity is regulated by circulating oestrogen through feedback mechanisms acting on the hypothalamic–pituitary axis. GnRH analogues (agonists and antagonists) are synthetic medications that suppress gonadotrophin release when given continuously, leading to reversible suppression of sex hormone production.
- GnRH agonists produce a transient increase in sex hormones but with continued non-pulsatile stimulation FSH and LH synthesis is inhibited, and oestrogen levels fall.
- GnRH antagonists inhibit release of FSH and LH without an initial surge. Ultimately the effect of GnRH agonists and antagonists is similar.
- In order to improve the symptoms of these conditions, GnRH analogues can be used in the management of:
    - adenomyosis
    - endometriosis
    - uterine fibroids
    - menorrhagia
    - pelvic pain
    - severe premenstrual disorders, such as PMDD
    - hormone-sensitive cancers such as breast cancer: where ovarian suppression is needed to reduce circulating oestrogen as part of treatment or adjuvant therapy.
- They can also be used as part of gender-affirming hormone therapy to suppress endogenous ovarian hormones prior to, or alongside masculinising hormones therapy.
- Common side-effects include menopausal symptoms such as vasomotor symptoms, mood swings and vaginal dryness. If these treatments are taken for more than 6 months, bone health can be affected, with increased risk of osteoporosis.
- To help reduce side-effects of their use, a small-dose HRT or tibolone can be used alongside these treatments (which will not affect the effectiveness of the GnRH analogue). This is known as 'add-back HRT'. Some GnRH analogue preparations are available in products combined with oestrogen and progestogen; an example is Ryeqo, which is a combination pill containing relugolix (a GnRH receptor antagonist), estradiol and norethisterone acetate.
- Use of GnRH analogues can cause periods to stop or lighten. They do not provide contraception (although Ryeqo is an effective contraceptive after 1 month, provided it is used consistently and regularly, as advised). When GnRH analogues are stopped, periods usually return after 6–10 weeks.

Chemotherapy- and radiotherapy-induced menopause

- Chemotherapy can affect ovarian function temporarily or permanently, leading to symptoms of menopause. This can be very distressing for women, who not only are going through treatment for cancer but their treatment produces symptoms of menopause, which can significantly affect their quality of life (see *Section 6.11*).
- Radiation therapy to the pelvic area can impair ovarian function by damaging ovarian tissue. It can be used in the management of some pelvic cancers.

6.10 Surgical menopause

- Surgical menopause is when both ovaries are surgically removed (a bilateral salpingo-oophorectomy or BSO) before a woman goes through her natural menopause.

- This differs from a natural menopause, as oestrogen production is suddenly withdrawn, so symptoms can be sudden and may be more severe, especially in younger women.
- It is important that women discuss the implications of this surgery before the operation. They should be informed about the short- and long-term consequences of removal of their ovaries, and the treatment options available to them after the operation.
- For more information refer to: https://thebms.org.uk/wp-content/uploads/2024/10/13-BMS-TfC-Surgical-Menopause-SEPT2024-D.pdf and www.surgemenopause.com (for women).

6.10.1 Indications

- Both ovaries may be removed at the same time as a hysterectomy is performed, or as a stand-alone procedure, to manage several health conditions. For benign conditions and PMDD this would be considered after failure of conservative and medical treatments and following careful risk–benefit discussion.
    - Malignant:
        - As part of treatment for ovarian carcinoma, or as 'risk-reducing surgery' to lower the likelihood of developing ovarian cancer in women at high familial or genetic risk (e.g. those with Lynch syndrome or a *BRCA1/2* mutation).
        - Current guidelines advise that women with a *BRCA* gene mutation, who have no personal history of breast cancer, may use HRT after undergoing a BSO (provided there are no contraindications) until they reach the average age of menopause. Data is limited, but the use of HRT until age 51 is not thought to affect the reduction in breast cancer risk found after a BSO in these women. After the age of 51, current advice is that if they have ongoing symptoms, then non-hormonal treatments should be used.
    - Benign:
        - To manage conditions such as heavy menstrual bleeding, endometriosis, fibroids and chronic pelvic pain.
    - PMDD.
    - Gender reassignment.

6.10.2 Risks and benefits of surgical menopause

- Benefits include:
    - Reduced risk of ovarian cancer.
    - Relief of symptoms related to their medical condition, such as reduced PMDD symptoms or decreased pelvic pain in those with endometriosis.
- Risks include:
    - Postoperative complications such as bleeding, infection, pain, UTIs and thromboembolism.
    - Loss of fertility.
    - Menopausal symptoms, due to sudden loss of ovarian oestrogen production.
    - Reduction in libido, which could be due to loss of production of ovarian testosterone (although androgen precursors are still produced by the adrenal glands).
    - In premenopausal women, removal of the ovaries may be associated with an increased risk of future health problems such as coronary heart disease, cognitive impairment, dementia, osteoporosis and mental health problems such as anxiety and depression (see *Section 6.8*).

6.10.3 Management

- Holistic advice about lifestyle (see *Section 6.6.1*).
- See *Section 6.8* for advice about women who have a surgical menopause under the age of 40.
- Women planning to undergo surgical menopause should be offered the chance to discuss menopause and fertility (both before and after treatment) with a healthcare professional who has expertise in fertility.

- Current guidelines recommend that all women under the age of 45 who undergo surgical menopause should be offered HRT, to be continued until at least age 51, unless contraindicated.
- If there are no contraindications, women who have had a hysterectomy and do not require a progestogen can be offered oestrogen-only HRT. Women who do have a uterus must take combined HRT (using both oestrogen and a progestogen) to reduce the risk of endometrial cancer. Some women who have had a hysterectomy will be advised to take combined HRT, for example if they have a history of endometriosis (*see Section 6.10.4*).
- Women who have had a subtotal hysterectomy may retain some endometrial tissue, which could increase the risk of hyperplasia or malignancy if they use oestrogen-only HRT. In these cases, a progesterone challenge (two cycles of sequential HRT) can be given. If no bleeding occurs, or if pathology confirms no residual endometrium, oestrogen-only HRT can be used. Otherwise, continuous combined HRT containing both oestrogen and a progestogen should be prescribed.
- Tibolone can be considered for some women who have had a surgical menopause and can be helpful in women with low libido. It is a synthetic steroid hormone; its metabolites have oestrogenic, progestogenic and androgenic properties. It is not recommended for use in women with a history of breast cancer and should be used with caution in women over age 60 because of the increased stroke risk.
- Manage symptoms of GSM with vulval care, non-hormonal vaginal moisturisers and lubricants and, if eligible, low-dose localised vaginal oestrogen. Refer to the British Gynaecological Cancer Society and BMS guidelines (www.bgcs.org.uk/wp-content/uploads/2024/09/BGCS-BMS-Guidelines-on-Management-of-Menopausal-Symptoms-after-Gynaecological-Cancer-09.09.24.pdf).
- Testosterone can be added to systemic HRT to improve low libido for women with hypoactive sexual desire disorder (HSDD) (see *Section 7.18*).
- Alternative and complementary therapies or non-hormonal prescribable medications can be considered if HRT is contraindicated, or the woman chooses not to take it (see *Section 6.6.7*).

6.10.4 HRT after surgical menopause for endometriosis

- Current advice is that women who take HRT following a hysterectomy for widespread endometriosis should be given a continuous combined HRT (with both oestrogen and a progestogen) or tibolone to reduce the risk of stimulation and malignant changes in any remaining deposits of endometrium.
- An oestrogen-only HRT regime has a better breast safety profile, but seek advice from a menopause specialist before considering this as there is a risk of reactivating endometriosis and a potential malignant transformation of remaining endometrial deposits.
- If symptoms of endometriosis recur HRT should be reviewed, possibly stopped, and advice sought from Gynaecology.

6.11 Menopause after cancer

- Globally, 9 million women are diagnosed with cancer every year.
- Cancer treatments such as bilateral oophorectomy, chemotherapy, radiotherapy or hormonal therapy can affect ovarian function and induce a temporary or permanent menopause.
- Women taking HRT who are diagnosed with oestrogen receptor positive cancers will be advised to stop taking HRT. This can cause them to experience symptoms of menopause, which can be exacerbated by the use of treatments such as anti-oestrogen therapies.

- Multidisciplinary management of menopause after cancer is essential, including primary care and if appropriate other healthcare specialists who are experienced in managing menopause after cancer.
- Standard menopause diagnostic criteria may not be suitable to diagnose menopause after cancer, as ovarian function and periods may return years after cancer treatment finishes.

6.11.1 Managing menopause after cancer

- Offer clear, evidence-based information about the treatments and what to expect during and afterwards, including:
  - information about symptoms of menopause
  - side-effects of individualised cancer treatments, including how to manage these if they occur.
- Offer written advice about the range of treatments that may be taken both during and after the cancer treatment to ease the symptoms of menopause, including hormonal, non-hormonal, alternative and complementary treatments.
- Offer lifestyle advice as in *Section 6.6.1*.
- For many women with a history of cancer, HRT can be a viable option. However, in cases where HRT is contraindicated, such as with certain hormone-sensitive cancers, non-hormonal treatments are recommended (see *Section 6.6.7*).
- Manage symptoms including GSM and prescribe localised vaginal oestrogen, if there are no contraindications (see *Section 6.7*).
- During and after treatment for cancer women may struggle with body image, have less desire for sexual intimacy, find that penetration has become painful; they may be unable to have an orgasm or just do not find sex pleasurable. Refer to a menopause specialist with expertise in managing patients with these symptoms.
- Give advice about fertility and/or contraception, if appropriate.
- Menopause following cancer treatment may be associated with concerns about future health. Management should include supportive advice aimed at optimising cardiovascular health, maintaining bone health and supporting cognitive wellbeing.

6.11.2 Patient support

- This can include:
  - Managing emotions: coping with the diagnosis, managing stress, practising relaxation and breathing techniques, exploring spirituality, addressing changes in self-image, and dealing with fears related to cancer recurrence, mortality and emotional wellbeing.
  - Managing symptoms and side-effects.
  - Questions about treatments, and about the consequences of not being able to take treatments such as HRT.
  - Managing socially (personal relationships, relationships and sex, talking to children and loved ones, talking to people, talking to employers and colleagues, and healthcare professionals).
  - Managing practically (how to talk with the GP, including prescriptions, work, driving, travel, money and benefits, wills, insurance, nutrition and exercise).

Patient resources

- These include:
  - www.maggies.org
  - https://menopauseandcancer.org
  - https://futuredreams.org.uk
  - *Navigating Menopause After Cancer* by Dani Binnington.

6.11.3 Clinical resources

- The joint guideline with the BMS and British Gynaecological Cancer Society. This resource shows a useful table summarising recommendations for use of systemic HRT and vaginal oestrogen following treatment for gynaecological cancer:
  - https://thebms.org.uk/publications/bms-guidelines/management-of-menopausal-symptoms-following-treatment-of-gynaecological-cancer

6.12 Resources

6.12.1 Resources for clinicians

- https://thebms.org.uk/publications/tools-for-clinicians
- www.pcwhs.co.uk
- https://elearning.rcgp.org.uk/course/info.php?id=663
- www.nice.org.uk/guidance/ng23

6.12.2 Resources for women

- https://thebms.org.uk/wp-content/uploads/2023/08/MEN0921351544-005_Menopause-Support-Booklet-5-3.pdf
- Understanding the risks of breast cancer chart: www.womens-health-concern.org/wp-content/uploads/2019/10/WHC-UnderstandingRisksofBreastCancer-MARCH2017.pdf
- https://thebms.org.uk/education/principles-practice-of-menopause-care/bms-ppmc-resources-toolkit
- www.menopausematters.co.uk
- www.womens-health-concern.org/help-and-advice/factsheets
- Herbal medicine: more information about herbal medicine can be found at: *How to Harness the Power of Menopause with Natural Medicine*. Available at: https://subscribepage.io/Free_Guide
- National Institute of Medical Herbalists: https://nimh.org.uk.

6.13 Further reading

American College of Obstetricians and Gynecologists (2021) *Treatment of urogenital symptoms in individuals with a history of estrogen-dependent breast cancer*. Available at: https://www.acog.org/clinical/clinical-guidance/clinical-consensus/articles/2021/12/treatment-of-urogenital-symptoms-in-individuals-with-a-history-of-estrogen-dependent-breast-cancer

British Menopause Society (undated) *BMS Consensus Statements*. Available at: https://thebms.org.uk/members/consensus-statements

British Menopause Society (undated) *BMS Tools for Clinicians*. Available at: https://thebms.org.uk/publications/tools-for-clinicians

British Menopause Society (2025) *Managing sleep disturbance during the menopause transition*. Available at: https://thebms.org.uk/wp-content/uploads/2025/08/25-NEW-BMS-ToolsforClinicians-Managing-sleep-disturbance-AUGUST2025-A.pdf

CoSRH (amended 2025) *Aged Over 40*. Available at: www.cosrh.org/Public/Public/Standards-and-Guidance/Aged-Over-40.aspx

Department of Health and Social Care (updated 2025) *Guidance: Chapter 12: Alcohol*. Available at: www.gov.uk/government/publications/delivering-better-oral-health-an-evidence-based-toolkit-for-prevention/chapter-12-alcohol

Djapardy, V. and Panay, N. (2021) Alternative and non-hormonal treatments to symptoms of menopause. *Best Pract Res Clin Obstet Gynaecol*, **81:** 45–60.

ESHR (2024) *Premature Ovarian Insufficiency.* Available at: www.eshre.eu/Guidelines-and-Legal/Guidelines/Premature-Ovarian-Insufficiency

Harlow, S.D. and Paramsothy, P. (2011). Menstruation and the menopausal transition. *Obstet Gynecol Clin North Am*, **38(3):** 595–607.

International Menopause Society (2011) *Hot flushes and night sweats.* Available at: https://thebms.org.uk/wp-content/uploads/2015/10/Background-Oct2011.pdf

Leeds Teaching Hospitals NHS Trust (reviewed 2025). *GnRH therapy for gynaecological conditions.* Available at: www.leedsth.nhs.uk/patients/resources/gnrh-analogue-injections

Maki, P.M. and Jaff, N.G. (2022) Brain fog in menopause: a health-care professional's guide for decision-making and counseling on cognition. *Climacteric.* Available at: www.imsociety.org/wp-content/uploads/2022/10/IMS-White-Paper-2022-Brain-fog-in-menopause.pdf

McDougall, M. (2025) *How to Harness the Power of Menopause with Natural Medicine.* Available at: https://subscribepage.io/Free_Guide

Menopause Research and Education Fund (undated) *Resources.* Available at: https://mref.uk/mref-resources

Mullin, S. and Manley, K. (2025) Menopause care: alternatives to hormone replacement therapy. *The Obstetrician & Gynaecologist*, **27(4):** 308–20. Available at: https://obgyn.onlinelibrary.wiley.com/doi/10.1111/tog.70010

National Osteoporosis Guideline Group website: www.nogg.org.uk

NICE (revised 2022) CKS: *Vitamin D deficiency in adults.* Available at: https://cks.nice.org.uk/topics/vitamin-d-deficiency-in-adults

NICE (updated 2023) *Familial breast cancer: classification, care and managing breast cancer and related risks in people with a family history of breast cancer* [CG 164]. Available at: www.nice.org.uk/Guidance/CG164

NICE (2024) *HRT and the likelihood of some medical conditions.* Available at: www.nice.org.uk/guidance/ng23/resources/incidence-of-medical-conditions-with-and-without-hrt-a-discussion-aid-pdf-13553199901

NICE (updated 2024) *Menopause: identification and management* [NG23]. Available at: www.nice.org.uk/guidance/ng23

NICE (revised 2025) CKS: *Dementia.* Available at: https://cks.nice.org.uk/topics/dementia

NICE (revised 2025) CKS: *Osteoporosis – prevention of fragility fractures.* Available at: https://cks.nice.org.uk/topics/osteoporosis-prevention-of-fragility-fractures

Royal Marsden NHS Foundation Trust (revised 2023) *A beginner's guide to* BRCA1 *and* BRCA2. Available at: https://patientinfolibrary.royalmarsden.nhs.uk/brca1brac2

Chapter 7
Hormone replacement therapy

7.1 HRT summary

- Hormone replacement therapy (HRT), also known as menopause hormone therapy (MHT), is the use of a variety of hormone treatments to relieve the symptoms of perimenopause and menopause. It is also given to replace hormones in women who have a hormone insufficiency, such as those with premature ovarian insufficiency (POI).
- The BMS states that HRT should be considered a first-line treatment to prevent and treat osteoporosis in women with POI and in menopausal women below the age of 60, especially those who have menopausal symptoms.
- In the UK the term HRT is used, but internationally the term MHT is preferred.
- The perimenopause and menopause can have a significant impact on many women. More than 75% of women experience menopausal symptoms which can have a negative impact on their lives, whether at home, socially or at work. HRT is the most effective treatment and, compared with placebo, has been consistently shown to improve menopausal symptoms and is associated with a significant improvement in overall quality of life.
- The decision whether to take HRT, and the dose and the duration of its use, should be made on an individualised basis after discussing the benefits and risks to help women make an informed choice.
- HRT should be offered first-line for treatment of vasomotor symptoms and menopause-related low mood / anxiety, if there are no contraindications.
- HRT can be made of one hormone (oestrogen) or two hormones together (oestrogen and progestogen).
- Systemic HRT regimes involve the hormones being absorbed into the bloodstream. Oestrogen can be absorbed through the skin (transdermally) as a gel, patch or spray, taken orally as a tablet, or absorbed from a subdermal implant. Progestogen, if needed, can be given as a 52mg LNG-IUD (expiry 5 years), absorbed transdermally from a combined oestrogen and progestogen patch, or taken orally as a capsule or tablet. There are many different ways of prescribing HRT, and there is no 'one size fits all'.
- The hormone oestrogen (usually in the form of estradiol) forms the main part of HRT. The symptoms of menopause are caused by the ovaries producing less oestrogen as the number of follicles reduces and ovarian function declines. HRT is given to increase the level of oestrogen and relieve the symptoms.
- Taking oestrogen-only HRT can increase the risk of endometrial cancer, so adding a progestogen is necessary to reduce this risk for women who have a uterus. Progestogens may be added to an oestrogen for some days of the month (sequential combined HRT) or every day (continuous combined HRT).
- Testosterone can be added to systemic HRT in women who have persistent low sex drive (known as hypoactive sexual desire disorder, HSDD) once other causes for this have been explored. It is important that symptoms of vulvovaginal atrophy are treated as well, so that sex is comfortable. Currently there is no evidence to support use of testosterone to improve other symptoms such as brain fog, low energy and low muscle strength. More research is needed.
- Localised vaginal oestrogen (also called topical HRT) is a low-dose oestrogen treatment, given as a cream, gel, pessary or silicone ring, applied to the vagina and/or vulva, to relieve the symptoms of genitourinary syndrome of the menopause (GSM), which affect up to 80% of women. It can be used alone, or alongside systemic HRT in women with GSM symptoms. A DHEA vaginal pessary is an alternative option.
- Symptomatic patients in the perimenopause can take HRT; they do not have to wait until their periods stop.
- HRT taken by healthy women with menopause symptoms, under the age of 60, during a natural perimenopause and menopause, has the benefit of improving their symptoms and is associated with low risks.

- Women who go through menopause after the age of 45 usually do not need to take HRT if they are not bothered by their symptoms.
- Patients with POI should be started on HRT, to protect their future health, even if they do not have any menopause symptoms (unless there is a contraindication. CHC use is an alternative option for eligible women). HRT should be continued until at least the age of natural menopause (around age 51). The British Menopause Society (BMS) states that in clinical practice, women with early menopause <45 years should be given similar advice.
- HRT is important in managing surgical menopause, especially in women under the age of 45 (if there are no contraindications). All women having a surgical menopause should have counselling and be provided with information about the hormonal consequences of the surgery and the role of HRT for them. This should take place before the surgery, and before they leave the hospital they should have a clear plan for follow-up.
- HRT can be continued as long as needed; there is not a cut-off age, or a maximum time length for taking it. Patients should have an annual review, with shared decision-making, taking into account patient choice, to ensure there is a clear indication for taking HRT, the benefits outweigh the risks, and that there are no contraindications.
- HRT is not currently recommended solely to prevent aging, memory loss, cardiovascular disease or dementia.
- There has been confusion about HRT and breast cancer risk, which has led to fear in health professionals prescribing HRT and women being misinformed about the risks:
  - In otherwise healthy women, the overall risk of breast cancer associated with 5 years of HRT use in the early postmenopausal period is small.
  - After 5 years use of HRT to treat a naturally timed menopause, there is a small increased risk of a new breast cancer diagnosis. The relative risk relates to the HRT regime taken (oestrogen only < sequential combined < continuous combined) and increases with duration of HRT use.
  - Lifestyle factors play an important role in risk. In women aged 50–59, having obesity, or drinking ≥2 units of alcohol per day, is associated with a greater risk of developing breast cancer than using combined HRT for 5 years (see *Section 7.16.2*).
  - The risk of breast cancer with HRT should be considered alongside the benefits obtained from taking HRT, including improved quality of life, symptom management, cardiovascular and bone protective effects.
- HRT has changed in the last 20 years, with new formulations of estradiol and progestogen being used instead of oral conjugated equine oestrogens (CEE) and medroxyprogesterone acetate (MPA). The limitations of studies done in the past including the Women's Health Initiative (WHI) and the Million Women Study (MWS) are now recognised. The leaflets inside HRT/MHT products are still based upon the studies started in the 1990s.
- The Women's Health Concern fact sheet *HRT: the history* contains information for women on the important studies which have shaped the use of HRT since 1965: www.womens-health-concern.org/wp-content/uploads/2022/11/10-WHC-FACTSHEET-HRT-The-history-NOV22-A.pdf
- HRT prescriptions are free in Wales, Scotland and Northern Ireland. In England the HRT prescription prepayment certificate (HRT PPC) is a scheme designed to reduce the cost of HRT. It covers all eligible HRT products prescribed for a set cost for a 12-month period.

7.2 Types of oestrogen and progestogen used in HRT

7.2.1 Oestrogen

- The type of oestrogen used now in most systemic HRT products is 17β-estradiol (E_2) which is bioidentical / body identical (see *Section 7.3*).
- This form of oestrogen can be given continuously (taken orally or absorbed transdermally), and the dose can be adjusted to achieve symptom control.

7.2.2 Progestogen

- Oestrogen taken without a progestogen (unopposed oestrogen replacement) is associated with a significant increase in the risk of endometrial hyperplasia.
- A progestogen is needed alongside the oestrogen to minimise the risk of endometrial hyperplasia and endometrial cancer, in any of the following indications:
  - Women with a uterus.
  - After an endometrial ablation.
  - After subtotal hysterectomy, where the cervix is still present or with some remaining endometrium.
  - May be advised in women who have had a hysterectomy for endometriosis.

Table 7.1: Benefits and downsides of progestogens

Progesterone	
Micronised progesterone (MP)	Metabolites such as allopregnanolone act at GABA receptors (may cause sedation and reduce anxiety) Neutral effect on lipids and insulin sensitivity No increased risk of VTE Less effective at cycle control than other progestogens
Retroprogesterone	
Dydrogesterone (DYG)	Neutral effect on lipids and insulin sensitivity Unlikely to increase VTE risk compared to other progestogens Now available as a 10mg stand-alone tablet in the UK
C21 synthetics: structurally related to progesterone	
Medroxyprogesterone acetate (MPA)	Good for cycle control Consider VTE risk, especially with use of higher doses or when combined with oral estradiol Via its action on the glucocorticoid receptor it upregulates thrombin receptor expression
C19 synthetics: structurally related to testosterone	
Norethisterone (NET) Levonorgestrel (LNG) Norgestrel	Androgenic, may be good for libido Good for cycle control Unfavourable effect on lipids and insulin sensitivity NET: consider VTE risk, especially with use of higher doses or when combined with oral estradiol; NET is metabolised to ethinylestradiol VTE risk is not increased with use of combined estradiol/NET transdermal patch
All 52mg LNG-IUDs – 5 year expiry Lower dose LNG-IUDs cannot currently be used for endometrial protection as part of HRT	Low systemic hormone absorption Contraceptive, improves heavy menstrual bleeding, provides bleed-free option for perimenopause Androgenic No increased risk of VTE
Desogestrel Progestogen-only pill (consider UKMEC)	Less androgenic than NET/LNG As a POP (no oestrogen) no increased risk of VTE
Spironolactone derivative	
Drospirenone Progestogen-only pill (consider UKMEC)	Anti-androgenic – theoretically could be beneficial for PMS and acne Anti-mineralocorticoid – may improve bloating and BP As a POP (no oestrogen) no increased risk of VTE; refer to UKMEC 2025 Can cause hyperkalaemia; caution in renal disease

Table 7.2: Effects of individual progestogens on receptors

Progestogen	Progestogenic	Oestrogenic	Androgenic	Anti-andro-genic	Glucocorticoid	Anti-mineralo-corticoid
NET	+	+	+	–	–	–
LNG/norgestrel (including IUS)	+	–	+	–	–	–
Progesterone	+	–	–	+	+	+
MPA	+	–	*	–	+	–
DYG	+	–	–	–	–	*
Drospirenone	+	–	–	+	–	+
Desogestrel	+	–	*	–	–	–

+ effective; * weakly effective; – not effective

- A way to describe the need for progestogen to a patient, so that she understands the importance of taking both hormones, is that oestrogen helps to relieve menopausal symptoms, but is like 'a fertiliser on the lawn' and stimulates growth of the lining of the womb (endometrium). A progestogen is like 'a lawnmower' and helps to keep the endometrium thin and protect from endometrial hyperplasia and endometrial cancer. The fertiliser and lawnmower must balance, so with higher doses of oestrogen, progestogen dose may need to be increased.
- The benefits and downsides of progestogen are shown in *Table 7.1*.
- 'Progestogen' is an umbrella term which includes:
  - The natural hormone progesterone.
    - Natural progesterone is not well-absorbed orally because of its poor solubility (hence poor gastrointestinal absorption), first-pass liver metabolism and a short half-life.
    - To overcome this, micronised progesterone was developed (tiny progesterone particles are suspended in oil and packaged in gelatin) to enhance intestinal absorption. This is also known as a body-identical / bioidentical progesterone.
    - Examples are Utrogestan and Gepretix. They can be used as part of HRT. They do not provide contraception.
  - The synthetic progestogens (also known as progestins).
    - These are synthetic steroids designed to mimic the action of progesterone. They have different chemical structures which improve oral bioavailability (so they can be taken as tablets) and extend half-life. Depending on their chemical structure they can act on different receptors as well as the progesterone receptor, such as the androgen and glucocorticoid receptors. This can explain their side-effect profile as shown in *Tables 7.2* and *7.3*.
    - Examples are dydrogesterone, norethisterone, medroxyprogesterone acetate, levonorgestrel, drospirenone and desogestrel. They can be used clinically for contraception, as part of HRT and to manage gynaecological conditions such as heavy menstrual bleeding and endometrial hyperplasia.

Table 7.3: Common side-effects of progestogens

Receptors	Common side-effects by stimulation of receptors
Oestrogenic	Breast tenderness and enlargement, leg cramps, bloating, nausea, headache
Progestogenic	PMS-type symptoms, mood changes, somnolence
Androgenic	Oily skin, acne, hirsutism
Glucocorticoid	Dosage- and duration-dependent: oedema, fluid retention, weight gain
Mineralocorticoid	Oedema, weight gain, bloating and headache

- Dydrogesterone is a synthetic progestogen called a retroprogesterone.
  - It is similar to natural progesterone but has a slight difference in its structure (reversal of the hydrogen orientation at carbon-9 and carbon-10 of the steroid backbone, creating a bent formation compared with the straight formation of progesterone). It has good oral bioavailability, longer half-life and more stable serum levels than natural progesterone. It has a strong affinity for progesterone receptors and has no oestrogenic, androgenic or corticoid effects, meaning it has a better side-effect profile than other progestins.
  - It can be used as part of HRT and also to manage other conditions such as dysmenorrhoea, PMS, irregular menstrual cycles, dysfunctional uterine bleeding, secondary amenorrhoea and endometriosis. It does not provide contraception.
  - Nalvee became available in the UK in August 2025. It is a dydrogesterone-only tablet licensed for use in HRT. Dydrogesterone is also available in fixed dose oral tablets in combination with oestrogen.

7.2.3 Choice of progestogen for endometrial protection as part of HRT

- Progestogen is available as:
  - micronised progesterone (MP)
  - dydrogesterone (DYG)
  - norethisterone (NET)
  - medroxyprogesterone acetate (MPA)
  - levonorgestrel (LNG)
  - drospirenone (DRSP)
  - desogestrel (DSG).
- See *Tables 7.7* and *7.10* for the recommended doses of these progestogens (some of which can be considered for use, off-licence, if other progestogens are not tolerated) as part of HRT alongside various doses of oestrogen.
- MP and DYG are less androgenic than the other progestogens, so may cause fewer side-effects such as acne, oily skin, excess body hair and mood changes. Observational data suggests that they may be associated with a lower risk of breast cancer and VTE compared to that seen with other progestogens.
- One disadvantage of using MP is that it can be less effective for bleeding control, leading to breakthrough bleeding on HRT. Adjusting the dose, changing to a different progestogen or using a 52mg LNG-IUD can be helpful in this case.
- Some women have a severe intolerance to MP and/or synthetic progestogens, and struggle to take them due to side-effects. In some women these side-effects may settle over time with continued use. In clinical practice taking the progestogen daily can be helpful for some women, rather than using it cyclically (see *Section 7.16.9*).

7.3 Bioidentical HRT

- The term 'bioidentical' has caused confusion about the two types of HRT.
- Bioidentical hormones are exact duplicates of those made by the human body (such as estradiol (E_2), estriol (E_3), progesterone and testosterone). They are also known as 'body-identical' hormones.
- Compounded bioidentical hormone replacement therapy (cBHRT)
  - This type of HRT uses bioidentical hormones produced by specialist pharmacies and is not recommended for use. It is not evidence-based for safety and effectiveness and does not follow the MHRA regulatory pathway, in the UK. It is not available on the NHS. There is lack

of evidence to justify multiple, expensive serum and saliva hormone tests which claim to precisely individualise this type of HRT.

- Regulated bioidentical hormone replacement therapy (rBHRT)
  - This type of HRT uses bioidentical hormones produced by the pharmaceutical industry in a conventional way and is authorised by the MHRA, in the UK. It is recommended for use by the BMS, and is available on the NHS. This includes products containing 17β-estradiol and micronised progesterone, but does not include products containing the other synthetic progestogens, which have different chemical structures to progesterone.

7.4 Systemic HRT

- HRT in which the hormones are absorbed into the bloodstream and have an effect throughout the body to relieve the widespread symptoms of menopause.
- The HRT regime and dose can be individualised to the woman to control her symptoms. Women may need to try different combinations to find the regime that suits them best.

7.4.1 Types of systemic HRT

Oestrogen-only HRT

- HRT with only oestrogen, for those who have had a total hysterectomy, and who do not require a progestogen.

Combined HRT

- HRT with oestrogen and progestogen, for those who still have a uterus, and those who require a progestogen.

Sequential combined HRT (sHRT)

- Provides continuous systemic oestrogen with added luteal phase progestogen. The progestogen is usually taken for 12–14 days each month. This regime gives a withdrawal bleed, usually at the end of the progestogen phase, lasting 3–7 days.
- Is recommended for women with a uterus (and those who require a progestogen) who start HRT in perimenopause when they are still having periods in the 12 months before HRT is initiated.
- This regime does not suppress ovulation, so women may experience symptoms, including unscheduled bleeding, due to their own fluctuating ovarian function.
- For more information refer to *Section 7.15*.

Continuous combined HRT (ccHRT)

- Provides continuous systemic oestrogen with continuous, daily progestogen.
- Is recommended for women with a uterus (and those who require a progestogen) and is suitable for women who start taking HRT post menopause, and have had amenorrhoea for 12 months before HRT is commenced.
- This regime can also be used in women who have been amenorrhoeic for at least 12 months taking a progestogen-only method of contraception, or are post-ablation.
- Women are expected to be amenorrhoeic on this preparation 6 months after initiation. It is common to get some bleeding during the first 3–6 months.
- Taking progestogen continually, as in ccHRT, provides better endometrial long-term protection than sHRT in which progestogen is taken cyclically, but if ccHRT is used too soon in perimenopause, it may cause irregular bleeding.
- For more information refer to *Section 7.15*.

7.4.2 When to change from sequential to continuous combined HRT?

- Women over the age of 45, taking a sequential HRT regime, should be offered, after 5 years of use or by age 54 (whichever comes first), a change to a continuous HRT regime because, as discussed, ccHRT provides better endometrial protection.
- This change can take place earlier, and women who have used a cyclical preparation for over 12 months could be transferred to a continuous regime. If they start having unscheduled bleeding, then it may be sensible to revert them to sHRT and try again after 6–12 months.

7.5 Hormonal contraception and perimenopause

- Perimenopause is a time of fluctuating (high and low levels) of endogenous oestrogen and FSH. This can cause classical menopause symptoms (vasomotor symptoms, mood symptoms, worsening sleep and GSM symptoms) as well as unscheduled bleeding, worsening PMS and worsening migraine.
- Adding HRT in perimenopause does not provide hormonal stability, as the endogenous hormones are fluctuating and oestrogen levels can range from high to low.
- Hormonal contraceptives may have a beneficial role in perimenopause, if there are no contraindications (see UKMEC; www.cosrh.org/Common/Uploaded%20files/documents/fsrh-ukmec-summary-september-2019.pdf) to suppress ovulation and provide hormonal stability.

Table 7.4: Use of combined hormonal contraceptive and progestogen-only contraceptives in perimenopause

CHC in perimenopause	Progestogen-only contraception in perimenopause
Provides contraception Suppresses ovulation Menstrual cycle regulation, good for managing dysfunctional anovulatory bleeding Treatment of menorrhagia and dysmenorrhoea Reduction in vasomotor symptoms and menstrual migraine (contraindicated with migraine with aura) BMD protection For women with POI the oestrogen dose in COCs containing 1.5mg estradiol or 20mcg ethinylestradiol may be inadequate for bone health Reduction in ovarian, endometrial and colorectal cancer Tailored COCP regimes can be used, off-licence, to avoid symptoms occurring in the hormone-free interval; low-dose ethinylestradiol pills, estradiol or estetrol pills are preferred Consider risks, for example VTE	Provides contraception Can suppress ovulation (DMPA, IMP, some POPs (DSG/DRSP)) Reduces menorrhagia and dysmenorrhoea Possible reduction in menstrual migraine May be associated with irregular bleeding (e.g. the DRSP prevents ovulation but does not prevent follicular development; for this reason it may be associated with irregular bleeding) No reduction in vasomotor symptoms No BMD protection HRT can be taken alongside the POP, IMP, DMPA Any 52mg LNG-IUD can be used for endometrial protection as part of HRT, and must be replaced within 5 years The 52mg LNG-IUD plus continuous estradiol reduces/ eliminates bleeding but not cyclical symptoms See *Table 7.7* for information on drospirenone and desogestrel use as the progestogen part of HRT, off-licence. Note that 75mcg DSG does not provide endometrial protection as part of HRT

7.6 Tibolone

- Tibolone is a synthetic steroid which has oestrogenic, progestogenic and androgenic action.
- It can be used by postmenopausal women to relieve menopause symptoms and reduce bone loss and fracture.
- It can be used for prevention of osteoporosis in postmenopausal women at high risk of future fractures if other treatments for the prevention of osteoporosis are not tolerated, or are contraindicated.

- It can be considered as an alternative to conventional HRT for postmenopausal women if an improvement in libido is needed.
- Tibolone or ccHRT are options for treatment to relieve menopause symptoms in women with endometriosis:
  - After an induced menopause (using GnRH analogues or surgery involving bilateral oophorectomy).
  - If they have had a hysterectomy and bilateral oophorectomy but may have some endometriosis deposits remaining.
  - https://thebms.org.uk/wp-content/uploads/2022/12/10-BMS-TfC-Induced-Menopause-in-women-with-endometriosis-NOV2022-A.pdf
- Tibolone is not recommended for use in women who have a history of breast cancer.
- Tibolone can increase risk of stroke and should be used with caution in women at risk of stroke. For women older than about 60 years, the risks associated with tibolone start to outweigh the benefits because of the increased risk of stroke.
- Tibolone is not associated with an increased risk of VTE. It may increase blood fibrinolytic activity and enhance the effect of anticoagulants such as warfarin.
- Tibolone 2.5mg/day is approximately equivalent to 1mg oral estradiol.

7.7 Initiating HRT

- Take a full medical/family history as explained in *Section 6.4*.
- Exclude other causes for symptoms such as cardiac disease or thyroid disorders in women with palpitations.
- Ensure there are no contraindications to taking HRT, such as undiagnosed abnormal vaginal bleeding or an oestrogen-dependent cancer (see *Section 7.11*).
- Check if there are any cautions to prescribing HRT which might affect the HRT regime you advise, such as migraine or epilepsy (see *Section 7.17*).
- Assess individual risk factors including breast, VTE, endometrium, osteoporosis, CVD, chronic kidney disease (CKD), age of patient when deciding dose, and route of HRT.
- Ask about medication/supplements which may interact with HRT (such as St John's wort) or affect the choice of HRT regime (such as the incretin medications) (see *Section 7.8*).
- The choice of HRT products should consider patient preference as well as risk and benefit. Ask which regime she will be able to remember to take correctly, to avoid poor compliance.
- Ensure she understands the benefits, risks and possible side-effects.
- Explain what might happen to her bleeding pattern after HRT is initiated. Explain what type of bleeding is a concern and when she should seek medical advice about unscheduled bleeding (see *Section 7.15*).
- Explain when to book an HRT review appointment. This would usually be 3 months after initiation, 3 months after a dose or product change, and annually once stable on a regime.
- Consider the following:
  - Dose and route of oestrogen (see *Table 7.10*).
  - The need for a progestogen.
    - Ensure safeguards are in place so that women with a uterus are not prescribed oestrogen-only HRT.
    - Ask about her past experience with progestogen use in hormonal contraception, and history of postnatal depression or PMS, as this may influence the type and regime for progestogen (see *Section 7.2.3*).
    - Ensure the dose of progestogen is adequate to oppose the dose of oestrogen. Note that the dose of progestogen may need to be increased if high-dose oestrogen is used (see *Table 7.10*).

   - Can oestrogen and progestogen be prescribed as separate products (consider compliance of taking the hormones separately), or as a combined product (both hormones in the same product, for example a combined patch or oral tablet)?
- Assess the need for sequential combined HRT or continuous combined HRT (see *Section 7.3*).
- When initiating sequential HRT in perimenopause, aim if possible to time the start of HRT to the natural cycle (as long as this does not require a long delay in starting the hormones, if cycles are very infrequent).
   - This involves starting oestrogen on day 1 of the next menstrual cycle (continuous use).
   - Usually a progestogen is taken alongside the oestrogen on days 14–28 of the oestrogen cycle (2 weeks off, 2 weeks on). This aims to mimic the natural cycle to avoid unscheduled bleeding.
   - Compliance can be a problem for women taking cyclical progesterone, so advise a way to make it easier to remember. If a progestogen is started in a woman with irregular menstrual cycles, in perimenopause, then some women find it easier to remember to take it for the first 12–14 days of each calendar month.
      - It is important to advise women to continue to take the progestogen cyclically in the pattern prescribed, no matter what happens to their bleeding pattern.
      - Give written advice and only prescribe a type of regime a woman can remember to take correctly.
      - Her progestogen could be given as a 52mg LNG-IUD, or as part of a combined patch or combined oral tablet if risk of compliance is poor with oestrogen and progestogen given as separate products.
   - When prescribing HRT, if prescribing the hormones separately, write the progestogen instructions on the oestrogen prescription for safety-netting.
      - For example: *"Change the patch twice weekly. This patch must be used alongside your 52mg LNG-IUD, which expires for HRT use on 12 September 2030."*
- Consider the need for contraception. Options include:
   - If eligible, under the age of 50, offer the choice of CHC instead of HRT.
   - Any 52mg LNG-IUD (replaced within 5 years).
   - A progestogen-only contraceptive method alongside her HRT, such as the POP, DMPA or IMP.
- Document your assessment and advice given.

7.7.1 Oral or transdermal oestrogen preparations and VTE risk

- Every woman should have a VTE risk assessment prior to initiating HRT.
- Risk factors for VTE include prior VTE, genetic causes (such as factor V Leiden and prothrombin gene mutation), BMI >30kg/m^2, immobility, smoking, age >55, cancer and cancer treatments, metabolic syndrome, hypertension and dyslipidaemia.
- VTE risk associated with HRT use depends upon the route of oestrogen (oral/transdermal; see *Table 7.5*) and the type of progestogen used.
- Oral oestrogen increases the risk of VTE (2–4-fold) compared to women not using HRT.
   - Oral oestrogen undergoes first-pass hepatic metabolism, activating the coagulation system and increasing liver biosynthesis of procoagulant factors. The effects of transdermal oestrogen on the liver proteins are neutral.
   - Many women can still take oral oestrogen, but it is not suitable for every woman.
- For women with risk factors for VTE, transdermal estradiol is the first-choice route, as it is vascular risk-neutral and does not appear to increase VTE risk. If a progestogen is required, oral micronised progesterone or a 52mg LNG-IUD are preferred options, as they also do not appear to increase VTE risk and are also vascular risk-neutral.

Table 7.5: Consider oral or transdermal HRT

Consider oral oestrogen if:	No risk factors for VTE Healthy women <60 years If there is poor absorption of transdermal oestrogen (which can be affected by skin conditions, hydration, perfusion, ethnicity and BMI) Patient preference: • Once-daily treatment, so easy to use • Fixed tablet doses, but a range of doses are available • May provide better bleeding control
Consider transdermal oestrogen if:	Patient preference Stroke risk: BMI >30, age >60, medical risks, smoker/sedentary Initiating or continuing after 60 years Poor control or side-effects on oral HRT Variable BP control High triglyceride levels Family history or personal history of VTE; consider Haematology advice History of, or risk of CVD; consider specialist advice Bowel disorder which may affect absorption of oral therapy/bariatric surgery Migraine Lactose sensitivity (all tablet preparations contain lactose) Taking interacting drugs (hepatic enzyme inducers), e.g. anticonvulsants Severe liver disorder Diabetes Gallbladder disease

7.8 Injectable weight-loss drugs, contraception and HRT

- Many women are using weight-loss medication, some of which can potentially reduce absorption of oral contraception and oral progestogens in HRT. It is important to ask about their use, as patients may be obtaining them privately.
- There are two areas to consider in patients who take GLP-1 agonists:
  - The need for effective contraception in patients using GLP-1 agonists (they are not recommended in pregnancy).
  - The concern about absorption of oral hormonal contraceptives and oral progestogens in HRT when some weight-loss drugs are used.
- Patients may be using oral hormonal contraception alongside HRT. If they experience severe diarrhoea or vomiting during use of GLP-1 agonists, they should follow CoSRH Clinical Guidance on drug interactions with hormonal contraception: www.fsrh.org/Public/Public/Documents/ceu-clinical-guidance-drug-interactions-with-hormonal.aspx

7.8.1 Contraception and GLP-1 agonist use

- Gastrointestinal side-effects (including nausea, vomiting and diarrhoea) are common side-effects of GLP-1 agonists. Diarrhoea and vomiting can affect the absorption of oral hormonal contraception. Refer to the CoRSH Clinical Guidance on drug interactions with hormonal contraception: www.cosrh.org/Common/Uploaded%20files/documents/drug-interactions-with-hormonal-contraception-5may2022.pdf

- Patients under the age of 55 who are at risk of pregnancy must be advised to use an effective method of contraception whilst using a GLP-1 agonist.
  - If they use tirzepatide alongside an oral hormonal method of contraception, they should add a barrier method of contraception, or switch to a non-oral contraceptive method, for 4 weeks after tirzepatide is initiated, and for 4 weeks after each tirzepatide dose increase.
  - They do not need to add a barrier method of contraception when using semaglutide, dulaglutide, exenatide, lixsenatide or liraglutide (see *Section 3.2.12*).

7.8.2 HRT and GLP-1 agonist use

- There is limited evidence regarding how GLP-1 agonists interact with progestogens used in HRT. Transdermal and vaginal routes are unlikely to be affected, but because GLP-1 agonists slow gastric emptying, there is concern that they may impair the absorption of oral progestogens in HRT.
  - The BMS released a guideline in April 2025 implying that both semaglutide and tirzepatide can affect absorption of oral progestogens, while the CoSRH only recommends changes in contraception with tirzepatide.
  - An option for HRT if semaglutide or tirzepatide are used, is to switch the oral progestogen to a non-oral progestogen (such as a combined patch or a 52mg LNG-IUD), while the GLP-1 agonist is being used.
  - Vaginal use of some micronised progesterone products (see *Table 7.7*) could be considered (off-licence) but there is no recommended guidance about this.
- If the patient prefers to continue with an oral progestogen, the dose of this should be increased for 4 weeks following initiation of the GLP-1 agonist and after each subsequent GLP-1 agonist dose escalation.
  - The BMS has not recommended a specific dose increase but the Primary Care Women's Health Society (PCWHS) has suggested that those women increase their progestogen dose to the dose suggested by the BMS for women taking high-dose oestrogen (but not taking a GLP-1 agonist), as shown in *Table 7.10*. There is no guidance for those women already taking a higher dose of oestrogen and already taking a higher dose of progestogen. A 52mg LNG-IUD may provide the best endometrial protection.
- To ensure patient safety and safe prescribing, the PCWHS has produced a leaflet, including a primary care action plan, which can be followed upon receipt of information that a patient is taking a GLP-1 agonist. This includes:
  - A template which can be sent to private providers of GLP-1 agonists.
  - A template which can be sent to patients under the age of 55 explaining how to manage contraception whilst they take a GLP-1 agonist.
  - They recommend arranging a review for all patients taking a GLP-1 agonist and HRT to ensure safe prescribing.
  - For details about how to manage patients on GLP-1 agonists refer to:
    - www.pcwhs.co.uk/_userfiles/pages/files/resources/glp1_contraception_hrt_article.pdf
    - https://thebms.org.uk/wp-content/uploads/2025/05/23-BMS-TfC-Use-of-incretin-based-therapies-APRIL2025-E.pdf

7.9 HRT products and doses

- This section shows the available products (in the UK) and recommended doses.
- When prescribing oestrogen and progestogen products separately, ensure the patient understands the importance of taking both hormones and how to use them.
- Oestrogen-only products – doses range from 'low-dose' oestrogen (25mcg patch or equivalent) to 'high-dose' oestrogen (100mcg patch or equivalent); see *Tables 7.6* and *7.10*.
- Adjuvant progestogen products can be used alongside oestrogen-only products in women who require a progestogen.

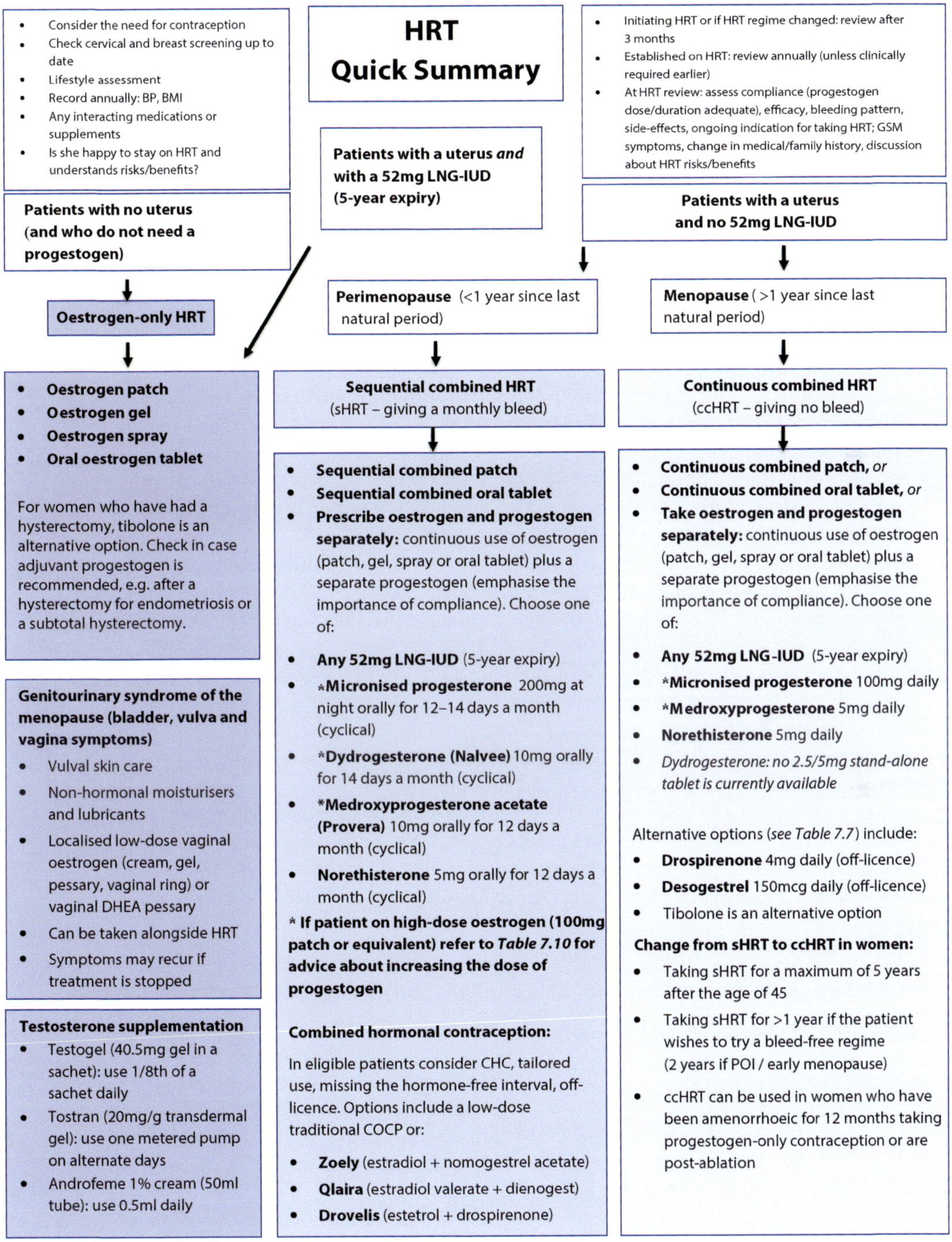

HRT Quick Summary

- Consider the need for contraception
- Check cervical and breast screening up to date
- Lifestyle assessment
- Record annually: BP, BMI
- Any interacting medications or supplements
- Is she happy to stay on HRT and understands risks/benefits?

- Initiating HRT or if HRT regime changed: review after 3 months
- Established on HRT: review annually (unless clinically required earlier)
- At HRT review: assess compliance (progestogen dose/duration adequate), efficacy, bleeding pattern, side-effects, ongoing indication for taking HRT; GSM symptoms, change in medical/family history, discussion about HRT risks/benefits

Patients with no uterus (and who do not need a progestogen)

↓

Oestrogen-only HRT

↓

- **Oestrogen patch**
- **Oestrogen gel**
- **Oestrogen spray**
- **Oral oestrogen tablet**

For women who have had a hysterectomy, tibolone is an alternative option. Check in case adjuvant progestogen is recommended, e.g. after a hysterectomy for endometriosis or a subtotal hysterectomy.

Patients with a uterus *and* with a 52mg LNG-IUD (5-year expiry) → (arrow to oestrogen-only options)

Patients with a uterus and no 52mg LNG-IUD

↓

Perimenopause (<1 year since last natural period)

↓

Sequential combined HRT
(sHRT – giving a monthly bleed)

↓

- **Sequential combined patch**
- **Sequential combined oral tablet**
- **Prescribe oestrogen and progestogen separately:** continuous use of oestrogen (patch, gel, spray or oral tablet) plus a separate progestogen (emphasise the importance of compliance). Choose one of:

- **Any 52mg LNG-IUD** (5-year expiry)
- ***Micronised progesterone** 200mg at night orally for 12–14 days a month (cyclical)
- ***Dydrogesterone (Nalvee)** 10mg orally for 14 days a month (cyclical)
- ***Medroxyprogesterone acetate (Provera)** 10mg orally for 12 days a month (cyclical)
- **Norethisterone** 5mg orally for 12 days a month (cyclical)

*** If patient on high-dose oestrogen (100mg patch or equivalent) refer to *Table 7.10* for advice about increasing the dose of progestogen**

Combined hormonal contraception:

In eligible patients consider CHC, tailored use, missing the hormone-free interval, off-licence. Options include a low-dose traditional COCP or:

- **Zoely** (estradiol + nomogestrel acetate)
- **Qlaira** (estradiol valerate + dienogest)
- **Drovelis** (estetrol + drospirenone)

Menopause (>1 year since last natural period)

↓

Continuous combined HRT
(ccHRT – giving no bleed)

↓

- **Continuous combined patch,** *or*
- **Continuous combined oral tablet,** *or*
- **Take oestrogen and progestogen separately:** continuous use of oestrogen (patch, gel, spray or oral tablet) plus a separate progestogen (emphasise the importance of compliance). Choose one of:

- **Any 52mg LNG-IUD** (5-year expiry)
- ***Micronised progesterone** 100mg daily
- ***Medroxyprogesterone** 5mg daily
- **Norethisterone** 5mg daily
- *Dydrogesterone: no 2.5/5mg stand-alone tablet is currently available*

Alternative options (*see Table 7.7*) include:

- **Drospirenone** 4mg daily (off-licence)
- **Desogestrel** 150mcg daily (off-licence)
- Tibolone is an alternative option

Change from sHRT to ccHRT in women:

- Taking sHRT for a maximum of 5 years after the age of 45
- Taking sHRT for >1 year if the patient wishes to try a bleed-free regime (2 years if POI / early menopause)
- ccHRT can be used in women who have been amenorrhoeic for 12 months taking progestogen-only contraception or are post-ablation

Genitourinary syndrome of the menopause (bladder, vulva and vagina symptoms)

- Vulval skin care
- Non-hormonal moisturisers and lubricants
- Localised low-dose vaginal oestrogen (cream, gel, pessary, vaginal ring) or vaginal DHEA pessary
- Can be taken alongside HRT
- Symptoms may recur if treatment is stopped

Testosterone supplementation

- Testogel (40.5mg gel in a sachet): use 1/8th of a sachet daily
- Tostran (20mg/g transdermal gel): use one metered pump on alternate days
- Androfeme 1% cream (50ml tube): use 0.5ml daily

Figure 7.1: Flow chart for prescribing HRT. NB: this provides general advice only – some women need individualised regimes due to risk factors for VTE, or to manage unscheduled bleeding on HRT.

- The BMS recommends the monthly progestogen dose is in proportion to the oestrogen dose in people who have a uterus, to reduce the risk of unscheduled bleeding and endometrial cancer. Women taking 'high-dose' oestrogen usually need to take a higher dose of progestogen, and doses are shown in *Tables 7.7* and *7.10*.
- When prescribing combination products containing fixed doses of oestrogen and progestogen, the dose can be adjusted to achieve symptom control; for example, Femoston 1/10mg can be increased to Femoston 2/10mg.
- In most women it is best to start at a low/standard dose oestrogen and titrate up, to achieve symptom control and minimise side-effects.
- Many women find a standard dose of estradiol is adequate for symptom relief, but some do require higher doses.
- It is recommended that younger women under the age of 40, either after surgical menopause or with POI, are given higher doses of oestrogen (75–100mcg patch or equivalent). See *Section 6.8* for more information.
- Older women who are started on HRT and those with migraine may benefit from starting with a low dose of oestrogen and slowly titrating up to achieve symptom control, to avoid side-effects.
- The dose of estradiol needed to provide bone protection is a 50mcg patch or equivalent, according to the International Menopause Society white paper, *Menopause and MHT* in 2024, but benefit can be seen with lower oestrogen doses.
- Any dose of HRT should ideally be tried for 3 months before considering if a change in dose is needed, but in clinical practice there is some flexibility. It is common to increase from a dose of 25–50mcg more quickly if the symptoms are not improved after 6 weeks, for example.
- Before increasing the dose consider if there may be other factors contributing to symptoms, such as incorrect use of the HRT product, an alternative diagnosis, or lifestyle factors such as diet, smoking, alcohol, caffeine, lack of exercise or life stressors.
- Absorption through transdermal estradiol products can vary individually, due to a range of factors including hydration, ethnicity and circulation.
- It may be necessary to change the HRT product if symptoms are not improving despite increasing the oestrogen dose. For some women, taking oral oestrogen gives much better symptom control due to poor absorption through the skin (see *Section 7.6.1*).
- Consider adding non-hormonal options such as CBT alongside HRT.

7.9.1 Oestrogen-only products

Table 7.6 shows examples of oestrogen-only products and advice about how to use them.

Table 7.6: Routes of administration of oestrogen in HRT

Transdermal estradiol patches Estradot, Evorel, Estraderm Mx (patches changed twice a week) Femseven (patches changed once a week)	Stuck to the skin below the waist (usually on the buttock) Available in a variety of strengths (releasing 25–100mcg estradiol/24hrs) Absorption is proportional to surface area of the patch stuck to the skin If not sticking well, or causing skin irritation, try a different brand (adhesives differ) or consider gel or spray

Table 7.6 *cont'd*	
Transdermal estradiol gel Oestrogel pump dispenser, contains 64 doses (estradiol 0.06% gel, 750mcg per actuation) Sandrena (estradiol single-dose sachets, 0.5mg and 1mg)	Daily application Allow 2–5 minutes to dry. Wash hands. For 2 hours after application avoid showering, applying other creams and direct contact with others/pets to the area of application If using moderate- or high-dose oestrogen, the dose can be divided if the patient prefers (half taken in the morning and half in the evening)
Transdermal estradiol spray Lenzetto 1.53mg/dose transdermal spray	Daily application Prime (prepare) each new carton, by pressing 3 sprays into the cover. Each carton then contains further 56 sprays; advise the patient to calculate how long the canister will last, according to their dose, and document this, so they avoid using an empty carton Hold the spray upright and spray daily to forearm or inner thigh, allow 2 mins to dry Do not overlap the circular areas of spray application Spray onto the same position(s) along the forearm each day; do not rub Keep the skin dry and avoid showering and applying other creams to the area, and close contact with others including pets to that area for 1 hour after application 17β-estradiol and octisalate form a reservoir depot underneath the skin – slow diffusion through the skin and into the microcirculation occurs at a steady rate over 24hrs, before it declines
Estradiol oral tablets Brands/doses include: • Elleste Duet 1mg/2mg • Elleste Solo 1mg/2mg • Zumenon 1mg/2mg	Taken daily Available in 1mg or 2mg tablets Some patients may be taking oral conjugated equine oestrogen, such as Premarin (300mcg, 625mcg, 1.25mg) but estradiol is preferred now
Subdermal oestrogen implant	Not used routinely but available in some clinics

7.9.2 Adjuvant progestogen preparations and recommended doses (to be used cyclically or continuously, alongside an oestrogen product) in HRT

- *Table 7.7* shows examples of progestogens which can be used, if required, alongside the oestrogen products in *Table 7.6*.
- Doses of adjuvant progestogens shown in *Table 7.7* are usually recommended for use alongside low/moderate doses of oestrogen. If higher doses of oestrogen are used, or if there is unscheduled bleeding on HRT, the dose of progestogen may need to be increased (refer to *Table 7.10* and *Section 7.14*).

Table 7.7: Adjuvant progestogens used as part of HRT

Micronised progesterone	Oral progesterone: available as capsules (Utrogestan 100mg, Gepretix 100mg and 200mg, and generic MP 100mg). Take at bedtime, with or without food (better absorbed with food but can lead to side-effects including somnolence/dizziness). Vaginal progesterone (limited evidence about effectiveness/best regime): oral progesterone capsules are not licensed for vaginal use. Utrogestan or Cyclogest 200mg vaginal pessaries and Lutigest 100mg vaginal pessaries are not licensed for endometrial protection as part of HRT. If there are progestogenic side-effects and other progestogens are not suitable, the BMS advises to consider off-label use of Cyclogest, Lutigest or Utrogestan vaginal pessaries or vaginal use of Utrogestan oral capsules. Vaginal dose = oral recommended dose. The BMS does state in its article that generic MP oral capsules or Gepretix oral capsules can be used vaginally. Licensed recommended doses to be used alongside low–moderate-dose oestrogen: • Sequential combined (cyclical) regime: 200mg for a minimum of 12–14 consecutive days per month. In clinical practice is often given 14 days off and 14 days on, or for the first 12–14 days of each calendar month to make it easier to remember • Continuous combined (daily) regime: 100mg daily from day 1–25 of each cycle. In clinical practice as ccHRT, 100mg is used daily without a break. Often better tolerated than other progestogens with fewer side-effects, but not in all women Both Utrogestan and Gepretix capsules contain soya bean lecithin (possible relationship with soya and allergy to peanut, so avoid in patients with peanut allergy)
Dydrogesterone	Available as Nalvee 10mg oral tablets (not available in the UK as 5mg or 2.5mg stand-alone tablets) Recommended dose to be used alongside low–standard-dose oestrogen: • Sequential combined (cyclical) regime: 10mg for a minimum of 14 consecutive days per month
Medroxyprogesterone acetate	Available as Provera Recommended doses to be used alongside low–moderate-dose oestrogen: • Sequential combined (cyclical) regime: 10mg for a minimum of 10–12 consecutive days per month • Continuous combined (daily) regime: 2.5–5mg daily – see *Table 7.10* Note that Provera is not licensed as part of HRT. It may be used, off-licence, but is not available on the HRT prepay certificate in England. MPA in fixed combination products such as Indivinia is licensed for use as HRT and is available on the HRT prepay certificate
Norethisterone	The generic norethisterone is widely used Recommended doses to be used alongside low–moderate-dose oestrogen (see *Table 7.10*): • Sequential combined (cyclical) regime: 5mg for a minimum of 10–12 consecutive days per month • Continuous combined (daily) regime: 5mg daily Note that stand-alone norethisterone is not licensed as part of HRT. It may be used, off-licence, but is not available on the HRT prepay certificate in England. NET in fixed combination products such as Evorel Sequi or Elleste Duet are licensed for use as HRT and available on the HRT prepay certificate NB: 1mg provides endometrial protection for ultra-low to standard dose oestrogen, but the lowest stand-alone dose currently available in the UK is 5mg (off-licence use of three Noriday, i.e. 1.05mg, could be considered if 5mg is not tolerated).
52mg levonorgestrel IUD	All 52mg LNG-IUDs can be used for endometrial protection for up to 5 years, releasing levonorgestrel 20mcg/24hrs

Table 7.7 *cont'd*	
Drospirenone	Can suppress endogenous ovarian activity The BMS states that this can be considered as an equivalent alternative for women who have progestogenic side-effects with other preparations, off-licence; the dose would be 4mg daily, omitting any placebo tablets in the packet
Desogestrel	Can suppress endogenous ovarian activity Desogestrel 75mcg daily (one tablet) cannot be used as the endometrial component of HRT If desogestrel 75mcg is used as contraception in women taking HRT, then the addition of further progestogen (e.g. alongside low-/moderate-dose oestrogen, micronised progesterone 100mg daily, or 200mg for 12/14 days a month) would give adequate endometrial protection The BMS states that earlier studies have shown that desogestrel 150mcg (two tablets daily) is effective as the progestogen component of ccHRT with no increase in the risk of endometrial hyperplasia. Note: some generic versions of desogestrel contain soya bean oil and it is recommended that these products should not be taken by patients who have soya or peanut allergy. For these patients prescribe by brand name and consider Cerelle or Cerazette, neither of which contain soya bean oil

7.9.3 Sequential combined oestrogen and progestogen products

Table 7.8 shows examples of sequential combined HRT products which can be taken transdermally or orally, containing both oestrogen and progestogen.

Table 7.8: Sequential combined oestrogen and progestogen products

Transdermal patches	Evorel Sequi: (four estradiol 50mcg/24hr patches and four estradiol 50mcg/24hr + norethisterone 170mcg/24hr patches). Eight patches in each pack to be taken in order. Patches changed twice a week. Advise patients the patches must be taken in the correct order to avoid unscheduled bleeding.
Oral tablets	Femoston: 1/10mg or 2/10mg • 1/10mg: 14 estradiol 1mg tablets and 14 estradiol 1mg/dydrogesterone 10mg tablets • 2/10mg: 14 estradiol 2mg tablets and 14 estradiol/dydrogesterone 10mg tablets Elleste Duet: 1mg +1mg/1mg or 2mg + 2mg/1mg • 1mg +1mg/1mg: 16 estradiol 1mg tablets and 12 estradiol 1mg/norethisterone 1mg tablets • 2mg + 2mg/1mg: 16 estradiol 2mg tablets and 12 estradiol 2mg/norethisterone 1mg tablets Trisequens: estradiol (varying doses) + 1mg norethisterone • The hormone levels change three times within each packet of tablets and a bleed should occur once a month. 12 blue tablets (estradiol 2mg), 10 white tablets (estradiol 2mg/norethisterone 1mg) and 6 red tablets (estradiol 1mg), during which a bleed should occur.

7.9.4 Continuous combined oestrogen and progestogen products

Table 7.9 shows examples of continuous combined HRT products which can be taken transdermally or orally, containing both oestrogen and progestogen.

Table 7.9: Continuous combined oestrogen and progestogen products

Transdermal patches Patch changed twice a week:	Estradot Conti 30/95 (estradiol 30mcg/24hr + norethisterone 95mcg/24hr) Estradot Conti 40/130 (estradiol 40mcg/24hr + noerethisterone 130mcg/24hr) Evorel Conti patches (estradiol 50mcg/24hr + norethisterone 170mcg/24hr). Eight patches in each pack
Patch changed once a week:	Femseven Conti patches (estradiol 50mcg/24hr + levonorgestrel 7mcg/24hr). Four patches in each pack
Oral tablets	Femoston Conti • Estradiol 500mcg/dydrogesterone 2.5mg tablets • Estradiol 1mg/dydrogesterone 5mg tablets Elleste Duet Conti • Estradiol 2mg/norethisterone 1mg Angeliq • Estradiol 1mg/drospirenone 2mg Indivinia • Estradiol valerate 1mg/MPA 2.5mg • Estradiol valerate 1mg/MPA 5mg • Estradiol valerate 2mg/MPA 5mg Kliofem • Estradiol 2mg/norethisterone 1mg Kliovance • Estradiol 1mg/norethisterone 500mcg Novofem • Estradiol 1mg/norethisterone 1mg Premique low-dose • Conjugated oestrogen 300mcg/medroxyprogesterone 1.5mg modified-release tablets
Oral capsules	Bijuve • Estradiol 1mg + micronised progesterone 100mg
Tibolone	Livial 2.5mg tablets

7.9.5 HRT doses

HRT doses are individualised to each woman; there is no 'one size fits all' and a number of factors will guide which dose of oestrogen and progestogen is recommended. For some women, lower or moderate doses of oestrogen are adequate, but for other women higher doses are required. If a woman increases the dose of oestrogen it is important to make sure that she is taking enough progestogen to provide endometrial protection. To ensure the dose of progestogen is adequate to oppose the dose of oestrogen, the BMS has produced guidance (see *Table 7.10*) which shows a range of oestrogen doses (ultra-low to high) and suggested doses of progestogen, if required, to be used alongside the increasing doses of oestrogen to provide adequate endometrial protection.

The information in *Table 7.10* is a guide only. HRT prescribing must be individualised, and there are some situations clinically where you might consider increasing the dose of progestogen in women who use a moderate dose of oestrogen (for example a woman with risk factors for endometrial cancer, such as obesity). Also if a woman is experiencing unscheduled bleeding on HRT, her HRT regime may need to be changed (see *Section 7.15*).

7.9.6 High-dose oestrogen

- Some women may require higher doses of oestrogen to relieve their symptoms. They may try a variety of different oestrogen products up to the maximum licensed doses and still have difficulty absorbing enough oestrogen to provide relief of their symptoms.
- Evidence is lacking to provide safety data about the optimal dose of progestogen required for endometrial protection to balance high-dose oestrogen (including above licensed doses), and about the effect on breast tissue of taking higher doses of progestogen.
- There are an increasing number of women being prescribed high-dose oestrogen, outside of the product licence. In some women this is reasonable; however, in some women this will result in their serum estradiol levels being very high, and well above those needed to control their menopause symptoms. This can lead to a condition known as tachyphylaxis in which women with high levels of estradiol continue to have menopausal symptoms. They can feel that they need more oestrogen to improve their symptoms, but, in fact, the high serum levels of estradiol may actually be causing the symptoms (including low mood or anxiety) and they need to slowly reduce the dose of oestrogen to improve their symptoms.

Table 7.10: Doses of oestrogen and progestogen in HRT

Oestrogen doses					
	Ultra-low dose	**Low dose**	**Standard dose**	**Moderate dose**	**High dose**
Oestrogel	½ pump	1 pump	2 pumps	3 pumps	4 pumps
Sandrena	0.25mg (½ of a 0.5mg sachet)	0.5mg	1.0mg	1.5–2mg (licensed up to 1.5mg)	3mg (off-licence)
Lenzetto spray	1 spray	2 sprays	3 sprays	4–5 sprays (off-licence)	6 sprays (off-licence)
Patch	12.5mcg/d (½ of a 25mcg/d patch)	25mcg/d	50mcg/d	75mcg/d	100mcg/d
Oral estradiol	0.5mg	1mg	2mg	3mg (off-licence, rarely used)	4mg (off-licence, rarely used)

Progesterone/progestogen doses – the dose may need to be adjusted if there is unscheduled bleeding on HRT								
Oestrogen dose	**Micronised progesterone (oral or vaginal)**		**MPA**		**Dydrogesterone**	**Norethisterone**		**52mg LNG-IUD**
	Continuous	**Sequential**	**Continuous**	**Sequential**	**Sequential**	**Continuous**	**Sequential**	**One for up to 5 years of use for all doses**
Ultra/low	100mg	200mg	2.5mg	10mg	10mg	5mg†	5mg†	
Standard	100mg	200mg	2.5mg/5mg	10mg	10mg	5mg†	5mg†	
Moderate	100mg	200mg	5mg	10mg	20mg*	5mg	5mg	
High	200mg	300mg	10mg	20mg	20mg*	5mg	5mg	

*Dydrogesterone – there are no current guidelines from the BMS about recommended doses to use alongside higher doses of oestrogen. The POI Guideline HCP Toolkit 2024 recommends a dose of 20mg to be used with moderate/high-dose oestrogen cyclically, and for ccHRT it recommends a dose of 5mg daily alongside low/standard doses of oestrogen and 10mg daily alongside moderate- to high-dose oestrogen. A 5mg stand-alone tablet of dydrogesterone is not currently available in the UK.

†1mg provides endometrial protection for ultra-low to standard dose oestrogen but the lowest stand-alone dose currently available in the UK is 5mg (off-licence use of three Noriday i.e. 1.05mg, could be considered if 5mg is not tolerated).

NB: This table is based on information from https://thebms.org.uk/wp-content/uploads/2024/12/01-BMS-GUIDELINE-Management-of-unscheduled-bleeding-HRT-NOVEMBER2024-A.pdf and the POI Guideline HCP Toolkit 2024. It should be used for guidance in conjunction with individualised HRT prescribing.

- In 2023, the BMS and RCGP were co-signatories to a safety alert about the use of high doses of oestrogen, which states that oestrogen should not regularly be prescribed in doses higher than the upper limit listed on the Summary of Product of Characteristics, as shown in *Table 7.10*.
- Some women do require higher doses, and in exceptional cases where higher doses are needed, informed consent should be obtained from the patient, and they should be informed that this is off-licence, and the progestogen should be increased proportionately.
- Consider early referral to a menopause specialist if symptoms are not being adequately managed with licensed doses of oestrogen (having tried a range of products), exclude alternative diagnoses and ensure patient expectations are appropriate.
- The clinician who signs a prescription takes full medical legal responsibility for the effect and adverse effects of that medication. A GP can prescribe on behalf of a specialist if they are happy that it is safe to do this. If this is not the case, they can ask the specialist to continue prescribing.
- Refer to the GMC guidance on prescribing unlicensed medication: www.gmc-uk.org/professional-standards/the-professional-standards/good-practice-in-prescribing-and-managing-medicines-and-devices/prescribing-unlicensed-medicines.

7.10 Testing oestrogen levels

- The aim of HRT, taken by women aged 45 and over, is not to restore the physiological serum levels occurring in ovulatory cycles of fertile women, but to improve the menopausal symptoms.
- It is rarely necessary to measure oestrogen levels, but it can be helpful in some cases. If you do feel it necessary, consider the reason you are checking it and how you will approach the result. Consider testing in the following circumstances:
  - If there is poor symptom relief as dose of estradiol increases, it can be helpful to aid the decision to discuss other causes for symptoms. However, if a patient has ongoing symptoms, then listening to their symptoms, providing holistic care and changing their HRT regime may be more helpful than measuring a serum estradiol level.
    - A very low/unmeasurable level suggests no absorption through a product.
  - In women with POI there is no HRT monitoring strategy, but testing can be helpful in women with POI and early menopause if they have poor symptom relief or there are concerns about adequate bone protection.
- Advise women who are having hormone blood tests to avoid contamination of the result, by avoiding applying any hormone gel/spray to the arm from which the blood will be taken, in the days preceding the blood test.
- When interpreting results consider that serum estradiol levels fluctuate slightly, even when using the same oestrogen regime, after long-term use, and in individual women.
- Estradiol levels do not reflect how a woman might feel. Some women feel very well with lower estradiol levels and others feel well with higher ones. Blood levels cannot reliably predict symptom control.
- Estradiol levels vary between different laboratories because of different methods of testing, so results from different labs cannot be compared. Mass spectrometry is the best method for measuring estradiol levels.
- Try not to test serum estradiol in perimenopause because assays do not differentiate between endogenous or exogenous estradiol and free or protein-bound oestrogen, and endogenous oestrogen levels fluctuate wildly.
- The level of serum estradiol to prevent loss of bone density or prevent osteoporotic-related fractures is not known.
- If a patient is taking oral estradiol, a significant percentage is metabolised to estrone, so checking serum estradiol is not helpful.

- Refer to the BMS Tool for clinicians: *Measurement of serum estradiol in the menopause transition:* https://thebms.org.uk/wp-content/uploads/2025/07/24-NEW-BMS-ToolsforClinicians-Measurement-of-serum-estradiol-JULY2025-B.pdf.

7.11 Contraindications to HRT

There are very few women who cannot take HRT. If a woman has menopausal symptoms and there are contraindications or cautions to prescribing HRT, or if there is any uncertainty about the most appropriate management options, advice should be sought from a healthcare professional with expertise in menopause.

Refer to NICE guidance *Menopause: identification and management* [NG23] for a list of conditions stated as contraindications or cautions to prescribing HRT. NICE states that HRT should not be prescribed in women with:

- Current, past or suspected breast cancer. It also states that in exceptional circumstances women with severe menopause symptoms (and a history of breast cancer) can be offered HRT (off-label) after a discussion about the associated risks. Seek advice from oncology and a healthcare professional with expertise in menopause.
- A known or suspected oestrogen-sensitive cancer (such as some endometrial or ovarian cancers).
- Undiagnosed abnormal vaginal bleeding (investigate and manage first).
- Untreated endometrial hyperplasia.
- Previous idiopathic or current VTE (seek advice from Haematology).
- Active or recent thromboembolic disease, such as angina or myocardial infarction (seek advice from Cardiology).
- Thrombophilic disorder (seek advice from Haematology and see *Section 7.17.2*).
- Active liver disease with abnormal LFTs.
- Pregnancy.

There are some medical conditions where HRT can be prescribed, but you need to consider the HRT regime prescribed (e.g. oral or transdermal oestrogen and type of progestogen), and you may need to monitor the medical condition or seek advice from a specialist before prescribing. See *Section 7.17.1*.

NICE states to prescribe HRT with caution in women with: acute porphyrias; diabetes mellitus (increased risk of CHD); risk factors predisposing them to VTE; history of breast nodules or fibrocystic disease (risk of breast cancer); history of endometrial hyperplasia; hypophyseal tumours, increased risk of gallbladder disease, migraine, epilepsy; increased risk of breast cancer (consider family history of breast cancer), endometriosis (due to the potential risk of disease reactivation and malignant transformation); uterine fibroids (may increase in size).

7.12 Managing patients taking HRT

- Review 3 months after initiation of HRT, after dose or product change and once stable, annually thereafter.
- Help women to make informed choices about whether to continue or change HRT, based on their individual risk profile, considering how this may change over time.
- As a woman ages, her risks change, particularly with thrombotic risk and risk of breast cancer. Rather than stopping HRT she may prefer to change the preparation of HRT to one that is safer for her (such as from oral oestrogen to transdermal oestrogen).
- Assessment includes:
  - HRT compliance, symptom control, side-effects, bleeding pattern, new health concerns, change in family history, medication and OTC treatments, contraception needs; reassess BP and weight.

   - Adjust dose, route and hormone choice, as needed.
   - If she is having any unscheduled bleeding on HRT, after an assessment it may be necessary to adjust her HRT regime or arrange for an examination and further tests to investigate the cause; see *Section 7.15*.
   - Ensure monthly progestogen dose is adequate for oestrogen, both in dose and duration.
   - Check a 52mg LNG-IUD has been fitted within the last 5 years, if being used as part of HRT for endometrial protection.
   - Check if a sequential regime should be changed to a continuous regime; see *Section 7.4.2*.
   - Ask about libido, consider the need for testosterone therapy. If taking testosterone, arrange any recommended monitoring blood tests. See *Section 7.18*.
   - Ask about symptoms of GSM, consider the need to add localised vaginal oestrogen (see *Section 6.7*).
- Advise about national screening programmes, including cervical and breast.
- Remind about the importance of healthy lifestyle choices. Advise about bone health, including dietary calcium, adequate vitamin D and exercise for bone health.
- Manage other health conditions and risk factors.

7.12.1 How long does it take for HRT to work?

- Vasomotor symptoms: 1–3 months.
- Urogenital symptoms: 3–6 months.
- Psychological symptoms: variable response.

7.12.2 Poor response to HRT

There are several reasons for this; consider:
- Too soon for symptom response.
- Oestrogen dose not high enough, or too high.
- Poor compliance with HRT.
- Absorption poor from one product, try an alternative product.
- Symptoms not due to menopause.
- Discuss lifestyle pillars in detail; consider their effect upon symptoms.

7.13 Stopping HRT

- There is no limit on the length of time a woman can use HRT. Some women use it for a few years, others may need it for longer.
- If a decision is made to stop HRT it may be best to withdraw it slowly, reducing the dose to reduce risk of recurrent symptoms, and if symptoms do recur then recommence treatment.
- Some data suggests an increased risk of death from cardiac causes and stroke in women who stop HRT under the age of 60, which was not seen if HRT was stopped after the age of 60. For this reason, it may be best not to stop HRT unnecessarily before the age of 60; however, there is currently no specific guidance on this.
- If HRT is stopped, discuss the importance of healthy lifestyle choices to protect from future health conditions including cardiovascular disease, osteoporosis, genitourinary syndrome of the menopause and dementia.
- If a woman has GSM symptoms, then continuing low-dose localised vaginal oestrogen, if systemic HRT is stopped, should be advised.
- If symptoms return, and are affecting quality of life, HRT can be restarted.

7.14 Side-effects of HRT

- Both oestrogen and progestogen can cause side-effects in some women. *Table 7.11* explains some of the side-effects and how to manage them.

Table 7.11: Side-effects of oestrogen and progestogen and ways to manage these

Oestrogen	
Side-effects	• Headache • Nausea/dyspepsia • Bloating / fluid retention • Breast tenderness or enlargement • Leg cramps (may be continuous or randomly throughout the cycle) • Anxiety • Bleeding • Oral oestrogen increases SHBG levels, which can result in lower free testosterone concentrations. This may be a benefit if women are noticing postmenopausal hirsutism, but a problem if women experience a low libido whilst taking oral oestrogen
How to manage side-effects	• Reduce the dose of oestrogen • Change the route or type • Wean up slowly • Exclude other causes for symptoms
Progestogen	
Side-effects	• Bloating / fluid retention • Breast tenderness • Headaches • Acne • Mood symptoms • Drowsiness (with MP)
How to manage side-effects	• Change the type of progestogen, consider the receptor activity which could cause side-effects (see *Section 7.2.2*) • MP is generally better tolerated than other progestogens; consider vaginal use of some micronised progesterone products if oral use causes mood or GI side-effects (see *Table 7.7*) • DYG can also be better tolerated • In eligible women consider a CHC method • Change to ccHRT (which can be better tolerated than a cyclical progestogen regime in some women) • Consider tibolone (may reduce progestogenic adverse effects for postmenopausal women) • Consider DRSP as an alternative progestogen • For women with severe progestogen intolerance refer to a menopause specialist clinic if symptoms persist despite trial of alternative progestogens. Depending on the woman, here they can discuss use of alternative HRT regimes (with progestogens used in different doses and durations, with appropriate endometrial monitoring) or use of GnRH agonists with add-back HRT, or tibolone. For some women, surgical removal of the ovaries with use of add-back HRT is needed • Refer for mental health support as needed (see *Chapter 8*), particularly consider hormone sensitivity in women with a history of PMS, PMDD and PND

- Research suggests a complex relationship between oestrogen and histamine systems, though direct evidence for oestrogen causing histamine intolerance (HIT) is currently limited.
  - Oestrogen may stimulate histamine release (and influence histamine metabolism), and in turn, histamine can also stimulate oestrogen release.
  - Susceptible women in their 40s in perimenopause (with fluctuating high/low oestrogen levels) may develop new allergies or intolerances (often to alcohol or certain types of food) or may find atopic symptoms worsen, such as hayfever, asthma or eczema.
  - Adding HRT may improve some menopause symptoms but may worsen symptoms related to histamine, which can include a variety of symptoms including gastrointestinal issues, headaches (including migraine), skin reactions, and respiratory problems such as asthma.
  - This can be managed by supporting gut health and making dietary modifications, reducing stress, making adjustments to HRT, and some women benefit from taking antihistamines. Specialist dietary advice may be helpful for some women.
- Many women are concerned about weight gain during perimenopause and menopause. There is no evidence that HRT causes weight gain.

7.15 Unscheduled bleeding on HRT

- What is unscheduled bleeding on HRT?
  - Irregular bleeding which occurs after initiating or changing a 'bleed-free' HRT – continuous combined HRT (ccHRT).
  - Irregular bleeding which occurs in addition to the expected monthly withdrawal bleed in women taking sequential combined HRT (sHRT).
- It is common to have unscheduled bleeding within the first 6 months of initiating HRT, or within 3 months of a change in HRT dose or preparation in women who are already taking HRT. This can affect up to 38% of people using sHRT and 41% using ccHRT. It can lead to repeated GP consultations and to women stopping their HRT.
- In order to provide recommendations for management of unscheduled bleeding according to risk of endometrial cancer, the following joint guideline has been produced on behalf of the BMS: *Management of unscheduled bleeding on HRT* (https://thebms.org.uk/publications/bms-joint-guidelines/management-of-unscheduled-bleeding-on-hormone-replacement-therapy-hrt/). This section covers some of the recommendations in the guideline.
- When HRT is initiated, it is important to advise women of the bleeding pattern to expect with their HRT regime, what constitutes unscheduled bleeding and when to seek medical advice.

Normal bleeding pattern expected with sequential combined HRT

- This regime of HRT should give a regular withdrawal bleed at or towards the end of the progestogen phase, usually lighter or similar to the woman's previous bleeding. It can take 6 months to settle into this bleeding pattern when sHRT is commenced, and 3 months after a dose adjustment.
- Abnormal bleeding on this type of HRT is persistent irregular bleeding, prolonged bleeding, intermenstrual bleeding, postcoital bleeding, the development of pain with bleeding or bleeding that becomes increasingly heavy.
- Advise women given an sHRT regime that they must take their progestogen, as prescribed, no matter what happens to their bleeding pattern, and they must not 'cut short' their time taking progestogen.

Normal bleeding pattern expected with continuous combined HRT

- With this regime of HRT women should be amenorrhoeic after 6 months.

7.15.1 Assessment of women who have unscheduled bleeding on HRT

- This should aim to consider all the causes for abnormal vaginal bleeding. Review their HRT regime, their bleeding pattern before and while taking HRT, and their risk factors for endometrial cancer.
- Ask about other symptoms including pelvic pain, vaginal discharge and symptoms of GSM.
- Include in the history:
  - Bleeding history – how often, duration of bleeding, regularity (such as mid cycle or prior to a withdrawal bleed), type of bleeding (light, heavy, flooding) or postcoital bleeding.
  - Duration since initiation of current HRT regime / prior use of HRT / changes in HRT preparation.
    - Treatment change: an increased oestrogen dose may trigger bleeding due to increased endometrial stimulation.
  - Compliance: exactly how has she been using HRT (both hormones)?
    - Missed doses of progestogen can trigger an unscheduled bleed (consider holidays, when there is a time change or medication can be forgotten).
    - If using a patch, where is it stuck, does it stick well / cause skin irritation?
    - If using an oestrogen gel/spray, are they being applied correctly?
    - Is her 52mg LNG-IUD correctly sited, has it been fitted within the last 5 years?
    - Has she adjusted her HRT herself?
  - Check that the monthly progestogen dose is proportionate to oestrogen dose and taken for the correct duration each month. In women using sHRT, ensure a minimum of 10 days NET or MPA, 12 days of micronised progesterone, or 14 days of dydrogesterone per month is being taken.
  - If taking high-dose oestrogen, is she taking adequate progestogen? There is limited evidence about the optimal dose of progestogen required for endometrial protection when high-dose oestrogen is used, but *Table 7.10* summarises the current recommendations.
  - Is she taking sHRT or ccHRT? If sHRT, are the pills or patches being taken in the correct order? Women >45 years taking sHRT should be offered a change to ccHRT after 5 years of use or by the age of 54 (whichever comes first).
  - Are there endometrial cancer risk factors other than HRT? These can be divided into minor risk factors (including BMI >30kg/m^2, diabetes and PCOS) and major risk factors (including BMI ≥40, Lynch/Cowden's syndrome).
  - Family history: including Lynch/Cowden's syndrome.
  - Contraception use (consider pregnancy risk).
  - Sexual history.
  - Cervical screening history.
  - Drug interactions (GLP-1 agonists, anti-epileptics, anti-fungals, Covid vaccinations, herbal medicines such as St John's wort / other sources of oestrogen such as compounded bioidentical hormones).
  - Gastrointestinal upset (which can interfere with absorption).
- Offer an examination:
  - Abdominal and pelvic: assessing for pain, bulky uterus (fibroids) or an ovarian mass.
  - Vulval and vaginal examination, looking for atrophy, ulceration, skin lesions and prolapse.
  - Visualise the cervix, looking for abnormal features, a polyp, an ectropion, and checking IUD threads are in place. This is particularly important in women who are not up to date with the cervical screening programme, or who have had previous abnormal cytology or a polyp.
  - Where relevant, consider investigations including cervical screening; lower genital tract swabs; BMI and a pregnancy test.
- Offer vaginal oestrogen if there are symptoms of GSM or atrophic findings on examination.

7.15.2 Managing HRT after unscheduled bleeding

- The BMS guideline (available at https://thebms.org.uk/publications/bms-guidelines/management-of-unscheduled-bleeding-on-hormone-replacement-therapy-hrt) advises to assess cancer risk factors and bleeding pattern, to identify the HRT regime, duration and compliance, to offer an examination and investigations such as cervical screening or genital swabs if indicated.
- It advises what major and minor risk factors for endometrial cancer are, and a flow chart considers these with the time of taking HRT and bleeding pattern; it then advises if HRT can be optimised and when a review might be advised, or if an urgent transvaginal scan is advised to investigate further. This is a live document so it is not included here, but please refer to it to help with managing cases of unscheduled bleeding on HRT.
- It advises that persistent unscheduled bleeding continuing for more than 4–6 months after initiation of HRT requires investigation.

7.15.3 Adjusting HRT to reduce episodes of unscheduled bleeding

- The BMS guideline recommends that in some cases HRT can be optimised to manage the unscheduled bleeding; if this is the case, *Table 7.12* includes options to consider. More detail is included in the BMS guideline.

Table 7.12: Some recommendations for reducing and managing unscheduled bleeding on HRT, summarised from the BMS guidance

General advice	If compliance is a problem with hormones prescribed separately, then consider a combined preparation (which might be easier to remember than taking the hormones separately) Offer the 52mg LNG-IUD, if appropriate*, to women initiating HRT, particularly if contraception is also required Offer change of 52mg LNG-IUD if new-onset unscheduled bleeding at 4 years of use and investigations are normal (particularly if BMI ≥40). In women with a BMI >30, offer weight management support, the 52mg LNG-IUD; increase MP to 200mg continuous or 300mg sequential; reduce oestrogen dose and consider non-hormonal options
Unscheduled bleeding on sHRT in women in perimenopause	Offer a 52mg LNG-IUD* Add desogestrel, which can suppress endogenous ovarian activity If <50 years, and low risk for VTE, consider switching HRT to a COC If low risk for VTE, consider changing to an oral HRT preparation Increase the MP dose to 300mg for 12 days a month from 200mg, or increase the duration of MP use from 14 days to 21 days a month, or change to a synthetic progestogen 3-month trial of an additional progestogen on top of the current preparation (this can also be done in women using the 52mg LNG-IUD) Reduce the oestrogen dose and use non-hormonal alternatives
Unscheduled bleeding on ccHRT in women in perimenopause	Offer a 52mg LNG-IUD If low risk for VTE, consider changing to an oral HRT preparation Increase the MP dose or change to a synthetic progestogen 3-month trial of an additional progestogen on top of the current preparation (this can also be done in women using the 52mg LNG-IUD) Consider switching back to sHRT for 6 months, in women who are recently postmenopausal Reduce the oestrogen dose and use non-hormonal alternatives

*May not be suitable for women who have a uterine malformation, submucosal fibroids >3cm, a history of trauma or endometrial ablation.

7.16 Benefits and risks of taking HRT

- When counselling women about the risks and benefits of taking HRT it is important to consider that the menopause transition can have a significant impact on many women, with 75% experiencing menopausal symptoms and 25% experiencing severe symptoms. The average duration of menopausal symptoms is 7 years, but around 30% of women experience long-term symptoms.
- HRT has been shown to improve quality of life and it is the most effective treatment for menopause symptoms.
- Informed consent involves discussing the overall benefits associated with HRT use, including relief of menopausal symptoms, improved quality of life, the long-term impact on cardiovascular and bone health balanced by the risks, including risk of breast cancer. The decision whether to take HRT, the dose and how long HRT is taken for must be individualised to the woman, discussing benefits and risks.
- When HRT is used for a clear reason and commenced within a few years of menopause, in most women the benefits outweigh the risks.
- Benefits and risks are summarised in the NICE guidelines, which were updated in 2024 (*Menopause: identification and management* [NG23]). Some of its recommendations were controversial and the BMS produced a response upon its release to discuss the limitations of the guideline: https://thebms.org.uk/2024/11/bms-statement-in-response-to-the-publication-of-the-updated-nice-menopause-guideline-ng23.

7.16.1 Benefits of HRT

- The benefits, in healthy women who have a naturally timed menopause and do not have contraindications or a hormone-related cancer, depend on the type of HRT taken, the duration of use and the woman's medical history.
- It is the most effective treatment to relieve menopausal symptoms, such as VMS, fatigue, sleep and mood changes, and GSM.
- Oestrogen therapy in HRT reduces the risk of hip, vertebral and other fractures in women with normal bone density, osteopenia and osteoporosis, and improves bone density. This benefit is maintained while HRT is being taken but decreases once HRT is stopped.
- Cardiovascular protection in healthy younger and midlife women:
  - The timing of initiation of HRT is referred to as the 'cardiovascular window of opportunity' and the 'timing hypothesis' and may have an impact on the risk of CVD in women who take HRT.
  - Cochrane data analysis shows that HRT initiated within 10 years of the menopause is likely to be associated with a reduction in both coronary heart disease (CHD) and cardiovascular mortality. This reduction was not seen in women who initiated HRT more than 10 years after menopause. However, both the WHI long-term follow-up and Cochrane analysis showed that there was no significant increase in the risk of cardiovascular events, cardiovascular mortality or all-cause mortality in women who started HRT more than 10 years after menopause, or beyond the age of 60. Otherwise healthy women beyond the age of 60 or more than 10 years after their menopause can benefit from taking HRT to relieve ongoing menopausal symptoms, if there are no contraindications and the benefits outweigh the risks.
- Additional potential benefits include reduced risk of colorectal cancer (with combined HRT), and oestrogen may benefit sarcopenia.
- See *Sections 6.8* and *6.10* for the benefits of taking HRT in POI / early menopause and surgical menopause.

7.16.2 Risks of HRT

- As with all medicines, there are risks associated with taking HRT. The risks in healthy women with a naturally timed menopause, without contraindications or a hormone-related cancer depend on the type of HRT taken, the duration of use and the woman's medical history and include:

Venous thromboembolism (VTE)

- Route of oestrogen: compared with women not taking HRT:
  - The risk of VTE is increased (2–4-fold) by use of oral HRT (oestrogen alone or oestrogen with progestogen).
  - Evidence shows that the use of transdermal oestrogen is unlikely to increase the risk of VTE.
- Type of progestogen:
  - Evidence shows that micronised progesterone, dydrogesterone and the 52mg LNG-IUD are unlikely to increase risk of VTE compared to the risk of using other oral progestogens.
- Tibolone is not associated with an increased risk of VTE. The main vascular concern with tibolone is the increased risk of stroke.

Breast cancer

- Misinformation about the risks of breast cancer and HRT over the past 20 years has resulted in a fear to prescribe among health professionals and fear among women who do not have a true understanding of the possible risks and benefits of HRT.
- Breast cancer affects 1 in 7 women in the UK in their lifetime. Risk of developing breast cancer rises slowly with age, whether HRT is taken or not. 80% of breast cancers are diagnosed over the age of 50.
- The baseline risk of breast cancer for women varies according to their age, their inherited genetic susceptibility and their environmental and lifestyle risk factors.
- Evidence which should be taken into account when discussing HRT and breast cancer risk with women is summarised in this BMS consensus statement (https://thebms.org.uk/wp-content/uploads/2025/09/08-BMS-ConsensusStatement-Benefits-risks-of-HRT-before-after-a-breast-cancer-diagnosis-SEPT2025-B.pdf).

Keep it simple summary

When discussing the association between HRT and breast cancer it is helpful to consider advice which can be given to women who have a low (baseline population) risk of breast cancer (most women) and to those at higher risk of breast cancer (who may have a strong family history of breast cancer or carry a genetic mutation).

1. You can advise all women that their individual risk of breast cancer is influenced by a range of factors, including their age, family history, age at puberty and number of pregnancies. Lifestyle factors also play a significant role: obesity, smoking, drinking ≥2 units of alcohol per day can increase breast cancer risk, while engaging in regular moderate-intensity exercise (at least 2.5 hours per week) helps to reduce it. It is important to be breast aware and attend mammography screening.
2. HRT is the most effective treatment to relieve the symptoms of menopause and it is important to balance the benefits of taking HRT (improving symptoms and quality of life, providing protection against cardiovascular disease and osteoporosis) with the risks of taking HRT (small increased risk of breast cancer).
3. In women with a low baseline risk of breast cancer (most women), the benefit of using HRT for up to 5 years to relieve their symptoms is greater than any potential risk.
4. The type of HRT regime and the duration it is used for can affect risk of breast cancer:
   - Use of oestrogen-only HRT is associated with little or no change in breast cancer risk.

- Use of combined HRT (oestrogen plus a progestogen) can be associated with a duration-dependent increase in risk of breast cancer. Currently it is thought combined HRT (used for up to 5 years) is not associated with a significant increased risk of breast cancer, but if it is used for longer than 5 years it is associated with a small increase in risk of breast cancer. This increase in risk is less than the risk associated with being overweight in women over 50 years, or with drinking ≥2 units of alcohol a day. When HRT is stopped the risk of breast cancer reduces, but may rise again a number of years after stopping HRT due to the effect of HRT on the growth of microscopic (undetectable) cancer cells in the breast. When HRT is started the rate of growth of these cancers could increase (so they are discovered sooner), but when HRT is stopped, the rate of growth slows, but they still continue to grow slowly, so can be discovered years after HRT is stopped.

5. The dose of oestrogen in HRT does not affect risk of breast cancer.
6. Choice of progestogen may affect risk; evidence suggests that micronised progesterone and dydrogesterone are associated with a lower risk of breast cancer compared to that of other progestogens.
7. Vaginal oestrogen is not associated with an increased risk of breast cancer.
8. In women with POI or early menopause, their years of HRT exposure is counted from age 50.

How does taking HRT impact upon the risk of breast cancer in a woman with no personal history of breast cancer, but who has a family history of breast cancer?

- It is important to take a family history of cancer before prescribing HRT (see *Section 6.4*). It may be that a woman needs to be referred to secondary care or for genetic screening, depending on the age and number of relatives with breast or ovarian cancer, to find out her own risk of breast cancer.
- Refer to *Section 12.4,* which discusses risk of breast cancer and explains baseline risk (low underlying risk of breast cancer, i.e. most of the population), moderate risk and high risk of breast cancer.
- Inherited genetic susceptibility can increase the likelihood of a diagnosis at any age, but contributes to a higher proportion of cases in younger women.
- Only 5–10% of breast cancers are caused by having an inherited faulty gene such as a *BRCA* mutation. *BRCA1* and *BRCA2* are genes that produce proteins that help to repair damaged DNA. Mutations in these genes disrupt their normal function and can lead to an increased risk of cancer, particularly breast and ovary. One in 450 people in the UK carries a *BRCA* mutation (one in 40 women of Ashkenazi Jewish descent), and men can be carriers.
- The BMS states that, *"there is no strong evidence that taking HRT further increases risk of breast cancer in women with a family history of breast cancer or personal diagnosis of a high-risk benign breast condition (i.e. lobular carcinoma* in situ, *atypical hyperplasia)".*
- However, it also recommends that in high-risk women (with a familial risk or a high-risk benign breast condition), lifestyle and non-hormonal treatments are used first-line to manage vasomotor symptoms. HRT can be considered in individual women suffering from persistent symptoms, following a discussion with a menopause specialist.
- High-risk women with *BRCA1* and *BRCA2* mutations and who have had prophylactic risk-reducing bilateral salpingo-oophorectomy can use HRT to manage menopause symptoms until the age of 50, without increasing their risk of breast cancer. After age 50, lifestyle changes and non-hormonal alternatives should be used.

Coronary heart disease (CHD)

- CHD is a leading cause of death in women. The risk of CHD for women around the age of menopause varies according to their individual cardiovascular risk factors.
- Hormonal changes, particularly involving sex hormones, influence the risk of acute coronary artery disease. Oestrogen has protective effects on the cardiovascular system, including vasodilation, anti-inflammatory properties and favourable lipid profiles.

- Having cardiovascular risk factors, such as hypertension, is not a contraindication to taking HRT, if they are optimally managed.
- HRT should not be used for primary prevention of cardiovascular disease in asymptomatic women who go through a natural menopause after the age of 45. HRT should not be used for secondary prevention of cardiovascular disease.
- For women with established ischaemic heart disease who continue to experience vasomotor symptoms despite non-hormonal treatment, decisions about using HRT should be made through a shared decision-making approach. Consider seeking advice from a healthcare professional with expertise in menopause, and if HRT is initiated, then the BMS recommends a transdermal route with low-dose oestrogen and a non-androgenic progestogen when necessary (see *Section 7.16.3*).
- Refer to the BMS consensus statement *Primary prevention of coronary heart disease in women*: https://thebms.org.uk/wp-content/uploads/2024/12/22-BMS-TfC-Management-of-menopause-for-women-with-CVD-DEC2024-A.pdf.

Stroke

- Oral oestrogen is associated with a slight increase in the risk of stroke. Transdermal oestrogen does not appear to increase the risk of stroke above the baseline risk for that woman. Transdermal oestrogen at the lowest effective dose is preferred for women who have an increased risk of stroke.
- Women under the age of 60 have a very low risk of stroke so can consider taking HRT with an oral oestrogen, if there are no risk factors for VTE. Women >60 years have a higher baseline risk of stroke, so transdermal oestrogen is preferred.
- Micronised progesterone or dydrogesterone are the preferred progestogen choices in women who are at increased risk of stroke.
- Tibolone has been shown to increase the risk of stroke (2-fold). For women older than about 60 years, the risks associated with tibolone start to outweigh the benefits because of the increased risk of stroke.

Endometrial cancer

- Oestrogen-only HRT given to women with a uterus increases the risk of endometrial hyperplasia and endometrial cancer.
- The risk is reduced by addition of a progestogen. The dose of progestogen must be proportionate to the dose of oestrogen (see *Table 7.10*).
- The progestogen must be used for the correct duration each month to provide adequate endometrial protection (see *Table 7.7*).
- Consider risk factors for endometrial cancer, such as BMI >30kg/m^2, PCOS and diabetes when prescribing, and encourage the use of the 52mg LNG-IUD in women at higher risk.
- Follow advice about changing from sequential HRT to continuous combined HRT (see *Section 7.3.5*).

Ovarian cancer

- There may be a small increase in the risk of developing ovarian cancer (serous and endometrioid) associated with the use of HRT.

T2DM

- Taking HRT is not associated with an increased risk of developing diabetes.
- In women with diabetes, HRT is not associated with an adverse effect on their blood glucose.
- The progestogen choice can affect insulin sensitivity and lipids (see *Section 7.16.3*).

Dementia

- NICE NG23 states that dementia risk may increase with combined HRT if started above age 64.
- HRT started in women under the age of 60 is unlikely to increase risk of dementia.

7.16.3 Individualising HRT for metabolic health

- The menopausal transition is linked to a rise in cardiometabolic risk, primarily driven by central obesity, diabetes, hypertension and dyslipidaemia.
- Some HRT regimes, when given to perimenopausal or early postmenopausal women, have been shown to have beneficial effects on lipid profiles, insulin sensitivity, body composition, arterial stiffness and chronic inflammation, contributing to a positive overall risk–benefit profile.
- Effect of HRT on lipids:
    - Evidence shows that generally, HRT is associated with favourable changes in lipids.
        - Oral oestrogen can lower LDL cholesterol and increase HDL cholesterol.
        - MPA and NET can lower lipoprotein(a).
        - Transdermal oestrogen is more lipid-neutral.
        - Adding an oral androgenic progestogen can reduce the benefit oestrogen has on lipids. Non-androgenic progestogens (such as micronised progesterone and dydrogesterone) have a neutral effect on the lipid profile.
- Effect of HRT on insulin resistance:
    - Oestrogen improves insulin sensitivity (oral oestrogen is better than transdermal).
    - Androgenic progestogens can worsen insulin resistance. Non-androgenic progestogens have a neutral effect.
- Micronised progesterone and dydrogesterone have neutral effects on lipids and insulin resistance when compared to androgenic progestogens.
- When considering individualising HRT in women with cardiometabolic/vascular risk factors, transdermal oestrogen is preferred.
- Micronised progesterone, dydrogesterone and the 52mg LNG-IUD are preferred progestogen options where there is increased vascular risk (e.g. T2DM, CVD and women >60).

7.17 Prescribing HRT in certain groups

7.17.1 Migraine

- Migraine attacks can be more prevalent in perimenopause, associated with oestrogen fluctuations. Prevalence of migraine improves over time after the menopause.
- Women with migraine, including migraine with aura, can take HRT. CHC is contraindicated in women with migraine with aura, if it is taken for the purpose of contraception.
- HRT uses estradiol, producing similar levels to the oestrogen during the menstrual cycle, so women with migraine, including those with aura, can consider taking oral HRT. However, aura can occur for the first time or can worsen after starting HRT, and this is more likely to occur with oral rather than transdermal oestrogen. For this reason, if HRT is initiated in women with migraine with aura, the transdermal route is the preferred first option.
- If HRT is given to women with migraine (with or without aura), transdermal oestrogen preparations, favouring a patch or gel, starting with low-dose oestrogen gradually increasing to control symptoms without exacerbating migraine, are preferred. Some women benefit from starting with a quarter of a 25mcg oestrogen patch and weaning up very slowly, for example.
- Use of vaginal oestrogens may cause a temporary increase in migraine during the first few weeks, but this usually quickly settles.
- Ensure information is provided about triggers, acute migraine attacks, supplements, preventer treatment, and new treatments.
- Resources include:
    - www.nationalmigrainecentre.org.uk/understanding-migraine/what-is-migraine
    - https://thebms.org.uk/wp-content/uploads/2022/12/06-BMS-TfC-Migraine-and-HRT-NOV2022-A.pdf

HRT and migraine in perimenopause

- HRT started in perimenopause, when oestrogen levels are fluctuating, can lead to a worsening of migraine.
- Sequential HRT use in perimenopause does not provide hormonal stability. In women with migraine without aura, hormonal stability in perimenopause can be provided by use of continuous combined hormonal contraception until age 50 in eligible women. Consider the oral COC with estradiol or estetrol, given continuously, with no hormone-free interval, if there are no contraindications, and refer to UKMEC.
- Alternative HRT options for women with migraine (with or without aura) include the use of transdermal estradiol and if progestogen is required, taking it continuously is recommended, with preparations such as:
  - A 52mg LNG-IUD (replaced within 5 years).
  - Transdermal norethisterone (as continuous combined patches).
  - Micronised progesterone daily.
  - Drospirenone 4mg daily, omitting the 4 hormone-free pills in the pack, off-licence.
  - Desogestrel 75mcg daily plus 100mg Utrogestan daily (or 150mg desogestrel daily, off-licence). DRSP and DSG POPs suppress ovarian activity, which can benefit some women with migraine.
- Seek advice from a menopause specialist with expertise in migraine if symptoms are not controlled.

7.17.2 Women with a personal history of VTE or an inherited thrombophilic disorder

- Having a heritable/acquired thrombophilia or a previous history of VTE is not an absolute contraindication to HRT. Alternative treatments should be offered first and if HRT is considered, a clear discussion about the risks and benefits of using HRT should be well documented. The use of transdermal oestrogen and micronised progesterone is unlikely to significantly increase the VTE risk above the individual's own risk.
- Refer to haematology for advice about women who are particularly high risk for VTE before considering HRT. HRT can be considered after haematology review. Concomitant use of anticoagulation may be required in some cases. Use of CHC is contraindicated.
- If HRT is initiated, avoid oral oestrogen. Low-dose transdermal oestrogen, with oral micronised progesterone, dydrogesterone or a 52mg LNG-IUD, where required, are the preferred options.
- Identify and address ongoing risk factors.

7.17.3 Women with a personal history of coronary disease or stroke

- NICE NG 23 advises that for women with a personal history of coronary heart disease or stroke, ensure that HRT is discussed with and offered, if appropriate, by a healthcare professional with expertise in menopause.
- Refer to: https://thebms.org.uk/wp-content/uploads/2024/12/22-BMS-TfC-Management-of-menopause-for-women-with-CVD-DEC2024-A.pdf.

7.17.4 Women over 60, or more than 10 years after menopause

- 30–40% of women in their 60s and 70s have ongoing VMS. Investigate new-onset VMS, considering diagnoses such as hyperthyroidism and phaeochromocytoma.
- HRT can be initiated in women over the age of 60 who have ongoing symptoms of menopause, if there are no contraindications, and the benefits outweigh the risks.
- Lower doses should be started and slowly increased to achieve symptom control, preferably with a transdermal oestrogen and if required, micronised progesterone, considering individual benefit vs. risk.

7.17.5 History of fibroid

- Both oestrogen and progesterone can contribute to fibroid growth, but many women with fibroids can take HRT. If there is concern seek advice from secondary care.

7.17.6 Epilepsy

- Epilepsy may be affected by hormone fluctuations in perimenopause.
- HRT can be used in patients with epilepsy, but their epilepsy should be monitored when HRT is initiated or changed in case the anti-epileptic drugs need to be adjusted.
- It is thought that oestrogen increases seizure risk and that progesterone may have anti-seizure effects.
- In women with epilepsy use of transdermal oestrogen is preferred and if a progestogen is required, oral micronised progesterone may have benefits for epilepsy (more research is needed).
- Lamotrigine does not affect the levels of HRT, but HRT can decrease blood levels of lamotrigine, which consequently may affect epilepsy control.
- Some other anti-epileptic medication can reduce the effect of HRT, so higher doses of HRT may be required to achieve symptom control.
- Consider seeking the advice of a neurologist.
- Consider interactions with HRT and epilepsy medications when prescribing. Refer to:
  - *WHC fact sheet: Epilepsy, the Menopause and HRT* (www.womens-health-concern.org/wp-content/uploads/2024/01/32-WHC-FACTSHEET-Epilepsy-the-menopause-and-HRT-JAN2024-A.pdf).

7.17.7 Thyroid disorder

- Transdermal HRT is preferred. Oral oestrogens, due to interactions in the liver, can result in reduced levels of free serum thyroxine, and may affect the dose of levothyroxine required.

7.17.8 Induced menopause in women with endometriosis

- Women who have treatment for endometriosis which induces menopause, including GnRH analogues or surgery involving removal of the ovaries, should be offered HRT, if there are no contraindications, until at least the age of 51.
- Continuous combined HRT (or tibolone) is usually advised, even in women who have had a hysterectomy, to avoid malignant transformation of any remaining endometriosis deposits.
- Refer to https://thebms.org.uk/wp-content/uploads/2022/12/10-BMS-TfC-Induced-Menopause-in-women-with-endometriosis-NOV2022-A.pdf.

7.17.9 PMS / PMDD / PME

- Symptoms can worsen in perimenopause as hormones fluctuate. Offer advice including lifestyle, stress management, counselling/support; complementary therapies, antidepressants and CBT.
- Cycle suppression to help manage moderate/severe PMS, in eligible women:
  - Using the COCP (such as Yasmin/Yaz or Zoely).
  - Using HRT with a transdermal oestrogen dose for cycle suppression (equivalent to a 100mcg patch) plus a progestogen (such as a 52mg LNG-IUD or micronised progesterone at a dose adequate to provide endometrial protection with high-dose oestrogen for a minimum of 12 days a month; see *Table 7.10*).
- Women who have a severe intolerance to progestogens and struggle to take them can try different routes of progestogen, e.g. some micronised progesterone products can be used, off-licence (see *Table 7.7*), vaginally instead of orally, at equivalent dose. Taking progesterone daily rather than cyclically can be better tolerated, or an alternative progestogen can be tried (see *Table 7.7*).

- Some women are advised to use lower doses of progestogen, for shorter durations or extended/long-cycle HRT regimes (the progestogen is taken less frequently than every month, typically every 3 months). This should not be done without medical guidance, as it may lead to bleeding problems and increase the risk of endometrial hyperplasia. If these regimes are used, you should have a low threshold for pelvic ultrasound scanning to check the endometrial thickness and for endometrial biopsy, if it is clinically indicated.
- Refer to:
  - www.pms.org.uk/app/uploads/2018/06/guidelinesfinal60210.pdf.
  - www.rcog.org.uk/guidance/browse-all-guidance/green-top-guidelines/premenstrual-syndrome-management-green-top-guideline-no-48.
- In severe cases refer to a menopause specialist with expertise in this area for advice.
- Refer also to *Chapter 8* on female mental health.

7.17.10 HRT and surgery

- Advising about HRT and surgery should be individualised depending upon the patient's medical history, the type of surgery, their risk factors for VTE, whether they are taking oral or transdermal oestrogen, and use of thromboprophylaxis. The BMS advises that women who are admitted to hospital for elective surgery, acute surgery or who have a medical illness and who are using HRT, should receive thromboprophylaxis (as appropriate) and do not need to discontinue their HRT. Women who have additional risk factors for VTE and who take oral oestrogen can switch to transdermal oestrogen.

7.17.11 HRT after risk-reducing surgery

- For full details see *Section 6.10* on surgical menopause.

7.17.12 Early menopause (40–45 years)

- There is limited research data in women with early menopause, but BMS guidance recommends that this is managed in a similar manner to those with POI.
- Women should be offered HRT, unless contraindicated, at least until the average age of the menopause.

7.17.13 Menopause after cancer

- Women with menopause after cancer usually say that these symptoms are worse than those they experienced during their cancer treatment. A discussion between the patient, her oncologist and a health professional with expertise in menopause after cancer is essential, as menopause symptoms are often undertreated.
- Women may be able to use HRT or low-dose localised vaginal oestrogen, or a non-hormonal alternative, and it is vital she is offered the right advice for her particular cancer.
- Refer to:
  - the British Gynaecological Cancer Society and BMS guidelines: *Management of menopausal symptoms following treatment of gynaecological cancer* (www.bgcs.org.uk/wp-content/uploads/2024/09/BGCS-BMS-Guidelines-on-Management-of-Menopausal-Symptoms-after-Gynaecological-Cancer-09.09.24.pdf)
  - NICE *Genitourinary (GU) symptoms associated with menopause in women with a history of breast cancer* [NG23] (www.nice.org.uk/guidance/ng23/resources/visual-summary-on-genitourinary-gu-symptoms-associated-with-menopause-pdf-13553202493)
  - The benefits and risks of HRT before and after a breast cancer diagnosis (https://thebms.org.uk/publications/consensus-statements/risks-and-benefits-of-hrt-before-and-after-a-breast-cancer-diagnosis)

  - Managing menopause after cancer (www.thelancet.com/journals/lancet/article/PIIS0140-6736(23)02802-7/fulltext).
- Refer also to *Section 6.11*.
- Refer to:
  - The Menopause and Cancer Podcast: https://menopauseandcancer.org/podcast
  - *Navigating Menopause after Cancer* by Dani Binnington.

7.17.14 Learning difficulties

- People with learning difficulties have an increased risk of osteoporosis, CVD and dementia.
- At their annual health check ask about menopause symptoms and educate the patient, carers and family members. Provide written information and choice. Consider ease of taking HRT products when prescribing.

7.17.15 Transgender gender-affirming hormone therapy: past use

- Trans men are female at birth and transition to the male gender. This usually involves taking testosterone and may involve having surgery.
- Trans men of menopausal age may experience menopausal symptoms. The management of this is complex and there is very little guidance or licensed products. It is generally not appropriate to give an oestrogen product.
- Ensure that trans men or non-binary people registered female at birth who have taken gender-affirming hormone therapy in the past and have symptoms associated with menopause can discuss these with a healthcare professional with expertise in menopause.
- Some trans men will have a vulva and may need reassurance that a low-dose topical oestrogen is unlikely to have any systemic feminising effect.
- It is important to:
  - Encourage healthy lifestyle choices and consider menopause-specific CBT for VMS, difficulties with sleep or depressive symptoms.
  - Consider contraception, if required.
  - Monitor cardiovascular risk factors, lipid profile, BP, insulin sensitivity and body weight.
  - Ensure they are referred for cervical and breast screening, if appropriate.

7.18 Sexual desire and testosterone

- As women age, there can be a decline in sexual function, including libido, arousal, orgasm and sexual satisfaction, and there may be a significant decrease in these around the time of menopause. This can have a significant impact upon the woman and her relationship. Women not in relationships also often value their sexual selves and should be offered a chance to talk about this, too.
- Androgens including testosterone have an important role in development of female sexual anatomy, physiology and in sexual behaviour. Testosterone levels fall with age, and levels can be particularly affected in women who have a medical or surgical menopause.
- Female sexual desire is not linked with serum testosterone levels. Many women with low serum testosterone levels do not report low libido or other related symptoms. It is possible that intracrinological metabolism of testosterone in the cells, particularly the conversion of DHEA within the brain, may play a more significant role than circulating testosterone levels.
- See also *Chapter 4* on sexual health.

7.18.1 Talking about libido and sex

- Encourage an open conversation using a biopsychosocial model.
- Sex is complex; there are many reasons for change in sexual desire including relationship problems, pain, difficulties with arousal, history of trauma, psychosocial factors, wider health issues, partner's health issues and medications including SSRIs, antihistamines and antihypertensives.

- Everyone has a different view on sex and what they consider to be normal.
- Desire often reduces in long-term relationships and may be low if emotional needs are not being met. Consider psychosexual therapy referral.
- Discuss vulval and vaginal pain, pelvic health, whether there is tightness or weakness of the pelvic floor giving constipation and vaginismus or leakage, weak orgasm and stress incontinence and GSM.
- Use of hormones in HRT can be helpful for some women. Systemic oestrogen replacement can improve sexual desire and low-dose localised oestrogen can improve dyspareunia caused by vaginal atrophy. If a woman is taking HRT and it has not improved sexual desire, then consider her HRT regime. Oral oestrogen can increase SHBG levels, which can result in lowering free testosterone levels – this may affect libido, so switching to a transdermal oestrogen may be helpful.

7.18.2 When is testosterone indicated?

- Testosterone treatment can be added to HRT, in women who are experiencing low libido (described as hypoactive sexual desire disorder, HSDD) which is causing them distress, after other causes have been excluded.
- It is important they are taking adequate oestrogen, and also that their symptoms of GSM are managed. Being well-oestrogenised will improve genital arousal and ensure sex is comfortable, but they do not need to be on a specific dose of oestrogen for testosterone to be added to their HRT regime.
- Testosterone replacement can result in a significant improvement in sexual function (desire and orgasm) for some women, but there is currently insufficient evidence to support its use for other indications such as enhancing cognitive function, musculoskeletal health, bone density, or reducing fracture risk. Further research is ongoing in these areas.

7.18.3 Investigations

- Before initiating testosterone therapy, a total testosterone level should be checked to ensure it is low enough to safely prescribe a therapeutic trial of testosterone supplementation. Ideally the total testosterone should be measured by liquid/gas chromatography and tandem mass spectrometry, but direct assays can be used in clinical practice.
- If the total testosterone baseline level is already in the upper range, supplementing with testosterone could lead to supra-physiological levels and increase the risk of side-effects.
- There is no blood level below which a woman is considered to have a low, or an insufficient, testosterone, so testosterone should not be measured to diagnose a testosterone insufficiency.
- The BMS recommends that a total testosterone assay is needed, instead of measuring free testosterone and a free androgen index. It does not recommend testing SHBG. It may be helpful to check SHBG for the following reasons:
    - Testosterone supplementation may be less effective when SHBG levels are elevated.
    - If a woman is experiencing androgenic side-effects despite having a normal total testosterone level, a low SHBG may be the cause, since it results in a higher proportion of free, active testosterone.

7.18.4 Prescribing testosterone

- Depending on local protocols, testosterone may be prescribed in primary care.
- The BMS recommends a trial of conventional HRT is given for at least 3 months, before testosterone is initiated.
- In 2025 the MHRA approved AndroFeme 10mg/ml cream (1ml contains 10mg testosterone) for the treatment of HSDD in postmenopausal women on optimised HRT, after a review of psychological and social factors and other treatable causes have been managed.
- Other testosterone preparations, such as Tostran and Testogel, are not licensed for use in women. Prescribing them in women is 'off-licence' (because the licence is only for male hypogonadism) but is accepted practice in line with BMS guidance.

- Testosterone is contraindicated in:
    - Pregnancy/breastfeeding, active liver disease, hormone-sensitive breast cancer.
    - Care needs to be taken with competitive athletes because of anti-doping regulations.

7.18.5 Possible side-effects of testosterone

- The commonest are excess hair growth, acne and weight gain, which are usually reversible with reduction in dosage or discontinuation.
- Alopecia, deepening of voice and clitoral enlargement are rare with physiological testosterone replacement. If these occur testosterone should be stopped immediately.

7.18.6 Testosterone treatment options

- Gel can be rubbed onto the skin, rotating the site to avoid localised hair growth. Hands should be washed after applying gel.
- *Table 7.13* shows examples of testosterone products and dosing guidance.

Table 7.13: Examples of testosterone products

Tostran 20mg/g transdermal gel (60g canister)	Dose: one metered pump of 0.5g (10mg of testosterone) on alternate days
Testogel 40.5mg transdermal gel in sachet	Dose: ⅛th of a sachet daily (5mg of testosterone) Each sachet should last 8 days
AndroFeme cream 1% testosterone cream (50ml tubes with screw cap)	Initiation dose: 0.5ml (5mg of testosterone) daily to the upper outer thigh or buttock The dose can be increased to a maximum of 1ml (10mg of testosterone) after 3 months if there is no improvement in symptoms and the total serum testosterone level is within the premenopausal range 6-monthly reviews to check for side-effects and to measure serum testosterone are required

7.18.7 Ongoing monitoring and follow-up

- A positive improvement in symptoms can take 3–6 months. Absorption, metabolism and individual response to treatment can vary between women.
- The balance between benefits and side-effects is highly individual. If symptoms do not improve sufficiently by 6 months, testosterone supplementation should be discontinued.
- It is recommended to check total testosterone levels at 3–6 weeks after treatment is initiated, to ensure they remain in accepted female physiological range. The dose of testosterone does not need to be titrated up to achieve a target testosterone level.
- A total testosterone level should ideally be tested in the morning. Samples should not be taken for patients receiving high biotin doses (i.e. >5mg/day) until at least 8 hours following the last biotin dose, as high-dose biotin can interfere with immunoassays.
- Counsel patients about the risk of falsely elevated serum testosterone measurements resulting from testosterone gel contamination of the venepuncture site (this can also occur in capillary samples).
- Older immunoassays for testosterone can cross-react with other medicines (such as norethisterone) and produce a falsely high testosterone result. Discuss with the laboratory, or consider re-testing the testosterone level off norethisterone.
- Currently it is recommended to monitor total testosterone levels every 6–12 months to ensure levels remain in range, and review annually.
- There is no established guidance on the duration of treatment; current safety data supports use for up to 24 months.

7.18.8 Patient information

- www.womens-health-concern.org/wp-content/uploads/2022/12/22-WHC-FACTSHEET-Testosterone-for-women-NOV2022-B.pdf
- Offer reading material such as:
  - *Mind the Gap* by Dr Karen Gurney.
  - *Come As You Are* by Emily Nagroski.
  - *Better Sex Through Mindfulness: how women can cultivate desire* by Lori A. Brotto.
  - OMGYES: www.omgyes.com/doctors is an evidence-based resource about women's sexual pleasure. Clinicians and therapists are able to request permanent free access. It can be recommended to women for their personal use.

7.19 Referral to a menopause specialist

When to refer:

- Persistent side-effects to HRT.
- Inadequate control of symptoms despite changes in HRT.
- Complex medical history.
- In women with current or a history of hormone-dependent cancers.
- Women with high-risk cancer gene variants.
- Premature ovarian insufficiency.
- Bleeding problems.
- Women with menopausal symptoms and contraindications to HRT.

There are some situations where the risks of using HRT outweigh the benefits and HRT is not recommended. However, some women whose quality of life is significantly affected may choose to use HRT despite these risks, and should be referred to a menopause specialist for advice about individual risks and benefits.

7.20 Resources for clinicians

- BMS Tools for Clinicians: https://thebms.org.uk/publications/tools-for-clinicians
- BMS & WHC's 2020 recommendations on HRT in menopausal women: https://thebms.org.uk/wp-content/uploads/2025/09/02-BMS-ConsensusStatement-BMS-WHC-2020-Recommendations-on-HRT-in-menopausal-women-SEPT2025-A.pdf
- NICE guidelines NG23: www.nice.org.uk/guidance/ng23
- Primary Care Women's Health Society resources: www.pcwhs.co.uk/resources
- International Menopause Society: www.imsociety.org
- European Menopause and Andropause Society: https://emas-online.org
- Menopause Research and Education Fund Resources: https://mref.uk/fast-facts-resources

7.21 Further reading

Australian Menopause Society (2025) *Tibolone as menopausal hormone therapy*. Available at: https://menopause.org.au/hp/information-sheets/tibolone-as-menopausal-hormone-therapy

BMS (2022) *Progestogens and endometrial protection*. Available at: https://thebms.org.uk/wp-content/uploads/2026/02/14-NEW-BMS-TfC-Progestogens-and-endometrial-protection-FEB2026-B.pdf

BMS (2022) *Testosterone replacement in menopause*. Available at: https://thebms.org.uk/wp-content/uploads/2026/02/08-NEW-BMS-TfC-Testosterone-replacement-in-menopause-JAN2026-C.pdf

BMS (2023) *BMS & WHC's 2020 recommendations on hormone replacement therapy in menopausal women.* Available at: https://thebms.org.uk/wp-content/uploads/2025/09/02-BMS-ConsensusStatement-BMS-WHC-2020-Recommendations-on-HRT-in-menopausal-women-SEPT2025-A.pdf

BMS (2024) *HRT preparations and equivalent alternatives.* Available at: https://thebms.org.uk/wp-content/uploads/2024/02/15-BMS-TfC-HRT-preparations-and-equivalent-alternatives-JAN2024-B.pdf

BMS (2024) *Management of unscheduled bleeding on hormone replacement therapy (HRT).* Available at: https://thebms.org.uk/publications/bms-guidelines/management-of-unscheduled-bleeding-on-hormone-replacement-therapy-hrt/

Cockrum, R.H., Soo, J., Ham, S.A., Cohen, K.S. and Snow, S.G. (2022) Association of progestogens and venous thromboembolism among women of reproductive age. *Obstetrics & Gynecology,* **140(3):** 477–87.

Collaborative Group on Hormonal Factors in Breast Cancer (2019) Type and timing of menopausal hormone therapy and breast cancer risk: individual participant meta-analysis of the worldwide epidemiological evidence. *Lancet,* **394(10204):** 1159–68.

Gillies, K. (2025) *Genitourinary syndrome of the menopause (GSM).* PCWHS. Available at: www.pcwhs.co.uk/resources/57/genitourinary_syndrome_of_the_menopause_gsm

Goldhaber, S.Z. (2010). Risk factors for venous thromboembolism. *Journal of the American College of Cardiology,* **56(1):** 1–7.

Hamoda, H., Davis, S.R., Cano, A. *et al.* (2021) BMS, IMS, EMAS, RCOG and AMS joint statement on menopausal hormone therapy and breast cancer risk in response to EMA Pharmacovigilance Risk Assessment Committee recommendations in May 2020. *Post Reproductive Health,* **27(1):** 49–55.

Hillard, T., Abernethy, K., Hamoda, H. *et al.* (2017) *Management of the Menopause,* 6th edition. BMS.

Lambrinoudaki, I. and Armeni, E. (2023) Understanding of and clinical approach to cardiometabolic transition at the menopause. *Climacteric,* **27(1):** 68–74.

Maki, P.M. and Jaff, N.G. (2022) Brain fog in menopause: a health-care professional's guide for decision-making and counseling on cognition. *Climacteric,* **25(6):** 1–9.

Menopause Matters website: www.menopausematters.co.uk

Menopause Matters (undated) *HRT: Risks.* Available at: www.menopausematters.co.uk/risks.php

Mukherjee, A. and Davis, S.R. (2025) Update on menopause hormone therapy; current indications and unanswered questions. *Clin Endocrinol (Oxf)* [online ahead of print].

My Menopause Centre (2024) *Hormone replacement therapy for vegans and vegetarians.* Available at: www.mymenopausecentre.com/gp-resources/hormone-replacement-therapy-for-vegans-and-vegetarians/#fc-hrt-options-if-you-are-vegan-vegetarian

PCWHS (2025) *10 top tips on testosterone use for women.* PCWHS. Available at: www.pcwhs.co.uk/resources/7/10_top_tips_on_testosterone_use_for_women

PCWHS (2025) *HRT & breast cancer risks.* Available at: www.pcwhs.co.uk/resources/65/hrt_breast_cancer_risks

Shaw, I. (2020) *Menopause – guidance on management and prescribing HRT for GPs.* PCWHS. Available at: www.pcwhs.co.uk/_userfiles/pages/files/pcwhf_prescribinghrt1.pdf

Terral, C., Godard, P., Michel, F.B. and Macabies, J. (1981) Influence of estrogens on histamines liberation induced by allergens in vitro. *C R Seances Soc Biol Fil,* **175(2):** 247–52. Available at: https://pubmed.ncbi.nlm.nih.gov/6166357

Vinogradova, Y., Coupland, C. and Hippisley-Cox, J. (2019) Use of hormone replacement therapy and risk of venous thromboembolism: nested case–control studies using the QResearch and CPRD databases. *BMJ,* **364**: k4810.

Chapter 8
Female mental health

8.1 Introduction to the premenstrual disorders

8.1.1 What are premenstrual disorders and who is affected?

- Premenstrual disorders (PMDs) is an umbrella term for several distinct conditions, including the widely-recognised premenstrual syndrome (PMS) and the most severe form of premenstrual dysphoric disorder, PMDD.
- Most women are aware of physical and/or psychological changes that occur during their menstrual cycle. The exact nature of the symptoms experienced physically and mentally varies.
- Despite the prevalence of the premenstrual disorders, they remain poorly recognised and undertreated.
- The impact of premenstrual disorders varies in severity.
  - Severe premenstrual disorders (including PMDD) have an enormous impact on women's physical, social, psychological and economic wellbeing.
  - In contrast, women who experience minor, transient premenstrual symptoms that do not impair their activities or affect their quality of life are described as having physiological premenstrual 'symptoms' rather than premenstrual 'syndrome'.
- A recent meta-analysis suggests that PMS affects approximately half of women of reproductive age worldwide.
- PMDD is thought to affect between 3.2 and 7.7% of women of reproductive age worldwide.
- Women with PMDD are almost seven times more likely to attempt suicide and almost four times as likely to exhibit suicidal ideation than women without the condition.
- Women with PMS are also at higher risk of suicidal ideation, but not suicide attempts.
- The key to effective management of the premenstrual conditions lies in symptom recognition and accurate diagnosis.
- **Many women who are susceptible to hormone-related mood change will have vulnerability across their reproductive lives.**
- Susceptibility to PMDs and other forms of reproductive depression seems more prevalent in women who are neurodivergent, e.g. with autistic spectrum disorders or ADHD. History of exposure to trauma is also more common in women with PMDs. There is also diagnostic overlap with joint hypermobility and autonomic dysfunction.

8.1.2 What causes the premenstrual disorders?

- Understanding the aetiology of the PMDs remains an ongoing area of research.
- It is clear that ovulation, and therefore the presence of luteal phase hormones, is a key factor in the premenstrual disorders, as symptoms of PMDs do not occur prior to menarche, during pregnancy or after menopause.
- The exact cause remains uncertain, however. **Research shows hormone levels are not distinguishable between women with and without PMDs** – showing it is not hormones per se that are responsible for the condition, rather that individuals with PMD have an atypical response to them.
- Overlapping genetic and environmental factors seem to feed into a state of neurobiological vulnerability to PMDs. Research is focused in four main areas:
  - **Genetic susceptibility**
    - Studies suggest some heritability in PMDD.
  - **Dysregulation in the serotonergic system**
    - Changing hormone levels may impact the serotonin system. Depletion of tryptophan, the main precursor of serotonin, has been shown to worsen premenstrual symptoms. The efficacy of SSRIs in treatment of the PMDs also supports this theory.
    - Oestrogen and progesterone levels also affect the dopamine system.
  - **The effect of progesterone and its metabolite, allopregnanolone, on the GABAergic system**

    - In people with PMDs there appears to be increased sensitivity to changes in allopregnanolone levels.
    - Allopregnanolone works as an agonist at the GABA-A receptor to enhance the neurotransmitter's calming effect on mood.
    - SSRIs may also alter allopregnanolone levels, which may explain how they can be effective treatment in PMD.
  - **Stress and inflammation**
    - Stress seems to have a role through amplifying sympathetic activity.
    - **There may also be an exaggerated immune–inflammatory response.**

8.1.3 Making the diagnosis

- **In order to diagnose a premenstrual disorder, we must demonstrate the following:**
  - Cyclicity with respect to luteal phase.
  - Relief of symptoms after onset of menses, with a symptom-free period.
  - Impact on daily functioning.
  - Presence of symptoms over at least two consecutive cycles (useful menstrual diaries for patients can be downloaded from www.IAPMD.org).
- Symptom persistence and severity can fluctuate: one study showed that only 36% of women who met the diagnostic criteria for PMS continued to meet the diagnostic criteria one year later.
- Postmenopausal women with previous PMDs may experience recurrence of psychological and physical symptoms when they receive progestogen therapy.
- Research indicates that reproductive steroids affect virtually every system implicated in the pathophysiology of depression. **Women who are susceptible to hormone-induced mood change may also show mood change with pregnancy, the postnatal period, infertility treatment, perimenopause and menopause, and when exogenous hormones are prescribed as contraception or HRT.**
- This susceptibility to sex-steroid-related mood change is widely recognised as creating a 'window of increased vulnerability' to mental health conditions during the reproductive years.

8.1.4 Classification of premenstrual disorders

- Historically, the nomenclature and definitions for the premenstrual disorders have been varied and confusing.
- The International Society for Premenstrual Disorders (ISPMD) produced the first consensus on definitions and diagnostic criteria. This now underpins the definitions in the *Diagnostic and Statistical Manual of Mental Disorders,* 5th edition (DSM-5) and the *International Classification of Diseases,* 11th revision (ICD-11). ISPMD also developed the clinical standards for managing PMDD which underpin the Treatment Guidelines released by the Royal College of Obstetricians & Gynaecologists (RCOG) in 2013.
- The ISPMD defined premenstrual disorders as core PMDs (associated with ovulatory cycles) or variant PMDs (see also *Table 8.1*).
  - **Core premenstrual disorders** (incorporating premenstrual syndrome and PMDD)
    - Symptoms occur regularly in ovulating women.
    - They are generally present during the luteal phase.
    - They generally resolve by the end of menstruation.
    - A key diagnostic point is that a symptom-free interval is present.
  - **Variant premenstrual disorders** include everything that does not meet the criteria for the core PMDs. There are four subtypes:
    - **Premenstrual exacerbation (PME):** where there is a physical condition (e.g. asthma, migraine, epilepsy) and/or a psychological condition (e.g. depression, anxiety, eating disorders or obsessive–compulsive disorder, OCD) which is present throughout the month but worsens cyclically (usually in the luteal phase).

Table 8.1: Differentiating between core and variant PMD

Core PMD	
Subclassified according to nature of symptoms: • Predominantly physical • Predominantly emotional • Mixed	Symptoms occur in ovulatory cycle Symptoms can be physical or psychological Symptoms absent after menstruation and before ovulation Symptoms must be prospectively rated for at least 2 cycles Symptoms must cause functional impairment
Variant PMD	
Premenstrual exacerbation	Exacerbation of an underlying somatic (e.g. asthma, migraine) or psychological disorder that is present throughout the month but worsens in the luteal phase
Non-ovulatory PMD	Poorly understood and rare; symptoms arise from follicular activity of the ovary
Progestogen-induced PMD	PMD symptoms arise from exogenous sources of progestogen in the COCP or HRT
PMD with absent menstruation	PMD arises from cyclical ovarian activity even though menstruation has been suppressed – e.g. in women who have had endometrial ablation, have a 52mg LNG-IUD or have had a hysterectomy

- **PMD with absent menstruation:** this may happen when amenorrhoea has been induced, e.g. following LNG-IUD insertion, endometrial ablation or hysterectomy with conservation of the ovaries. Symptoms are thought to arise from cyclical ovarian activity despite absence of ovulation.
- **Progestogen-induced PMD:** in susceptible women, the exogenous hormones in sequential HRT or hormonal contraceptives can induce symptoms. Progestogen-only contraceptives and continuous HRT can also cause PMD-like symptoms but as these are non-cyclical, they are not included in this definition and are considered as adverse effects of continuous hormonal therapies (colloquially this is often referred to as 'progestogen sensitivity').
- **Non-ovulatory PMD:** this disorder is poorly understood but it is thought that in some women, follicular activity can precipitate symptoms even if ovulation does not occur.

8.1.5 Premenstrual dysphoric disorder

- It was only in 2013 that PMDD was clearly defined and included as a distinct diagnosis in the DSM-5.
- In 2019 the ICD-11 also included PMDD as a distinct condition listed under genitourinary diseases but cross-listed in depressive disorders.
- This was considered a breakthrough for women's health, but also invited controversy regarding the purported pathologisation of 'normal hormonal changes' and risks of over-diagnosis.
- Since the inclusion of PMDD in the DSM and ICD there has been a significant increase in interest, funding and research into the condition.

How can we diagnose PMDD?

- The DSM-5 diagnostic criteria for PMDD require the following to be fulfilled:
  - **Cyclicity of symptoms**
    - Cyclicity is key, with definite temporal relationship to cycle.
    - Must be present in the final week before the onset of menses, start to improve within a few days after the onset of menses and become minimal or absent in the week post menses.

- **Presence of at least 5 of 11 symptoms as listed here:**
- **Core symptoms (of which at least one must be present):**
  - Marked affective lability (e.g. mood swings, feeling suddenly sad or tearful, increased sensitivity to rejection).
  - Marked irritability or anger and increased interpersonal conflicts.
  - Markedly depressed mood, feelings of hopelessness, or self-deprecating thoughts.
  - Marked anxiety, tension and/or feelings of being keyed-up or on edge.
- **Additional symptoms**
  - Decreased interest in usual activities.
  - Poor concentration.
  - Lethargy, reduced stamina.
  - Marked change in appetite, overeating or food cravings.
  - Sleep changes – hypersomnia or insomnia.
  - A sense of being overwhelmed or out of control.
  - Physical symptoms such as breast tenderness, joint pains, bloating or weight gain.
- **Severity of impact**
  - Clinically significant impact must be present (i.e. causing distress and interfering with work, school or usual social activities or relationships with others).
- **Exclusion of PME**
  - Often the hardest part of diagnosis.
  - Should not be an exacerbation of an underlying psychiatric disorder such as anxiety, depression or personality disorder.
  - PMDD can co-occur with these conditions.
- **Confirmation with prospective daily ratings**
  - Diagnosis requires cycle diaries for at least two consecutive cycles.
  - If one of these cycles is atypical, complete a third.
- **Symptoms are not attributable to drugs / other medical condition**
  - Take a careful drug history and medical history to exclude influences of medication, drug abuse or a medical condition such as hyperthyroidism.

Suicidality in PMDD

- Women with PMDD must be considered high-risk for suicidality. Loss of impulse control and impaired interpersonal functioning are likely to contribute to vulnerability to suicide in women with PMDD.
- Studies suggest that cycle diaries, though crucial to accurate diagnosis, are often not completed. Women are often desperate for help by the time they speak to a healthcare professional and if there is extreme distress or suicidal ideation, delaying treatment by 2 months may be unacceptable.

Differential diagnoses, variances and other associations in PMDD

- Distinguishing PMDD from premenstrual exacerbation or other mental health or physical conditions can be difficult. The presence of a symptom-free window for at least a few days after menstruation is crucial.
- Cycle diaries and a symptom-free interval are essential to separate PMDD from the premenstrual exacerbation of another condition.
- Particular care should be taken to distinguish PMDD from emotionally unstable personality disorder and understanding how it may relate to trauma-related conditions.
- A history of exposure to trauma is more likely in women with PMDD and there can be overlap between the diagnostic criteria for these conditions. Evidence also suggests women with trauma exposure may experience worsening of trauma-related symptoms during periods of reproductive shift, e.g. postpartum and in the perimenopause. Understanding the interrelated

nature of lived experience and physical/psychological symptoms allows us to take a holistic, biopsychosocial approach to management of these issues.
- PMDD is common in the neurodivergent population. Consider if 'missed' neurodivergence may be present when diagnosing PMDD. Look for the presence of cyclical exacerbation or symptoms in neurodivergent patients.
- Although the DSM-5 criteria focus on the classical late luteal pattern of symptoms, it is becoming increasingly evident that the PMDs encompass women with other patterns of cyclical symptoms, e.g. exacerbation during ovulation, or symptoms starting a few days after menses.
- Pragmatic questions should be asked, particularly whether this patient is likely to benefit from cycle control to manage her pattern of physical and psychological symptoms. The focus should be on identifying patterns that repeat from month to month, and on shared decision-making regarding treatments that may reduce the severity and impact of symptoms.
- Given the high risk of suicidal ideation and attempts in this population, patients with PMDD in primary care can be referred to secondary care for diagnosis and MDT management of symptoms, if the practitioner is not confident in management.

8.1.6 Management of the premenstrual disorders

Lifestyle and diet

- All women with premenstrual disorders should be advised that lifestyle modification has been shown to improve symptoms.
- General measures to improve symptoms include:
  - Eating regular balanced meals every 2–3 hours that are rich in complex carbohydrates (theorised to increase central serotonin availability via increased tryptophan, with some trial data to support this).
  - Regular moderate aerobic exercise.
  - Regular sleep.
  - Stress reduction.
  - Smoking cessation and alcohol restriction, where applicable.
  - Cognitive behavioural therapy (CBT) should be routinely offered and can be useful alongside pharmacological approaches as well as being an alternative to medication.

Supplements and complementary medicine

- Vitamin B6 has been extensively studied and 100mg has shown weak superiority to placebo in meta-analysis. Higher doses may lead to neurological side-effects.
- Calcium supplementation at 600mg twice daily has shown some benefit in RCTs. There is some additional evidence supporting vitamin D supplementation.
- Magnesium is recommended by the International Association for Premenstrual Disorders (IAPMD) at 500mg daily following evidence of benefit.
- Agnus castus is the best researched supplement for PMS with encouraging evidence of benefit. There is no consistent dose recommendation, although the National Association for Premenstrual Syndrome (NAPS) flow chart suggests 20–40mg daily. There is no standardised quality-controlled preparation available.
- Acupuncture, St John's wort, gingko, isoflavones and a number of other complementary and alternative medicines have a weak evidence base for efficacy but should currently not be recommended first-line.

Non-hormonal medications

- Menstrual cramping and joint pain can be managed with NSAIDs (unless contraindicated), e.g. ibuprofen, mefenamic acid or naproxen.
- SSRIs have a clear evidence base for efficacy and should be considered a first-line treatment.

- When used for PMDs, SSRIs seem to have a very rapid onset of action, with improvement seen within 24 hours and peaking at 48 hours. This suggests a different mode of action than when used in depression or anxiety.
- Starting doses are the same as for other indications and they appear equally effective when offered continually, or for the luteal phase only (i.e. given on days 15–28 of the cycle). Luteal phase dosing is off-licence.
- Adverse effects are present in around 50% of SSRI users, including sexual dysfunction, nausea, sleep disturbance and fatigue. Loss of libido can be particularly challenging for women with PMS/PMDD who may already be struggling in their relationships.
- Research is taking place into allopregnanolone modulators (blocking allopregnanolone at the GABA-A receptor). 5-alpha reductase inhibitors have also been studied, as they block the conversion of progesterone to allopregnanolone.
- Anecdotally, some women find antihistamines such as fexofenadine or H_2 antagonists such as famotidine helpful. There is currently no clear evidence to support their role in management. There are also potential overlaps between premenstrual disorders, hypermobility, mast-cell activation syndrome (MCAS) and autonomic nervous system dysfunction, e.g. POTS (postural orthostatic tachycardia syndrome), which may explain the efficacy of these medications in some patients.

Hormonal medications (including use of GnRH analogues)

- **Women with PMDs have usually experienced unwanted mood change with hormonal medications and are often nervous when a prescription is suggested.**
- It is important to reassure them that initial flare in symptoms is common with all options listed below but this usually settles within 6 weeks. **They should be reassured that they will be listened to if they wish to stop medication because they cannot tolerate it.**
- Patients may need to try several different options before finding one that suits them.
- Hormonal methods may be offered alongside, or as an alternative to, lifestyle and complementary therapies and SSRIs.
- Where hormonal medications fail to improve symptoms, patients should be referred to secondary care for consideration of GnRH analogues and/or surgery.

Combined oral contraceptives

- Ovarian suppression and modulation of hormonal fluctuations in the menstrual cycle are the main aims of hormonal therapies for PMDs.
- The combined oral contraceptive pill is an effective option when used in a tailored regimen. Evidence supports giving the COCP continuously (stopping only when breakthrough bleeding occurs) or bi-/tricycling (i.e. reducing the pill-free interval to every second or third pack).
- Breaks may need to be taken if persistent spotting occurs. When a break is taken, reducing this to 4 days rather than the typical 7 can minimise the risk of cycle-related symptoms.
- The best evidence base is for drospirenone-containing contraceptives, e.g. Yasmin / Lucette / Dretine / Yacella / Eloine.
- Evidence is increasing that Zoely, which contains estradiol and nomegestrol, is also well-tolerated in women with PMDs.

Estradiol

- **Inhibition of ovulation / cycle suppression can also be achieved with higher doses of transdermal oestrogen.**
- **This is particularly useful in women in whom the COCP is contraindicated, or in women at perimenopause who request HRT.**
- 100mcg patches of transdermal estradiol have been shown to be effective at suppressing ovulation and cycle-related symptoms.
- Contraception cannot be assumed.

- The endometrium requires protection. The following are all acceptable options to try – it is worth taking a detailed history of what previous synthetic and natural progestogens may have been tried and how they were tolerated. This may inform your choice of progestogen:
  - **A 52mg LNG-IUD** provides low-dose levonorgestrel. Around 10% of women with progesterone intolerance will not tolerate this device. Women should be advised that symptoms can flare initially but this generally settles within 6 weeks. They should be reassured the device can be removed if they remain intolerant, which should eliminate symptoms within 24 hours. Many women with history of mood change with contraception are fearful of a coil, as they cannot stop the treatment themselves – giving this clear reassurance often allows a woman to feel more comfortable in trying this method.
  - **Continuous Utrogestan** (micronised progesterone) is often better tolerated than synthetic progestins. 100mg nocte has historically been used – though the recent BMS Joint Guideline on Unscheduled Bleeding would now suggest that 200mg may be required to protect against endometrial hyperplasia with a dose of 100mcg of transdermal oestrogen.
  - **Sequential micronised progesterone** may be needed to ensure predictable bleeding in younger women. The NAPS and RCOG guidelines do not advise on dose, but usually this has been 200mg for 12 days. Again, recent BMS guidelines suggest 300mg may be required for adequate endometrial protection. Watch for flare of symptoms with progesterone initiation or withdrawal, which will make this pattern of prescribing unsuitable for many.
  - **Micronised progesterone** may be better tolerated vaginally as Cyclogest pessaries or 8% Crinone gel. Current evidence supports giving the same dose advised for the oral route. This route bypasses first-pass metabolism, avoiding conversion to allopregnanolone.
  - Some progestogen-intolerant women may struggle to take the higher doses of progesterone recommended by the most recent guidelines. **In these cases, consider referring to a specialist for further management**. The RCOG guidelines state: *"When using a short duration of progestogen therapy, or in cases where only low doses are tolerated, there should be a low threshold for investigating unscheduled bleeding."*
  - **Slynd** (drospirenone 4mg) is also now available and though off-licence, has been included by the BMS in acceptable options for endometrial protection (based on the fact that drospirenone-containing COCPs contain 3mg as adequate progestogenic opposition for up to 30mg of ethinylestradiol). This option has not been incorporated into PMD guidelines so far but has shown promising results in progestogen-sensitive women.

Danazol

- Danazol is an androgenic steroid which has been shown to be effective in cycle suppression but is rarely advised for use due to its potential for irreversible masculinising side-effects.

GnRH analogues

- **When simpler measures have failed, patients can be referred to secondary care for consideration of GnRH analogues.** These are not generally initiated by the non-specialist, but once commenced are often covered by shared care arrangements and administered in primary care.
- GnRH analogues produce profound ovarian suppression and effectively induce medical menopause.
- They induce hypo-oestrogenic side-effects which require treatment.
- GnRH analogues are usually reserved for severe PMDD where surgical management is being considered. If symptoms do not respond within 12 weeks, the diagnosis of PMDD may need reviewing.
- Significant bone loss begins within 6 months of use. GnRH analogues are therefore only licensed for 6 months of continuous use.
- Add-back hormones must be prescribed if use is to be extended beyond this. They are usually started much earlier to prevent bone loss and avoid troublesome vasomotor symptoms.

- Continuous combined HRT (the oestrogen dose does not need to be 100mcg in this situation as the ovaries are already suppressed by the GnRH analogue), usually with 100mg micronised progesterone orally or vaginally, is generally prescribed. An alternative is tibolone 2.5mg which is often well-tolerated.
- RCOG guidelines advise DEXA monitoring at least annually if on long-term GnRH analogues.
- Women may notice an initial flare in symptoms as the LH and FSH generally rise before being downregulated and therefore suppressing ovulation.

Surgical treatment of PMDD

- **When treating severe PMS or PMDD and other methods have failed, or long-term GnRH therapy is required, hysterectomy and bilateral oophorectomy has been shown to be of benefit.**
- Surgery is not usually considered without preoperative use of GnRH analogues to test cure and ensure that HRT will be tolerated.
- Occasionally oestrogen alone will be administered during this period if tibolone or progesterone are not tolerated. The RCOG guidelines state that this should be on an individual basis due to concerns regarding endometrial hyperplasia. This is usually only done with specialist initiation whilst considering surgical treatment.

8.1.7 Useful resources for professionals and patients

- www.PMS.org.uk – the National Association for Premenstrual Syndromes includes a PDF guideline for patients and professionals, cycle diaries and useful resources for managing the condition.
- www.IAPMD.org – the International Association for Premenstrual Disorders has information for professionals and patients, including webinars and cycle diaries, and online peer support for people with PMDD around the world.
- www.rcog.org.uk – the RCOG Green-top Guidelines for managing premenstrual syndrome.

8.2 Perinatal mental health

8.2.1 Definition and risk factors

- The DSM-5 criteria specify that peripartum depression onset is during pregnancy or within 4 weeks after delivery.
- It is generally agreed, however, that onset can occur at any time within the 12 months following childbirth. This contrasts with the 'baby blues', which affect between 3 and 8 out of 10 women and are usually mild and transient.
- Risk factors for perinatal depression include:
  - prior depression or anxiety, including during a previous pregnancy
  - life stress
  - prior history of premenstrual disorders or adverse mood reaction with hormonal contraceptives
  - lack of social support
  - relationship difficulties, e.g. poor partner support
  - domestic violence
  - unintended pregnancy
  - history of trauma, e.g. childhood abuse
  - complications at birth, e.g. preterm delivery, infant health problems or need for intensive care
  - antenatal thyroid dysfunction or pregestational/gestational diabetes
  - longer time to conception
  - having two or more children
  - history of substance misuse
  - discontinuation of psychotropic medication prior to / during pregnancy.

- Where there is a personal history of past or present severe mental illness, or a family history of severe perinatal illness, there is a higher chance of postpartum psychosis in the first 2 weeks after childbirth.

8.2.2 Prevalence and impact

- During pregnancy, 12% of women will be affected by depression and 13% of women will be affected by anxiety. In the first year after birth, 15–20% will be affected.
- First-time mothers, adolescent mothers and those who have had a traumatic delivery may benefit from proactive support. Studies have shown that home health visits, telephone peer support and psychotherapy can help prevent postpartum depression.
- Evidence suggests that perinatal depression is often missed or undertreated in general practice.
- Severe depression in pregnancy is associated with increased rates of obstetric complications, sudden infant death syndrome, low birthweight and preterm delivery, self-harm and suicide attempts.
- Suicide remains a leading cause of maternal death in the first postpartum year.
- There is an association between depression in pregnancy and depression in the adolescent and young adult offspring.
- There may also be impairment in cognitive, behavioural and emotional development of a minority of infants born to mothers with perinatal depression.
- There may be wider impacts within the family, including effects on the woman's partner and other children.
- Many women feel shame about these conditions and may benefit from psychological support to process their experience.

8.2.3 Prognosis

- If depression is untreated during pregnancy, women have a seven-fold increased risk of postpartum depression when compared to women without antenatal depression.
- Postpartum depression often improves spontaneously after 2–3 months. One-third of women remain unwell 12 months after childbirth, and 13% at 2 years.

8.2.4 Diagnosis

- **Mental health should be assessed during the pregnancy booking appointment, and in all contacts through the antenatal and postnatal period.**
- The postnatal check should include screening questions, such as the ones below, to elicit whether the baby blues resolved within 10–14 days of birth, or whether low mood has persisted:
  - *"During the past month, have you often been bothered by feeling down, depressed or hopeless?"*
  - *"During the past month, have you often been bothered by having little interest or pleasure in doing things?"*
- If there is a positive response to the depression screening questions, or the mother is at risk of a mental health problem, consider further evaluation using the Patient Health Questionnaire (PHQ-9) or the Edinburgh Postnatal Depression Scale (EPDS).
- Women should be assessed for level of risk. If there are severe symptoms, or you believe mother or infant to be at risk, refer to a mental health professional.
  - Consider whether there is adequate social support, and ensure the woman and her partner or other support know where to seek further help if things deteriorate.
  - You may need to follow local safeguarding protocols if you have any concerns about risk of child harm or maltreatment.
- Consider differential diagnoses, e.g. bipolar disorder and OCD.
- Ask about the presence of confusion, delusions or hallucinations, which may indicate the onset of postpartum psychosis.

8.2.5 Managing perinatal depression

Women on antidepressants prior to pregnancy

- **Where pregnancy is planned, advise women that antidepressants may be used at any stage of pregnancy where clinically indicated, including when trying to conceive.**
- The risk of destabilising the woman's condition should be weighed up against the wish to reduce, change or stop antidepressants.
- Aim for the lowest effective dose, and a single drug is preferable to polypharmacy. Where prescribing is complex, seek specialist advice.
- Antidepressants should not be stopped abruptly.
- No antidepressant has been proven to cause birth defects.
  - SSRIs:
    - SSRIs have the largest body of safety data and can be considered a first-line choice. There is no evidence one SSRI is safer than any other. Studies suggest a small risk of fetal heart defects (3 in 100 vs. 2 in 100 in the background population).
    - SSRI use in pregnancy may lead to transient neonatal withdrawal causing central nervous system, motor, respiratory and gastrointestinal symptoms. Hospital delivery is usually advised.
  - Tricyclic antidepressants (TCAs):
    - Although usually considered a second-line treatment in pregnancy, they are safe for use if clinically indicated (for example, where a patient is stable on them and may be at risk of relapse if treatment is withdrawn or changed).
    - Data is more limited than for SSRIs.
  - Serotonin–noradrenaline reuptake inhibitors (SNRIs):
    - Data is even more limited than for SSRIs and TCAs.
    - Where it is clinically indicated, they can be considered safe to use or continue, particularly where a woman is stable on treatment and at risk of relapse if treatment is stopped or changed.
- Consider her plans for breastfeeding, as there are some risks associated with psychotropic medications in this instance.
- Detailed information on risks of individual antidepressants is available from the UK Teratology Information Service (www.uktis.org). Prescribing should be a shared care decision, including the patient.
- Consider referring women with severe current or previous mental health issues, who are planning pregnancy, to secondary mental health service for preconception counselling. Pregnancy and the puerperium are vulnerable periods for relapse or destabilisation.

Managing new-onset antenatal depression

- Low-risk women with new onset of depression during pregnancy may be managed in primary care following the recommendations on treatment detailed at the start of *Section 8.2.5.*
- Consider urgent referral to secondary mental health services:
  - If there is evidence of risk of harm to the woman or other people.
  - If there is evidence (or history) of bipolar disorder.
  - If there is a history of severe mental illness, including previous perinatal depression or puerperal psychosis in the woman or a first-degree relative.

Managing postnatal depression

- Refer for immediate assessment by secondary mental health services (within 4 hours) if a woman has sudden onset of symptoms suggestive of postpartum psychosis or is at immediate risk of harm to herself or her baby.
- Refer urgently to secondary mental health services:
  - If she is severely depressed.

    - If she shows signs of self-neglect or being unable to look after her baby.
    - If there is a possible diagnosis of bipolar disorder.
    - If there is a history of severe mental illness, including perinatally.
- Where a woman is safe to be managed in primary care, take into account her preferences when prescribing.
- Information is available from the UK Drugs in Lactation Advisory Service (UKDILAS) on 0330 770 8564.
- An SSRI, TCA or SNRI can safely be used in the postnatal period.
- No psychotropic medication has a licence for use in breastfeeding mothers, so informed consent should be sought and documented.
- Paroxetine and sertraline are usually safer choices in breastfeeding mothers. The lowest effective dose should be used, and babies should be monitored for drowsiness, poor feeding and behavioural changes.

8.2.6 Postpartum psychosis

- Postpartum psychosis is rare, affecting 1–2 in 1000 women.
- It usually presents suddenly, within 2 weeks of delivery.
- Symptoms include severe mood swings, delusions, confusion and hallucinations. Distorted thoughts and behaviours may involve the baby and place it at risk.
- Recurrence in subsequent deliveries is common.

8.2.7 Bipolar postpartum depression

- Bipolar disorder may present postnatally, or an existing diagnosis may relapse in this period.
- 21.4–54% of women with postpartum depression have a diagnosis of bipolar disorder.
- These women are often younger in age, with earlier onset of symptoms after birth and some atypical depressive features.
- There may be a history of bipolar disease in first-degree relatives.
- It is important to identify bipolar symptoms, as treatment with antidepressants may trigger manic symptoms.
- These patients are usually managed by specialist mental health teams. Treatment often includes use of mood stabilisers, e.g. lithium, quetiapine and lamotrigine.

8.2.8 Perinatal obsessive–compulsive disorder

- Prevalence of obsessive–compulsive disorder (OCD) is higher in the perinatal population than in the general population.
- Clinical features in the perinatal period are likely to include concerns about harm to the infant, with contamination and cleaning/checking compulsions particularly common.
- Research suggests CBT with exposure and response prevention is particularly effective.
- There is also limited evidence for efficacy of SSRIs.
- Patients should be referred to specialist mental health services for assessment and treatment.

8.3 Hormonal contraception and mood disorders

- **Hormone-containing medications can often induce mood change in susceptible women.** Where cyclical, this falls under 'Variant PMDs – progestogen-induced' as detailed in *Section 8.1.4*.
- Where continuous administration of hormonal medication leads to mood change, this is usually considered an adverse effect rather than a form of premenstrual disorder. Colloquially, we often refer to this as progestogen intolerance or sensitivity.

- Management follows the NAPS and RCOG guidelines for PMS and PMDD. Many women will find they tolerate drospirenone- or nomegestrol-containing COCPs better or will improve when offered high-dose (100mcg) transdermal oestrogen alongside an LNG-IUD coil or anovulatory progestogen such as Slynd (drospirenone). Desogestrel is less often tolerated by progestogen-sensitive women, but may also be given. It can be used off-licence, in a double dose of 150mg, alongside transdermal oestrogen to provide both contraception and endometrial protection (though off-licence, this option is included in the BMS Joint Guidelines on Unscheduled Bleeding).
- Micronised progesterone is not contraceptive so is unsuitable for use for this indication.

8.4 Neurodiversity in women and girls

8.4.1 What is neurodiversity and who is affected?

- Neurodivergence is a term that describes the natural variation in human brain functioning and cognitive processing.
- Autism prevalence is estimated at 1–2% but is growing, likely due to improved recognition – especially amongst those with normal range IQ, and due to broadening of diagnostic criteria over time.
- Variations from the majority or 'neurotypical' population include:
  - autism spectrum disorder (ASD)
  - attention deficit hyperactivity disorder (ADHD)
  - dyslexia
  - dyspraxia (developmental coordination disorder)
  - Tourette syndrome
  - sensory processing differences.
- Diagnosis of neurodivergence is often missed or delayed in women and those assigned female at birth. Common symptom profiles were focused on male presentation, and biological and social factors can mean that the conditions present differently in females.
- A predictive model based on population data has suggested that 39% more women should be diagnosed with ASD than currently are.
- Diagnosis in adulthood is often more challenging, as there may be a lack of developmental history and individuals have learnt strategies to camouflage (mask) difficulties.
- Neurodivergent women and girls often mask more successfully than their male counterparts, but may struggle to continue to do so at reproductive milestones such as menopause.
- The considerable cognitive effort required to mask difficulties relating to neurodivergence leads to increased rates of stress, anxiety and depression.
- Individuals with 'milder' presentation may be more prone to late or missed diagnosis and have developed more coping strategies which 'hide' the diagnosis. For example, women with ADHD often become prone to work-related burnout, as challenges with executive function such as planning, prioritising, scheduling and multitasking can lead to overload and overwhelm. This may present clinically as anxiety, insomnia or depression, but deeper questioning may reveal relevant detail pointing to the need to consider neurodivergence.
- Consideration of the wider clinical picture can help in identifying possible 'missed' neurodivergence.
- Neurodivergent women and girls are more likely to also have:
  - Eating disorders (multiple studies reveal an overrepresentation of autism or autistic traits in the eating disorder population).
  - Premenstrual disorders such as PMS or PMDD (some research suggests that autistic individuals may be 2–3 times more likely to report cyclical mood change consistent with PMDD).

   - Heightened sensory sensitivity, emotional dysregulation and executive function challenges at certain points in their menstrual cycle or at reproductive milestones such as menopause.
   - Family members with existing ASD or ADHD diagnoses (heritability is estimated between 64% and 91%).
- Neurodivergence is not a mental health condition, but neurodivergent individuals are at a high risk of developing mental health problems, with depression and anxiety problems predominating, and suicide rates substantially increased.

8.5 Eating disorders and body dysmorphic disorder

8.5.1 Introduction

- Although eating disorders can present at any age, risk is highest between 13 and 17 years of age.
- It is estimated that over 725 000 people in the UK have an eating disorder. This is based on hospital admissions, so is likely to be a significant underestimate.
- The types of eating disorders as defined in the DSM-5 include the following:

Anorexia nervosa

- The lifetime prevalence of anorexia nervosa (AN) in females is between 2 and 4%.
- AN has a higher mortality rate than any other mental health disorder. 20% of deaths are due to suicide. The crude mortality rate is 5.1 deaths per 1000 person years.
- Clinical features of AN include:
   - Restricted energy intake or persistent behaviour which prevents weight gain and leads to a significantly low body weight.
   - Body image is disturbed, with denial of the seriousness of the current low body weight, or undue influence of body weight or shape on self-evaluation.
   - There is an intense fear of gaining weight, despite being underweight.
   - BMI specifiers were added in 2013:
      - Mild: BMI 17–18.5kg/m^2
      - Moderate: BMI 16–16.9kg/m^2
      - Severe: BMI 15–15.9kg/m^2
      - Extreme: BMI <15kg/m^2
      - The available evidence has questioned the reliability and clinical validity of these definitions.
- Although females with AN may present with hormonal disturbance and amenorrhoea, it is no longer included in the diagnostic criteria. However, periods and growth/puberty are often disturbed. Where amenorrhoea persists beyond 6 months there is risk of reduced bone density.
- Physical signs may include dry skin and hair loss, bradycardia, orthostatic hypotension, hypothermia, loss of muscle strength, constipation, fainting and fatigue.

Bulimia nervosa

- Recurrent (at least once weekly for 3 months) episodes of uncontrolled eating of an abnormally large amount of food.
- Binges are followed by inappropriate compensatory behaviours (induced vomiting, diet pill or laxative abuse) or excessive exercise.
- Self-evaluation is unduly influenced by body shape / weight, and often there is an intense fear of gaining weight.
- There may be persistent preoccupation with and cravings for food, then guilt and shame about bingeing and purging.

- Bulimia may go undiagnosed for years, as individuals may maintain a normal body weight and appear to eat normally in social situations.
- Physical signs may include knuckle calluses from recurrent induced vomiting (Russell's sign), salivary gland enlargement and dental enamel erosion.

Binge eating disorder

- Recurrent episodes of binge eating without any compensatory behaviours.
- Episodes associated with distress, guilt and marked loss of control.
- Individuals are often overweight or obese.

Avoidant/restrictive food intake disorder (ARFID)

- This is also referenced as 'selective eating disorder' in the DSM.
- Avoidance of food or restrictive pattern of eating based on certain food characteristics or aversive consequences.
- Leads to significant weight loss, nutritional deficiency, or dependence on supplements.

Pica

- Persistent eating of non-nutritive, non-food substances (for at least 1 month).
- Inappropriate to the developmental level.

Rumination

- Repeated regurgitation of food which may be re-chewed, re-swallowed, or spat out.
- Not due to a medical condition or better explained by another disorder.

Other specified feeding or eating disorder (OSFED)

- This is where there is clinically significant distress, but the full criteria for feeding and eating disorders are not met. Includes the following:
  - Atypical AN refers to restrictive disordered eating in people not at an extremely low body weight
  - Subthreshold bulimia or binge eating disorder
  - Purging disorder
  - Night eating syndrome.

Unspecified feeding or eating disorder (UFED)

- This covers disordered eating not more accurately captured by OSFED.

8.5.2 How can we diagnose eating disorders?

- **Eating disorders can be difficult to diagnose, especially in primary care.**
- Patients are often slow to present and may hide or fail to disclose symptoms. They may not think they have an eating disorder.
- The SCOFF questionnaire is a short, focused screening tool to identify anorexia nervosa or bulimia nervosa:
  - *"Do you ever make yourself feel* ***S****ick because you feel uncomfortably full?"*
  - *"Do you worry that you have lost* ***C****ontrol over how much you eat?"*
  - *"Have you recently lost more than* ***O****ne stone in a 3-month period?"*
  - *"Do you believe yourself to be* ***F****at when others say you are too thin?"*
  - *"Would you say that* ***F****ood dominates your life?"*
- Severe malnutrition and purging behaviours can cause cardiovascular instability or severe electrolyte disturbance – have a low index for assessing clinical signs. Emergency admission may be required; for example, where there is syncope, pre-syncope or severe abdominal pain. Check for risk of self-harm and suicide.

- Examination should ideally include calculation of BMI, temperature (hypothermia), BP (including lying/standing), hydration status, peripheral circulation. Look for muscle wasting (consider the Sit up-Squat-Stand (SUSS) test).
- Consider checking FBC, erythrocyte sedimentation rate (ESR), U&Es, LFT, blood glucose, creatinine and urinalysis and ECG if there is significant malnutrition or purgative behaviour. Calcium, magnesium, phosphate, thyroid function test (TFT), B12, folate and ferritin are sometimes also requested.
- Consider risk of insulin misuse in diabetic patients: often missing or reducing doses to induce weight loss. A high HbA1c, or history of recurrent diabetic ketoacidosis may raise suspicion of this.
- Differential diagnoses include inflammatory bowel disease, coeliac disease, mood disorders, drug misuse, thyroid disorders and malignancy.

How can we manage eating disorders?

- **Assess the need for emergency admission if there is serious medical or psychiatric risk.**
- Refer immediately to an eating disorder service for specialist assessment and management. Shared care agreements may be in place, particularly in chronic eating disorders.
- Whilst awaiting specialist assessment arrange regular review as appropriate.
- Have a low threshold for concern – people with eating disorders can appear deceptively well despite being medically unwell.
- Consider emergency admission if:
  - BMI or body weight rapidly falling (e.g. >1kg per week)
  - cardiovascular instability, e.g. bradycardia <40 bpm, tachycardia on standing, prolonged QT on ECG, or hypotension
  - hypothermia
  - reduced muscle power
  - concurrent infection
  - rapid deterioration
  - abnormal bloods
  - acute mental health risk, e.g. suicide attempt or serious self-harm.
- Compulsory admission may be required – seek specialist advice if you have serious concerns about a patient's safety but they do not consent to admission.
- The Royal College of Psychiatrists has released guidelines on assessing the impending risk to life in feeding and eating disorders. This document provides a red/amber/green rating to help us assess when urgent help may be needed. This is adapted from the previous MARSIPAN and JUNIOR MARSIPAN framework. The framework combines assessment of clinical risk factors with consideration of patient motivation, engagement with healthcare, and the presence of support around them.
- It is important to note that it is not only patients with AN who may present with immediate risk to life – for example, bulimic patients risk life-threatening electrolyte disturbances and gastrointestinal complications.

Bone health in eating disorders

- **Women with AN are 150–300% more likely to have fractures due to significantly lower bone mineral density than healthy control women.**
- Weight restoration is of key importance in the underweight to protect bone health.
- The long-term effects of bisphosphonates in this population are still unknown. The decision to start hormonal treatment for low bone density in a patient with an eating disorder should be taken with specialist advice.

Body image in women

- Body image is a frequent concern for women, with evidence that pregnancy, cancer and gynaecological conditions such as PCOS and reproductive milestones such as menopause are correlated with increasing body image concerns.
- Clinicians should be sensitive to the wider psychosocial pressures on women and consider referral for psychological support where women experience distress related to body image.

Body dysmorphic disorder in women

- Body dysmorphic disorder (BDD) is common but under-recognised. It affects women more than men. There is up to 49% heritability.
- BDD and OCD share genetic vulnerability. BDD may co-exist with OCD. There is also association with substance misuse and social anxiety disorder.
- Patients may not spontaneously disclose their concerns for fear of shame and negative judgement. Clinicians therefore may need to ask direct questions to identify the condition.
- It is defined in the DSM-5 as a preoccupation with perceived defects in one's physical appearance that to other people appear non-existent or only slight.
- The appearance preoccupation can trigger excessive repetitive behaviours (such as mirror checking, excess grooming, skin picking) or repetitive mental acts. To be diagnosed, the behaviours must cause impairment or distress.
- It is associated with marked functional impairment, poor quality of life and high rates of suicidality.
- Most women with BDD will seek cosmetic surgery treatment for their BDD concerns, but such treatment virtually never improves BDD symptoms and often makes them worse.
- Patients with suspected BDD should be referred to specialist mental health services for diagnosis and management. Treatment relies on psychotherapeutic approaches and pharmacotherapy, e.g. SSRIs.

8.6 Further reading

APA (2022) *Diagnostic and Statistical Manual of Mental Disorders, fifth edition, text revision (DSM-5-TR).* American Psychiatric Association. Available at: https://dsm.psychiatryonline.org

Baron-Cohen, S., Lombardo, M.V., Auyeung, B. *et al.* (2011) Why are autism spectrum conditions more prevalent in men? *PLoS Biol,* **9(6):** e1001081.

BMJ Best Practice (2022) *Postnatal Depression.* BMJ Publishing Group.

BMS (2024) *Management of unscheduled bleeding on hormone replacement therapy (HRT).* Available at: https://thebms.org.uk/wp-content/uploads/2024/12/01-BMS-GUIDELINE-Management-of-unscheduled-bleeding-HRT-NOVEMBER2024-A.pdf

Brady, M.J., Jenkins, C.A., Gamble-Turner, J.M. *et al.* (2024) "A perfect storm": autistic experiences of menopause and midlife. *Autism,* **28(6):** 1405–18.

Brown, L., Hunter, M.S., Chen, R. *et al.* (2024) Promoting good mental health over the menopause transition. *Lancet,* **403(10430):** 969–83.

Busse, J.W., Montori, V.M., Krasnik, C. *et al.* (2009) Psychological intervention for premenstrual syndrome: a meta-analysis of randomized controlled trials. *Psychother Psychosom,* **78(1):** 6–15.

Cary, E. and Simpson, P. (2024) Premenstrual disorders and PMDD – a review. *Best Pract Res Clin Endocrinol Metab,* **38(1):** 101858.

Cassidy. S. and Rodgers, J. (2017) Understanding and prevention of suicide in autism. *Lancet Psychiatry,* **4(6):** e11.

Cook, J., Hull, L. and Mandy, W. (2024) Improving diagnostic procedures in autism for girls and women: a narrative review. *Neuropsychiatr Dis Treat,* **20:** 505–14.

Craner, J.R., Sigmon, S.T. and McGillicuddy, M.L. (2014) Does a disconnect occur between research and practice for premenstrual dysphoric disorder (PMDD) diagnostic procedures? *Women Health*, **54(3):** 232–44.

Direkvand-Moghadam, A., Sayehmiri, K. and Sattar, K. (2014) Epidemiology of premenstrual syndrome (PMS) – a systematic review and meta-analysis study. *J Clin Diagn Res*, **8(2):** 106–9. Erratum in: *J Clin Diagn Res*. 2015, 9(7): ZZ05.

Epperson, C.N., Sammel, M.D., Bale, T.L. *et al.* (2017) Adverse childhood experiences and risk for first-episode major depression during the menopause transition. *J Clin Psychiatry*, **78(3):** e298–e307.

Feingold, K.R., Ahmed, S.F., Anawalt, B. *et al.* (eds) Table 2 Classification of premenstrual disorders (PMD). *Endotext*. Available at: www.ncbi.nlm.nih.gov/books/NBK279045/table/premenstrual-syndrom.table2clas

Grewal, J.K., Mu, E., Li, Q. *et al.* (2025) The prevalence of traumatic exposure in women with premenstrual dysphoric disorder (PMDD): a systematic review. *Arch Womens Ment Health*, **28(4):** 723–40.

Groenman, A.P., Torenvliet, C., Radhoe, T.A., Agelink van Rentergem, J.A. and Geurts, H.M. (2022) Menstruation and menopause in autistic adults: periods of importance? *Autism*, **26(6):** 1563–72.

Halbreich, U. (2003) The etiology, biology, and evolving pathology of premenstrual syndromes. *Psychoneuroendocrinology*, **28(suppl 3):** 55–99.

Hammarbäck, S., Bäckström, T., Holst, J., von Schoultz, B. and Lyrenäs, S. (1985) Cyclical mood changes as in the premenstrual tension syndrome during sequential estrogen-progestagen postmenopausal replacement therapy. *Acta Obstet Gynecol Scand*, **64(5):** 393–7.

Hudepohl, N., MacLean, J.V. and Osborne, L.M. (2022) Perinatal obsessive-compulsive disorder: epidemiology, phenomenology, etiology, and treatment. *Curr Psychiatry Rep*, **24(4):** 229–37.

Lai, M.C. and Baron-Cohen, S. (2015) Identifying the lost generation of adults with autism spectrum conditions. *Lancet Psychiatry*, **2(11):** 1013–27.

Lai, M.C., Kassee, C., Besney, R. *et al.* (2019) Prevalence of co-occurring mental health diagnoses in the autism population: a systematic review and meta-analysis. *Lancet Psychiatry*, **6(10):** 819–29.

Lai, M.C., Lombardo, M.V., Ruigrok, A.N. *et al.* (2017) Quantifying and exploring camouflaging in men and women with autism. *Autism*, **21(6):** 690–702.

Langan, R. and Goodbred, A.J. (2016) Identification and management of peripartum depression. *Am Fam Physician*, **93(10):** 852–8.

Moseley, R.L., Druce, T. and Turner-Cobb, J.M. (2020) 'When my autism broke': a qualitative study spotlighting autistic voices on menopause. *Autism*, **24(6):** 1423–37.

NHS Scotland (revised 2022) *Eating disorders* [SIGN164]. Available at: www.sign.ac.uk/media/1987/sign-164-eating-disorders-v2.pdf

NICE (updated 2020) *Eating disorders: recognition and treatment* [NG69]. Available at: www.nice.org.uk/guidance/NG69

NICE (revised 2024) CKS: *Eating disorders: How common is it?* Available at: https://cks.nice.org.uk/topics/eating-disorders/background-information/prevalence

NICE (revised 2025) CKS: *Depression – antenatal and postnatal.* Available at: https://cks.nice.org.uk/topics/depression-antenatal-postnatal

Obaydi, H. and Puri, B.K. (2008) Prevalence of premenstrual syndrome in autism: a prospective observer-rated study. *J Int Med Res*, **36(2):** 268–72.

Panay, N. NAPS *guidelines on premenstrual syndrome.* National Association for Premenstrual Syndrome. Available at: www.pms.org.uk/app/uploads/2018/06/guidelinesfinal60210.pdf

Panay, N. and Studd, J. (1997) Progestogen intolerance and compliance with hormone replacement therapy in menopausal women. *Hum Reprod Update,* **3:** 159–71.

Phillips, K.A. and Susser, L.C. (2023) Body dysmorphic disorder in women. *Psychiatr Clin North Am,* **46(3):** 505–25.

Prasad, D., Wollenhaupt-Aguiar, B., Kidd, K.N., de Azevedo Cardoso, T. and Frey, B.N. (2021) Suicidal risk in women with premenstrual syndrome and premenstrual dysphoric disorder: a systematic review and meta-analysis. *J Womens Health (Larchmt),* **30(12):** 1693–707.

RCGP/GPCPC (2023) *Antenatal and postnatal mental health NICE guideline CG192. Practical implications for GPs.* Royal College of General Practitioners and GPs Championing Perinatal Care.

RCOG (2016) *Premenstrual syndrome, management* (Green-top Guideline No. 48). Available at: www.rcog.org.uk/guidance/browse-all-guidance/green-top-guidelines/premenstrual-syndrome-management-green-top-guideline-no-48

Reilly, T.J., Patel, S., Unachukwu, I.C. *et al.* (2024) The prevalence of premenstrual dysphoric disorder: systematic review and meta-analysis. *J Affect Disord,* **349:** 534–40.

Robertson, E., Thew, C., Thomas, N., Karimi, L. and Kulkarni, J. (2021) Pilot data on the feasibility and clinical outcomes of a nomegestrol acetate oral contraceptive pill in women with premenstrual dysphoric disorder. *Front Endocrinol (Lausanne),* **12:** 704488.

Royal College of Psychiatrists (updated 2023) *Medical emergencies in eating disorders: guidance on recognition and management.* Available at: www.rcpsych.ac.uk/docs/default-source/improving-care/better-mh-policy/college-reports/college-report-cr233-medical-emergencies-in-eating-disorders-(meed)-guidance.pdf?sfvrsn=2d327483_63

Schiller, C.E., Johnson, S.L., Abate, A.C., Schmidt, P.J. and Rubinow, D.R. (2016) Reproductive steroid regulation of mood and behavior. *Compr Physiol,* **6(3):** 1135–60.

Schröder, S.S., Danner, U.N., Spek, A.A. and van Elburg, A.A. (2023) Exploring the intersection of autism spectrum disorder and eating disorders: understanding the unique challenges and treatment considerations for autistic women with eating disorders. *Curr Opin Psychiatry,* **36(6):** 419–26.

Sharma, V., Doobay, M. and Baczynski, C. (2017) Bipolar postpartum depression: an update and recommendations. *J Affect Disord,* **219:** 105–11.

Studd, J. and Nappi, R.E. (2012) Reproductive depression. *Gynecol Endocrinol,* **28(Suppl 1):** 42–5.

Toda, S., Tsushima, S., Takashio, O. *et al.* (2024) The repressed life of adult female patients with mild ADHD. *Front Psychiatry,* **15:** 1418698.

Toppino, F., Longo, P., Martini, M., Abbate-Daga, G. and Marzola, E. (2022) Body mass index specifiers in anorexia nervosa: anything below the "extreme"? *J Clin Med,* **11(3):** 542.

Werling, D.M. and Geschwind, D.H. (2013) Sex differences in autism spectrum disorders. *Curr Opin Neurol,* **26(2):** 146–53.

Witjes, H., Creinin, M.D., Sundström-Poromaa, I., Martin Nguyen, A. and Korver, T. (2015) Comparative analysis of the effects of nomegestrol acetate/17 β-estradiol and drospirenone/ethinylestradiol on premenstrual and menstrual symptoms and dysmenorrhea. *Eur J Contracept Reprod Health Care,* **20(4):** 296–307.

Wyatt, K.M., Dimmock, P.W., Jones, P.W. *et al.* (1999) Efficacy of vitamin B6 in treatment of premenstrual syndrome: systematic review. *BMJ,* **318:** 1375–81.

Chapter 9
Genitourinary issues

9.1 Pelvic organ prolapse

9.1.1 What is a pelvic organ prolapse and who is affected?

- NB: some publications and resources abbreviate 'pelvic organ prolapse' to POP; in this book we have spelt it out in full to avoid confusion with 'progestogen-only pill'.
- The term 'prolapse' refers to the downward displacement of a pelvic organ. This may be symptomatic, but many women with mild prolapse are not aware of the problem.
- Symptoms may include the following:
  - Vaginal bulging (a feeling of a 'bulge', 'something coming down' or 'falling out' through the vaginal introitus).
  - Pelvic pressure (feeling of heaviness or dragging discomfort).
  - Bleeding, discharge, infection (may relate to ulceration).
  - Splinting/digitation (the need to replace the prolapse manually, or apply pressure to void or defecate).
  - Low backache (often 'menstrual-like' backache which may be relieved when the prolapse is reduced).
  - Urethral prolapse (often a lump at the external urethral meatus).
  - Anorectal prolapse is also possible – usually with external protrusion of the rectum.
- Two-thirds of parous women have anatomical evidence of prolapse, but the majority of these are asymptomatic. 40% of women aged between 45 and 85 have an objective pelvic organ prolapse on examination but only around 12% of these will be symptomatic.
- Lifetime risk of prolapse is a little over 1 in 10. Risk factors include the following:
  - High BMI.
  - Increasing age.
  - Increasing parity / high birthweight babies / difficult vaginal birth.
  - Being postmenopausal.
  - Long-term constipation.
  - Chronic cough.
  - Jobs requiring heavy lifting.
  - Collagen disorder, e.g. Ehlers–Danlos or benign joint hypermobility syndrome.

9.1.2 Types and stages of pelvic organ prolapse

- The 2016 International Urogynaecological Association (IUGA) and International Continence Society (ICS) definitions are as follows:
  - **Central (uterine/cervical) prolapse:** clinically evident descent of the uterus or uterine cervix. Full eversion is often called procidentia.
  - **Anterior (vaginal wall) prolapse:** clinically evident descent of the anterior vaginal wall. Often referred to as a cystocele or urethrocele when it contains the bladder or urethra, respectively.
  - **Posterior (vaginal wall) prolapse:** clinically evident descent of the posterior vaginal wall. Often referred to as an enterocele or rectocele when it contains rectum or small bowel, respectively.
  - **Vaginal vault prolapse:** clinically evident descent of the vaginal vault.
- **Prolapse is graded according** to its current position with reference to a fixed point in the body (the hymen, usually situated 1–2cm inside the introitus). The NICE guidelines suggest the pelvic organ prolapse quantification (POP-Q) system should be used to help stage the degree of prolapse:
  - Stage 0: no prolapse.
  - Stage 1: >1cm above the hymen.
  - Stage 2: ≤1cm above or below the plane of the hymen.

- Stage 3: >1cm below the plane of the hymen, but no further than 2cm less than the total vaginal length.
- Stage 4: eversion of the lower genital tract is complete.

- When the prolapse is not clear on examination, it can help to ask the woman to stand or squat.
- Examination should assess for the presence of any pelvic mass or ascites, and for the health of the vulvovaginal tissues. Prolapse can become worse with loss of oestrogen around menopause.
- It can be helpful to organise assessment of the activity of the pelvic floor muscles (often performed by a gynaecological physiotherapist). Imaging is not routinely required.
- Women should be asked about symptoms associated with the prolapse, including impact on sexual function, and bladder and bowel function.

9.1.3 Preventing prolapse

- Caesarean section and smoking appear to be protective factors for primary prolapse.
- Vaginal birth is the biggest modifiable risk factor for prolapse, and is an important contributor to stress incontinence. Injuries to the levator ani muscle, perineal body and membrane occur in up to 19% of primiparous women. This injury is present in 55% of women with prolapse in later life.
- Risk factors for levator injury include forceps delivery. Vacuum delivery is protective. Early recognition of injury and attention to recovery is important.
- Pelvic floor exercises are often proposed as a measure to prevent pelvic organ prolapse. The evidence is strongest for improving symptoms once a prolapse has developed but exercising the pelvic floor, especially during pregnancy, seems to reduce the future likelihood of pelvic organ prolapse / urinary incontinence.
- Oestrogen has a profound effect on health of pelvic connective tissues and, as pelvic organ prolapse and urogenital atrophy are associated with menopause, may be expected to help prevent the condition. Although there is good evidence to support the use of oestrogen for urinary continence, there has been limited research regarding the role of androgens and oestrogens on pelvic organ prolapse, and their results have been contradictory.
- Modification of other risk factors could also reduce the risk of pelvic organ prolapse – for example, managing constipation to avoid straining. Weight loss or bariatric surgery has also been suggested as a preventative measure – studies support a reduction in symptom severity, but no change in POP-Q stage.

9.1.4 Treating prolapse

Non-surgical treatment

These options should be offered according to patient choice. They can, and often should, be offered in conjunction with one another.

Oestrogen

- Consider the use of topical oestrogens in women whose symptoms could be attributed to genitourinary syndrome of the menopause (GSM).
- An oestrogen-containing ring (e.g. Estring) is a good choice for women who may struggle with GSM but have cognitive or physical impairments that may make pessaries and creams difficult to use.

Modify lifestyle

- Women with a BMI >30kg/m^2 should be encouraged to lose weight.
- Treat constipation to minimise straining.
- Reduce heavy lifting where possible.

Support pessaries

- Consider vaginal support pessaries in women with symptomatic pelvic floor prolapse.
- Pessaries should be removed or replaced every 4–6 months (often fitting an Estring at the same time is useful, especially in older, less agile patients).
- It may take more than one fitting to correctly size a pessary. As well as rings (silicone and PVC), shelf and gelhorn pessaries, newer pessaries are available (e.g. Cube and Donut pessaries). A useful summary of the types of pessary available has been compiled by Pelvic, Obstetric and Gynaecological Physiotherapy (see https://thepogp.co.uk/_userfiles/pages/files/pessary_types_guide.pdf).
- Pessaries can cause local vaginal irritation or erosion, and can impact sexual activity. It is important that patients are offered a choice that suits them, and that topical oestrogen is also used if appropriate.
- If a pessary is not acceptable or tolerated by the patient, refer for surgery.

Pelvic floor muscle training

- Offer supervised physiotherapy with a women's health physiotherapist, for at least 16 weeks as a first option for women with stage 1–2 prolapse (evidence is less clear for stage 3 or 4 POP-Q).

Surgical treatment

Surgery should be offered to women whose symptoms are not well controlled with non-surgical measures.

Native tissue repair vs. mesh

- Mesh procedures were the subject of high-profile legal cases and much public concern. There is some evidence they remain of benefit for pelvic organ prolapse but there is limited evidence of long-term adverse effects.
- Women who have had previous mesh procedures may consider having mesh removed in view of the concerns. They should be referred to a gynaecological or urological surgeon who will discuss the case with the regional multidisciplinary team before proceeding, as there is limited evidence on the relative benefits of partial or total mesh removal vs. leaving *in situ*.

Uterine preservation

- Women can have the option of hysterectomy, or surgery that will preserve the uterus.
- If women express no preference, they should be offered vaginal hysterectomy with or without vaginal sacrospinous fixation (the top of the vagina is attached to the sacrospinous ligament) with sutures, or vaginal sacrospinous hysteropexy (the cervix is stitched to the sacrospinous ligament) with sutures, or a Manchester repair (where the cervix is shortened and the vaginal ligaments used to support the uterus).

Post hysterectomy vaginal vault prolapse

- These women are usually offered vaginal sacrospinous fixation, or sacrocolpopexy with mesh (mesh is used to attach the vagina to the sacrum).

Colpocleisis

- This procedure (surgery to close the vagina) is offered for vault or uterine prolapse where vaginal sex is not desired.

Surgery for anterior and posterior prolapse

- Women are offered anterior or posterior repair, without mesh.

Surgery for women with both pelvic organ prolapse and stress urinary incontinence

- Concurrent surgery should be considered, but women should be advised of a greater risk of complications, and longer-term efficacy of combined procedures is uncertain.

9.2 Urinary incontinence

9.2.1 What is urinary incontinence and who is affected?

- Urinary incontinence is defined as any involuntary leakage of urine.
- It is common, with possibly 40% of women experiencing urge incontinence and 24% with stress incontinence.
- Women tend to feel shame about admitting to the problem, meaning that only about 17% of those with urge incontinence had sought help in one study.
- The peak age for symptoms is around 35–44 years for urge incontinence, and 55–64 years for stress incontinence.
- Incontinence can lead to many complications that negatively impact a person's health and quality of life, e.g. low self-esteem, sexual problems, social isolation and sleep disturbance.
- There are two main types – stress and urge incontinence.
  - **Stress urinary incontinence**
    - Involuntary leak occurs with coughs, sneezing, exertion, coughing.
  - **Urge urinary incontinence (UUI)**
    - Leakage occurs just after the woman experiences a sudden urge to urinate (that is difficult to defer).
    - Urge incontinence is often accompanied by overactive bladder (OAB) which combines urgency, frequency and, often, nocturia.
    - OAB 'wet' occurs with associated UUI; OAB dry does not have an element of urge urinary incontinence.
  - **Mixed urinary incontinence**
    - Leak associated with symptoms of urgency, together with stress leakage on coughing, exertion or sneezing.
- Some women also experience overflow incontinence (chronic urinary retention) where a chronically over-distended bladder leaks.
- Continuous urinary incontinence is where involuntary urinary loss is constant.
- Situational urinary incontinence is where incontinence occurs only with specific triggers, e.g. during sex (or climax-specific, known as climacturia), or when changing body position.
- The main risk factor for developing any kind of urinary incontinence is aging, leading to:
  - Decreased bladder capacity and feeling of fullness.
  - Decreased rate of detrusor muscle contraction.
  - Decreased pelvic muscle resistance.
  - Increased residual urine volume.
- **Risk factors specific to stress incontinence:**
  - Pregnancy, parity and vaginal delivery.
  - Obesity.
  - High-impact activities.
  - Previous pelvic and vaginal surgeries.
  - Genetic and family history (including connective tissue disorders).
  - Constipation.
  - Smoking (likely due to chronic cough).
  - Menopause.
  - Certain medications, e.g. ACE inhibitors can relax the bladder outlet and urethra.
- **Risk factors specific to urge incontinence include:**
  - Neurological conditions such as Parkinson's, multiple sclerosis (MS), stroke or spinal cord injuries.
  - Recurrent UTI (seem to cause local irritation and involuntary bladder contractions).
  - Diabetes (often leads to OAB and sensory neurogenic bladder, predisposing to UUI).

- Menopause.
- Caffeine or alcoholic drinks (lead to polyuria, frequency, urgency and nocturia).
- High or low fluid intake.
- Smoking (irritants in cigarette smoke seem to irritate the bladder and worsen urinary tract symptoms).
- Certain medications – e.g. sympathomimetics, antidepressants and HRT can cause detrusor overactivity. Diuretics can also cause issues.

- **Risk factors for overflow incontinence:**
  - Occurs when there is an obstruction at the bladder neck and an impairment of detrusor contractility, e.g. neurological conditions, medications decreasing bladder contractility leading to retention then overflow.
- **Risk factors for continuous urinary incontinence include:**
  - Urethral diverticulae, genitourinary fistulae, congenital abnormalities in urological anatomy, e.g. ectopic ureters.

9.2.2 How do we diagnose and assess urinary continence issues?

- Take a detailed history around the symptoms, timing and nature of the symptoms being experienced, to help determine if this is urge, stress, OAB or mixed incontinence.
- Ask about voiding symptoms and the presence of any urinary symptoms such as haematuria, bladder or urethral pain, recurrent UTI or constant leakage that may suggest, for example, a fistula.
- Check for the presence of neurological conditions, urinary tract disorders, low spinal surgery, obstetric history, and medication that may cause or exacerbate urinary issues.
- Perform a general examination looking for:
  - Overweight or obesity.
  - Indicators of neurological disease, e.g. gait changes, muscle wasting, fasciculation.
  - Palpable bladder or any masses.
- Perform a pelvic examination to assess for masses, uterine enlargement, urethral diverticulae and/or vulvovaginal atrophy. Ask her to cough and assess for signs of leakage at the external urethral meatus.
- Assess pelvic floor muscle tone – grading scales exist, such as the Oxford grading system:
  - 0 = no contraction
  - 1 = flicker or pulsation under the examiner's finger
  - 2 = weak (some tension, but no lift)
  - 3 = moderate (lifting of the muscle belly and the posterior vaginal wall)
  - 4 = good (increased tension and a good contraction lifting the posterior vaginal wall against resistance by the examining finger)
  - 5 = strong (strong resistance which draws the examiner's fingers into the vagina).
- Consider further investigations, i.e. urine dipstick to check for blood, glucose, protein, leucocytes and nitrates. If positive, send mid-stream urine (MSU) sample and prescribe an antibiotic for presumed UTI whilst awaiting the result. Consider assessing renal function (urinary obstruction will require urgent management).
- Encourage the woman to keep a bladder diary for 3 days looking at quantity and type of fluids ingested, frequency of urination, volume voided (including overnight) and any episodes of urgency, incontinence or leak.

9.2.3 Managing urinary incontinence: when to refer?

- Patients require urgent referral on the suspected bladder cancer pathway if:
  - There is unexplained visible haematuria (without UTI) in a patient aged >45.
  - They are aged >45 and visible UTI persists despite treatment with antibiotics.
  - They are aged >60 with non-visible haematuria *and* dysuria / raised white cell count on a blood test.

- Refer to secondary care (urologist/urogynaecology/nephrology/neurology) if there is:
  - Persistent pain in bladder/urethra.
  - Voiding (outflow) difficulty.
  - Chronic urinary retention.
  - Palpable bladder on abdominal or bimanual examination after voiding.
  - A clinically benign pelvic mass.
  - Associated faecal incontinence.
  - Suspected neurological disease.
  - Suspected urogenital fistulae.
  - History of previous incontinence surgery / pelvic cancer surgery or radiotherapy.
  - Unexplained recurrent or resistant UTI in a woman over the age of 60.

9.2.4 General management of urinary incontinence within primary care

- All women should complete a bladder diary (this can be downloaded from www.baus.org.uk).
- Offer lifestyle advice where appropriate – for example weight loss where BMI is >30kg/m^2), modification of fluid intake, reducing caffeine, stopping smoking.
- Check for constipation and treat if present, as it can worsen urinary continence.
- Consider presence of diabetes and diabetic control where appropriate.
- Enquire about associated problems such as sleep disturbance, depression and anxiety. Offer support with these where possible.
- Consider urinary incontinence as an independent risk factor for falls.

9.2.5 Management of stress urinary incontinence

- Women should be offered referral to a pelvic floor physiotherapist or other trained specialist for at least 3 months of supervised pelvic floor muscle training (PFMT). The impact of PFMT seems to be improved where electromyographic biofeedback is used.
- If symptoms persist despite PFMT, consider referral to consider surgical treatment such as colposuspension, autologous rectus fascial sling or intramural bulking agents.
- Consider offering duloxetine – usually at an initial dose of 20–40mg bd. Duloxetine can cause problems where there is a history of cardiac disease, seizures, glaucoma or hypertension, and women should be appropriately counselled regarding side-effects. If ineffective, doses should be withdrawn slowly to avoid the risk of withdrawal reactions.

9.2.6 Management of urgency incontinence / overactive bladder

- Refer to local continence service for at least 6 weeks of bladder training.
- If symptoms persist or are troublesome, consider adding a medicine for OAB such as desmopressin.
- Consider a trial of oestrogen therapy intravaginally if the woman is peri- or postmenopausal. Some women additionally benefit from topical oestrogen on the urethral meatus.
- Evidence is emerging that CBT may also have a beneficial effect on symptom severity and quality of life.

9.2.7 Management of mixed urinary incontinence

- Women with mixed symptoms can be offered an anticholinergic medication, taking into account the associated risks of these (e.g. urinary retention, cognitive impairment and confusion). It is important to assess the total anticholinergic load to ensure prescribing does not leave patients at risk of falls or delirium.
- Antimuscarinics can take several weeks to work, and should be stopped if ineffective.
- Where antimuscarinics are ineffective or contraindicated, beta-3 adrenergic receptors (mirabegron, vibegron) may be considered.

- Where first-line treatments are ineffective after 4 weeks, consider an alternative antimuscarinic or proceed to a beta-3 adrenergic receptor agonist.
- Women who are not responsive to measures in primary care can be referred for specialist management; this may include the use of botulinum toxin type A into the bladder wall, percutaneous sacral nerve stimulation, augmentation cystoplasty or urinary diversion.

9.3 Faecal incontinence

- Faecal incontinence creates social stigma and is not always readily disclosed to clinicians. We therefore need to remember to enquire about the symptom in high-risk groups.
- It may relate to contributory factors including:
  - Structural or congenital changes / abnormalities in the anus/rectum.
  - Cognitive or behavioural issues.
  - Neurological conditions, e.g. MS, stroke, pudendal neuropathy, or cauda equina syndrome.
  - Abnormal stool consistency.
  - Chronic constipation, with overflow diarrhoea linked to faecal impaction.
  - Colorectal cancer.
  - Inflammatory bowel disease / coeliac disease / irritable bowel syndrome.
  - Gastroenteritis.
  - Pelvic surgery or radiotherapy.
  - Pelvic organ or rectal prolapse, or haemorrhoids.
  - General disability or aging.
  - Obstetric injury – especially following third- or fourth-degree tears.
  - Medication – including antibiotics, SSRIs, laxatives, digoxin or orlistat.
  - Obesity and diabetes mellitus (including associated autonomic neuropathy).
- Prevalence is estimated at 8–12% in the general population, and up to 60% of residents in nursing homes.
- Faecal incontinence can lead to skin irritation or breakdown, and depression, anxiety and social isolation. It also creates increased caregiver burden and financial pressure relating to continence products.

9.3.1 Assessment of faecal incontinence

- As the issue may not be readily disclosed, ask direct questions to patients in high-risk groups.
- Ask about timing, frequency, quantity and the circumstances of soiling.
- Ask about sensation – does the patient feel an urge to open the bowel before leakage? Is the sensation urgent? Classification is usually into urge, passive or combined subtypes. The Rome IV criteria state that a diagnosis of faecal incontinence can be made when symptoms have been present for over 3 months.
- What measures are being taken to help manage the issue – dietary, medication, and incontinence wear for example?
- Ask about bowel habit, including any recent changes that may need further investigation. What is the stool consistency? Is there pain and discomfort? Any abdominal symptoms such as bloating or nausea?
- Check for the presence of constipation, which can lead to overflow and leakage as well as reduced rectal sensation.
- Ask about obstetric history and history of weak pelvic floor: prolapse? Birth injury? Difficult/ prolonged labour, large birthweight or assisted delivery?

- Review medications, as many drugs may exacerbate faecal incontinence (for examples see https://cks.nice.org.uk/topics/faecal-incontinence-in-adults/diagnosis/assessment/#drugs-that-can-exacerbate-faecal-incontinence).
- Examination should include assessing perianal skin, assessment of perineal descent, a digital rectal examination including asking the patient to squeeze the examining finger to check anal tone. Check for faecal loading.

9.3.2 Management of faecal incontinence

- Women presenting with faecal incontinence require assessment of risk:
  - Where there is concern about cauda equina or stroke, emergency assessment should be arranged without delay.
  - Consider the possibility of colorectal cancer where women meet certain criteria (age ≥40 with unexplained weight loss and pain, aged ≥50 with unexplained rectal bleeding or aged ≥60 with iron-deficiency anaemia, changed bowel habit, or positive faecal occult bloods); urgent referral should be arranged.
  - Urgent suspected cancer (USC) referral is also required if there is an anal, rectal or abdominal mass or the woman is under the age of 50 with rectal bleeding **and** abdominal pain, changed bowel habit, weight loss or iron-deficiency anaemia.
- Treatment should focus on improving the underlying cause of soiling – for example, referral to optimise management of inflammatory bowel disease, treatment of chronic constipation or 3rd-/4th-degree haemorrhoids, or referral to neurology where there is evidence of a condition such as MS.
  - If faecal incontinence stems from obstetric injury, referral should be made to a specialist for consideration of surgical repair.
  - Refer patients to specialist continence services where possible – they will usually focus on conservative interventions such as PFMT, biofeedback and electrical stimulation devices and bowel retraining. Specialist assessment may include anorectal physiology studies, proctography and endoanal ultrasound. Surgery may be offered where prolapse, haemorrhoids or anal sphincter injury are contributing.
  - Non-surgical options include:
    - Dietary changes (a food diary is often advised, to look for triggers).
    - Bowel retraining (e.g. encouraging the person to empty the bowel after each meal to utilise the gastrocolic reflex), and the use of a squatting position (e.g. a Squatty Potty) to optimise bowel emptying whilst minimising straining.
    - Anti-diarrhoeal medication (first-line is loperamide, but where this is not tolerated codeine phosphate may be useful).
    - Continence products should be offered as needed.
    - Coping strategies (barrier creams, odour control, psychological support).

9.4 Recurrent UTI

9.4.1 Definitions

- Recurrent UTI is usually defined as two or more episodes of urinary tract infection in 6 months, or three or more episodes in 1 year.
- The episodes may represent relapse or reinfection.
- Studies based in primary care suggest about 2.6% of women over the age of 65 have recurrent UTI.
- It is important not to misdiagnose asymptomatic bacteriuria (the presence of bacteria in a sample without the presence of symptomatic infection) with recurrent UTI. Asymptomatic bacteriuria is more common in care home populations and in long-term catheter use: it is estimated that 1 in 5 women over age 80 have asymptomatic bacteriuria.

9.4.2 Aetiology of recurrent UTI

- Bacteria usually enter the urinary tract from the gastrointestinal tract – either by ascending into the urethra and up to the bladder, through haematogenous spread (more likely in immunocompromised or immunosuppressed), or through direct inoculation, e.g. via a catheter or surgery.
- The most commonly identified pathogen is *E. coli*, but less commonly identified organisms may include *Staphylococcus saprophyticus*, *Proteus mirabilis*, and *Pseudomonas*, *Enterococcus*, *Serratia* and *Klebsiella* spp.
- Candida can also cause UTI, though this is more unusual and usually associated with indwelling catheters or immunosuppression.

9.4.3 What puts some women at risk for recurrent UTI?

- Recent sexual intercourse or a new sexual partner are frequently associated with recurrent infections.
- A history of childhood UTI or a maternal family history increase risk of developing recurrent UTI in adulthood.
- Urinary tract obstructions, calculi or instrumentation.
- GSM is a common trigger for increasing susceptibility to urinary infections, and many women will notice a change in the frequency of UTI as they enter perimenopause. Early use of local oestrogen can have a huge impact on rate of infection.
- Women with urinary incontinence, incomplete bladder emptying and bladder prolapse (cystocele) may also be more vulnerable to recurrent infection, as are those with long-term catheters. Reduced functional status in older women also increases risk.
- Antibiotic resistance can be an issue where there is prolonged use of antibiotics or history of previous resistant infection.

9.4.4 Diagnosing recurrent UTI

- Recurrent cystitis is common. Most women will not require referral for management or investigations such as cystoscopy or imaging, as the diagnostic yield is low.
- It is important to check for red flag symptoms such as: being over 45 years with non-visible haematuria without UTI; visible haematuria persisting after antibiotic treatment; evidence of outflow obstruction; a pelvic mass; or age >60 with unexplained non-visible haematuria and with either dysuria or a raised white cell count on blood testing.
- Whilst MSU is used to diagnose UTI and to confirm the pathogen and antibiotic sensitivity, it is important to recognise the possibility of chronic embedded UTI (see *Section 9.4.6*), where pathogenic bacteria are hypothesised to have migrated into the bladder wall, creating symptoms without positive MSU. Urological opinion may be required in these cases.

9.4.5 Treatment and prevention of recurrent UTI

- Prevention of recurrent UTI requires avoidance of risk factors, non-antimicrobial measures, and antimicrobial prophylaxis. These interventions may be attempted in any order and in combination.
- Where there is significant residual urine, intermittent catheterisation or chronic indwelling catheterisation may need consideration by a specialist team.
- Behavioural modifications include:
  - Drinking adequate fluids (a study showed adding 1.5L fluid a day to postmenopausal women's intake of fluids reduced the number of episodes of cystitis over 12m).
  - Urinating after sex.
  - Wiping from front to back after defecation.

- Hormonal replacement:
  - Four meta-analyses show the efficacy of topical oestrogen therapy for prevention of recurrent cystitis. This is important and has been shown to help avoid urosepsis and hospital admissions in the elderly.
  - Oral oestrogen was not shown to be effective compared to placebo, suggesting that our first line should be offering local oestrogen to women struggling with this issue.
- Immunomodulation:
  - New 'vaccines' exist, such as StroVac and Solco-Urovac, which show patients are 50% more likely to remain recurrence-free with these agents. Currently access is limited to specialist care only.
  - Prophylaxis with probiotics (e.g. *Lactobacillus*) has not been shown consistently in trials to be beneficial.
  - Prophylaxis with cranberry has mixed evidence but the European Association of Urology (EAU) guidelines suggest recommending this, as some patient populations may find it beneficial and there has been little harm identified from use.
  - Prophylaxis with D-mannose showed it improves quality of life and significantly reduces infections in users, and prolongs cystitis-free periods, in both catheter users and non-catheter users.
  - Intravesical instillations with hyaluronic acid and chondroitin sulphate have been used to help repair and replenish the glycosaminoglycan (GAG) layer, which has helped in interstitial cystitis, OAB, radiation cystitis and for prevention of recurrent cystitis.
  - Methenamine hippurate, a chemical that increases the acidity of urine, has not been found to be helpful in treating UTI, but does appear to help reduce the frequency of recurrent infections.
  - Antimicrobial therapy remains the most effective approach to prevention of recurrent UTI. They may be given as continuous, low-dose courses or as postcoital prophylaxis. There is little difference in efficacy of these approaches, so patient preference is important. When the drugs are discontinued, infections tend to recur. Most studies suggest 3–12-month courses but there is no clear consensus on duration or frequency of such courses. Choice of antibiotic should reflect local resistance patterns – usually regimens include nitrofurantoin 50mg or 100mg daily, fosfomycin trometamol 3g once weekly, or trimethoprim 100mg daily. In pregnancy, cefalexin 125mg or 250mg daily is usually advised.
  - In women with a good history of accurate self-diagnosis, it is possible to prescribe short courses to be kept at home and started as needed.

9.4.6 Chronic embedded UTI

- This is a new diagnostic term which is still subject to controversy and not recognised universally.
- It describes the clinical situation of UTI symptoms (pain, frequency, discomfort in bladder or abdomen) persisting beyond a short-term antibiotic course. Urine tests such as mid-stream urinalysis do not show infection.
- It is hypothesised that bacteria may enter the lining of the bladder and then create a cycle, like herpes virus, of being dormant then producing a flare of symptoms. Chronic UTI is believed to be hard to diagnose, as traditional MSU samples may not identify the presence of bacteria.
- More specialists and research are recognising this condition and often, women are offered long-term antibiotics, bladder investigations such as cystoscopy and advice regarding bladder-friendly diet, pain control, antihistamines, antimuscarinics and bladder instillations.
- There are emergent immune-based treatments, including a vaccine, which show promise in reducing symptoms related to chronic UTI.
- Women with this clinical picture should be referred for specialist review.

9.5 Bladder pain syndrome / interstitial cystitis

- Both bladder pain syndrome (BPS) and interstitial cystitis (IC) are terms used to refer to a chronic pain syndrome where debilitating pain, lower urinary tract symptoms and pelvic pain result in a significant decline in quality of life.
- Current terminology, diagnostic processes and treatments often remain unsatisfactory and although the understanding of the aetiology and pathophysiology of BPS/IC is growing, the condition remains difficult to treat.
- Symptoms include frequency and urgency, together with chronic pelvic pain. There is often external genital pain, and it should be noted that there is significant overlap with vestibulodynia – thought to be due to the shared embryological origin of the tissues in these areas.
- The prevalence is thought to be between 0.01 and 6.5%.

9.5.1 Aetiology of bladder pain syndrome / interstitial cystitis

- Although the aetiology is still not fully understood, most evidence to date suggests a complex interplay of neurological, endocrine, immune and other mechanisms involving neurogenic inflammation, infection, autoimmunity, mast cell activation, defects in the GAG layer and increased permeability of the bladder epithelium.
- It is possible that BPS/IC is a systemic disease, as there is considerable overlap found with irritable bowel syndrome, vulvodynia, depression, migraine, sicca syndrome, systemic lupus erythematosus, allergy and asthma.

9.5.2 Diagnosis of bladder pain syndrome / interstitial cystitis

- There are no specific biomarkers for the diagnosis of BPS/IC, so confirming the diagnosis remains challenging. It is a diagnosis of exclusion and the recognition of key symptoms is key:
    - Exclude other conditions, e.g. infection, OAB, non-infectious cystitis, bladder calculi, pelvic floor disorders, vulvar disorders, gynaecological diseases, malignancy.
    - History will include pelvic pain and possible urinary frequency or urgency.
    - Previous medical history may include autoimmunity, pelvic surgery, vulvodynia.
    - Examination will include possible suprapubic tenderness, bladder neck point tenderness, normal urinalysis.
- Where BPS/IC is suspected, patients should be referred to secondary care for further assessment and management.

9.5.3 Management of bladder pain syndrome / interstitial cystitis

The therapeutic goal is to relieve bladder pain, reduce urgency and frequency and improve quality of life in patients. Treatment approaches usually include:

- Conservative treatment (e.g. patient education, mindfulness, CBT, online and family support).
- Avoidance of bladder irritants helps 90% of patients (e.g. coffee, wine, beer, tomatoes, sweeteners, acidic beverages and spicy foods).
- Massage, pelvic trigger point injections, myofascial therapy may help smooth the muscles and reduce pain. Kegel exercises may worsen pain and should be avoided.
- Regular, scheduled voiding helps improve bladder sensation and capacity.
- Pharmacological approaches include:
    - Amitriptyline (which has anticholinergic, antihistamine and sensitivity-reducing qualities and features in all guidelines for BPS/IC).
    - Other options initiated in secondary care include pentosan polysulphate, hydroxyzine, cimetidine, and an oral formulation of hyaluronic acid (guidelines vary slightly in which drugs they include).
    - Some patients find symptoms flare with systemic hormone therapies or cyclically, and may benefit from hormone manipulation.

- Intravesical instillations may be offered by secondary care.
- Surgical approaches may include low-pressure hydrodistension under cystoscopy. Botulinum neurotoxin A has proven effective when given intravesically.
- Sacral neuromodulation may also be effective.
- Small numbers of patients may proceed to cystoplasty or total cystectomy when symptoms are severe and refractory.
- Immunotherapies are an emergent field showing promise – monoclonal antibodies are being studied with promising results. Cannabinoids and stem cell therapies may also be more widely used for the condition in future.

9.6 Sexual pain / penetration disorders

9.6.1 Vulvar pain and vulvodynia

- Vulvar pain is the term used to describe pain in the vulval area caused by a specific disorder.
- Vulvodynia is the term used to describe vulvar pain of at least 3 months' duration without a clear identifiable cause. It often feels like a burning, stinging or raw sandpaper-like discomfort. It can occur spontaneously or only when the vulva is touched or penetrated.
- Vulvar pain and vulvodynia can both be debilitating, characterised by chronic pain which has a significant impact on quality of life. They often lead to painful sex, decreased libido and barrier with communication due to embarrassment about the condition. Lifetime prevalence of vulvodynia is estimated at 8%.
- The aetiology of vulvodynia remains incompletely understood and efforts are still being made to define and classify the condition. There are significant overlaps with other conditions such as chronic pain, fibromyalgia and bladder pain syndrome. It is likely these conditions share common aetiologies and over time definitions may shift to redefine or regroup symptoms. There is also overlap with pudendal neuropathy and persistent genital arousal disorder / persistent genital dysthesia (see *Section 9.7* for more information).
- A thorough assessment of symptoms, timing, triggers and comorbidities is therefore essential in understanding and managing the condition well.

Classification

In 2015 the International Society for the Study of Vulval Disease, the International Society for the Study of Women's Sexual Health and the International Pelvic Pain Society released a consensus statement (see *Further reading*) regarding terminology, classification of persistent vulvar pain and vulvodynia which helped unify and clarify this area.

Causes of vulvar pain

- Infection, e.g. recurrent candidiasis, herpes.
- Inflammation, e.g. lichen sclerosus, lichen planus, immunobullous disorders.
- Neoplasia, e.g. Paget's disease and squamous cell carcinoma.
- Neurological, e.g. post-herpetic neuralgia, nerve compression or injury, neuroma.
- Trauma, e.g. female genital mutilation, obstetrical.
- Iatrogenic, e.g. postoperative, chemotherapy, radiotherapy.
- Hormonal deficiencies, e.g. GSM, lactational amenorrhoea.

Types of vulvodynia

- Location, e.g. localised (vestibulodynia, clitorodynia) or generalised, or mixed.
- Provoked (e.g. insertional, contact) or spontaneous, or mixed.
- Onset (primary, with no known cause or secondary, and associated with another condition).

- Temporal pattern (intermittent, persistent, constant, immediate, delayed).

Women may have both a specific disorder (e.g. lichen sclerosus) and vulvodynia.

Potential aetiologies of vulvodynia

- Research has shown several possible underlying potential explanations for vulvodynia.
- Associations between vulvodynia and other common pain syndromes are frequent in at least 45% of patients: for example, orofacial pain, fibromyalgia, endometriosis, chronic fatigue syndrome and BPS/IC.
- Genetics seem to play a role, with at least three potentially overlapping genetic polymorphisms that increase the risk of candidiasis or other infections, changes promoting prolonged or exaggerated inflammatory responses, and changes that promote increased susceptibility to hormonal changes (e.g. relative androgen receptor insensitivity leading to pain with combined oral contraceptive use).
- Inflammation – various studies have demonstrated increases in inflammatory cells within painful regions of the vulvar vestibule. Other tissue changes have been demonstrated, such as hyperinnervation (increased numbers of nerve endings in affected tissue) and an inability to downregulate proinflammatory changes.
- Musculoskeletal – changes in pelvic floor tonicity have been shown to be associated with the presence of provoked vestibulodynia. Prolapse has also been shown to be associated, with studies suggesting resolution of pain after surgical correction of prolapse.
- Neurological – several studies have shown central sensitisation and peripheral neuro-proliferation in affected women.
- Psychosocial factors – population studies show that anxiety, depression, childhood trauma and post-traumatic stress are all risk factors for development of vulvodynia.

Diagnosis

- Diagnosis involves taking a thorough history of the onset, timing, triggers and location of the pain. Questions should be asked using the classification framework, to help identify known causes or triggers for vulvar pain (hormonal, iatrogenic, infective, inflammatory, etc.). The pain is usually described as rawness, stinging, burning or irritation, but not itch.
- Ask about the impact of the condition on sexual expression, confidence and relationships. Often there will be associated vaginismus (see below) and reduced arousal or ability to climax.
- Consider investigations to assess hormone status if appropriate, e.g. if there are symptoms or a story consistent with early menopause or premature ovarian insufficiency. There is some evidence that low ferritin may be associated with chronic vulval itch and pain. A lower vaginal swab may also help exclude infection, and if skin appears abnormal it may be necessary to refer to a vulval clinic for assessment and/or skin biopsy.
- It is important to perform an examination and inspect the tissues of the vulva and vagina, although there is frequently very little to see.
- Take care to create a safe environment: the examination should be done gently and in a trauma-informed way, as the prospect of examination may be distressing. A moist cotton bud can be used to help map areas of localised pain (e.g. clitoral or vestibular). Look for skin changes and adhesions, e.g. of the clitoral hood – clitoral phimosis is relatively common and poorly recognised. It can also be helpful to gently insert a gloved finger to test pelvic floor muscle tone and for tenderness.
- Check for ischial spine tenderness – a sign of pudendal neuropathy rather than vulvodynia.

Management of vulvar pain and vulvodynia

- There are many potential treatments but overall, the evidence is poor for efficacy in this area and there have been very few high-quality randomised controlled trials to guide treatment.

- The British Society for the Study of Vulval Diseases (BSSVD) Guidelines (at bssvd.org) are a useful summary and encourage a multidisciplinary approach. Combining treatments is often effective.
- Treatment may include pharmacotherapy, vibratory massage, psychosexual therapy, psychotherapeutic support, and pain management teams.
- Patient education is essential and has been shown to reduce distress. The Vulval Pain Society (https://vulvalpainsociety.org.uk) is another good resource for patients for this kind of support. Women are often fearful of pathology. Reassurance and education are important.
- Avoid contact irritants – wear cotton underwear, avoid underwear at night, consider avoiding fabric dyes and use non-biological washing products and unperfumed sanitary products. Soap is best replaced with gentle emollients or plain products such as coconut oil.
- Avoid overuse of antifungals topically.
- Topical treatment may be useful, including 5% lidocaine ointment or 2% lidocaine gel applied 20 minutes prior to intercourse and washed off prior to penetration. A condom may also be used to prevent penile numbness. These treatments may worsen contact irritation and of course, may reduce pleasure for the woman, so should only be considered when these issues have been discussed with the patient.
- Pharmacotherapy includes medications used in other neuropathic disorders such as:
  - Tricyclic antidepressants (TCAs) – frequently first-line, e.g. amitriptyline or nortriptyline. Evidence is lacking for efficacy at this time and side-effects can be considerable. Other antidepressants such as paroxetine and venlafaxine have been tried where TCAs cannot be tolerated.
  - Gabapentin is commonly tried but has a poor evidence base.
  - Consider a trial of local vaginal and vulval oestrogen cream/pessaries and gels where hormonal factors may be involved: e.g. around perimenopause or post menopause, when breastfeeding, or after cancer where there has been hormone deprivation (low-dose topical hormone use is often safe and appropriate for these women).
  - If the patient is using combined hormonal contraception (CHC), consider swapping to a non-hormonal method or LNG-IUD, as the loss of circulating androgens caused by CHCs has been shown to be associated with vestibular pain and interstitial cystitis in women who are less sensitive to testosterone.
- Physiotherapy can be hugely beneficial – early referral to a women's health specialist (gynae) physio should be considered. Pelvic floor muscle exercises, biofeedback training, TENS and vaginal trainers and massagers may be used.
- Vibratory massage has been shown to reduce the impact of vulval pain on sex by up to 73%. Patients can be shown pebble-shaped vibrators and encouraged to use these externally on the vulva for a minute once or twice daily. This has also been shown to help relax pelvic floor muscles.
- Psychological therapies are also very useful. CBT has been shown to reduce pain, as has mindfulness-based CBT.
- Partner attitudes to pain have been shown to impact wellbeing too – support may need to extend to the partner as well as the patient. Psychosexual therapy is often an essential part of supporting the patient to live with these conditions.
- Surgical treatment is occasionally recommended – usually a modified vestibulectomy, with the aim of removing hypersensitive tissue and replacing it with normal vaginal mucosa.
- There is very little data to support complementary or alternative medications.

9.6.2 Vaginismus

- The DSM-5 has changed the terminology to 'Genito-pelvic pain and penetration disorders', but most healthcare practitioners still refer to the reflex closure or hypertonicity of the pelvic floor muscles, preventing penetration or making it painful and difficult, as 'vaginismus'. This pelvic floor spasm or tightness commonly complicates other conditions causing painful sex, such as vulvodynia or BPS/IC.

- Vaginismus can be defined as "persistent or recurrent difficulties of the woman to allow vaginal entry of a penis, finger or any object – despite her expressed wish to do so". Some women have similar difficulty with anal penetration, where the condition is known as 'anodyspareunia'. Approaches to treatment are broadly the same.
- Vaginismus is common and can be thought of as a logical mechanism of self-protection in most cases. GPs can offer explanation, signposting and simple supportive interventions that can make a big difference to women struggling with the condition.
- Management of vaginismus is most successful when we take a multidisciplinary approach.
- Recent changes in definitions have made it difficult to accurately assess prevalence, although it is usually reported to affect 1–6% of women.

Aetiology

- Most researchers agree that vaginismus is a psychophysiological problem involving cognitive, behavioural and physiological factors.
- It is most easily understood using the 'fear avoidance' model (see *Fig. 9.1*).
- The woman will usually have had a negative experience or experiences of penetration, or perhaps been raised in sex-negative environments to fear pain or negative consequences as a result of being penetrated. Some women are unable to identify what may have triggered the fear of penetration. Others may have a clear history of sexual or medical trauma.
- There is then a vicious circle of defensive pelvic floor muscle contraction, leading to increased painful experiences of attempted penetration. The woman then usually learns to avoid penetration, and so the cycle continues.

Diagnosis

- Diagnosis of vaginismus can be challenging. A thorough history should be taken to identify the nature, site and triggers for pain. It is also important to rule out comorbidities.
- Vaginismus can be primary (penetration has never been possible or comfortable) or secondary (acquired only later in life). Ask questions to establish the onset of the condition, any particular triggering events and the extent of the difficulties being experienced. Can they accept a tampon / a finger? Is the issue present only in partnered sex, or also when they are on their own? What have they tried so far?
- It is important to establish if vaginismus sits alongside other causes of pelvic or genital pain, such as fibroids, endometriosis, inflammatory bowel disease or vulvodynia. Treatment approaches should include optimisation of these comorbid conditions.
- Ask about medical trauma, such as obstetric injury, upsetting gynaecological examinations or procedures, cancer treatment or surgery. How did these impact the timing or severity of the condition?

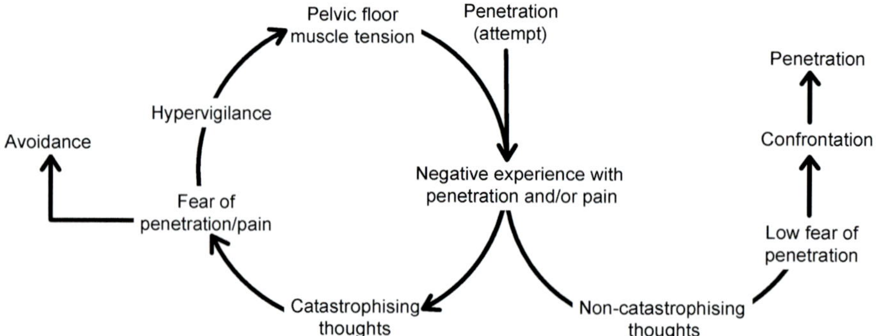

Figure 9.1: The fear avoidance model of vaginismus (reproduced from Binik, Y.M. and Hall, K.S. (eds) (2014) *Principles and Practice of Sex Therapy*, 5th edition, with permission from Guilford Publications).

- Assess hormonal status (on contraception? Breastfeeding? Menopausal?) and check for the presence of any dermatological conditions and/or STIs.
- Check for the presence of any voiding difficulties, and ask about medications, alcohol and drug use.
- What impact is this having on the patient's life? Often women are fearful they cannot maintain a relationship or have children as a result of the condition. Psychoeducation and information about anatomy can help, as many women are fearful they have an anatomical abnormality meaning penetration is impossible. Showing a diagram of the pelvic floor can help.
- A gentle, trauma-informed genital examination can be very helpful. External inspection for comorbid conditions and to check hormonal status is helpful. A lower vaginal swab may be useful, dependent on features of the history. A moist cotton bud pain-mapping exercise is likely to help reveal what is going on.
- A single digit vaginal examination can be helpful to palpate the pelvic floor muscles, which may be tender or tight. Watch the patient carefully during the examination – she may try to lift up her buttocks or close her thighs. Keep asking permission and checking she is comfortable for you to proceed. Where permission is not given, examination can safely be delayed until a later stage.

Implications

- Many women with vaginismus report not feeling heard, or being dismissed by medical professionals. Validation of a woman's concerns is therefore a vital first step in treatment.
- Cervical smear attendance can be impacted by vaginismus. It can help to offer a speculum to take home and try on her own, or for the woman to self-insert for the procedure. Positioning during the procedure is also important, as gluteal (and therefore pelvic floor) muscles can be activated – a couch positioned by the wall allows the knee to rest and if the other knee is gently supported by the clinician, this can aid muscle relaxation. It can also help to practise blowing the tummy up as if pretending to be pregnant – this softens the pelvic floor muscles, allowing easier penetration.

Treatment

- Treatment should be individualised and multidisciplinary – and incorporate management of any associated conditions such as endometriosis, vulvodynia or historic trauma.
- The evidence base supports the following interventions:
  - Patient education about anatomy, sexual arousal and mechanisms that create and prolong vaginismus can help.
  - Pelvic floor muscle relaxation using breathwork, electromyographic (EMG) biofeedback and the use of trainers. Early referral to a pelvic floor physiotherapist is very useful in supporting women with vaginismus.
  - Vaginal trainers have a less concrete evidence base but can be helpful to massage and learn to relax muscles around. Pairing this with breathwork and plenty of lubricant increases the success of the process of graded increase in trainer size. Patients may prefer to use their fingers or a small vibrator instead. Vibratory massage can be a helpful adjunct, using a flat or pebble vibrator. Arousal usually improves chances of success by increasing natural lubrication and the physiological process of vaginal tenting and uterine lifting that occurs when aroused.
  - Systemic desensitisation is a type of behavioural therapy which combines pelvic floor muscle relaxation and anxiety management strategies, such as breathwork.
  - CBT can help with graded exposure and cognitive restructuring to reduce fear avoidance behaviours.
  - Pharmacological approaches have limited evidence and are generally not recommended. Botulinum toxin A is increasingly used, but evidence for this remains minimal.

- Psychosexual therapy is a useful safe space to explore physical approaches together with a better understanding of how any underlying core beliefs or traumatic experiences may be contributing to the issue. The COSRT, Relate and the IPM all have lists of therapists able to help with this issue.

9.6.3 Pudendal neuralgia

- Pudendal neuralgia (PN) describes the pain caused by pudendal nerve entrapment and neuropathy. The pudendal nerve has sensory, motor and autonomic functions. When the nerve is damaged or irritated, it can create pain which is often misdiagnosed and poorly managed for many years before the cause is understood.
- The pain is usually bilateral and characterised by being aggravated by sitting.
- The pudendal nerve travels through a narrow gap between the piriformis and the coccygeus muscle, through the greater sciatic foramen and between the sacrotuberous and sacrospinous ligaments. This leaves it vulnerable to being pinched or impinged by its surrounding structures. It then travels through the pudendal canals where it divides to supply the clitoris and the perineum.
- PN is usually the result of cumulative microtrauma to the nerve. Indirect trauma, including from viral infections (herpes zoster, HIV, and herpes simplex infection), MS and diabetes can also cause pudendal neuralgia.
- Common causes also include:
  - Childbirth injuries (stretch and compression injuries from the fetal head passing through the pelvis).
  - Chronic constipation.
  - Direct trauma, including falls and road traffic accidents or pelvic surgeries.
  - Prolonged sitting.
  - Radiation therapy.
  - Repetitive hip flexion (exercise).
- True incidence is unknown, as the condition so often goes undiagnosed or misdiagnosed.
- Pain is characterised as burning, tingling, aching, stabbing or electric shock-like. In over half of patients pain is exacerbated by sitting and relieved by standing, lying down or sitting on a toilet.
- There may also be sciatic pain or medial thigh pain.
- Patients with PN also often complain of chronic perineal pain and bowel, bladder or sexual dysfunction. Pain in the coccyx or referred to calf, foot or toes is also common. Central sensitisation may be present with allodynia or foreign body sensation in the vagina or rectum (often described as sitting on a golf ball or a hot poker in the rectum).
- There may be associated urinary frequency, dysuria, urgency, and symptoms mimicking interstitial cystitis, painful nocturnal orgasms, persistent sexual arousal and dyspareunia. There is considerable clinical overlap with the presentation of PN and PGAD/GPD (see *Section 9.7*) and indeed, they may co-exist.
- Referral to a pain specialist is advised where PN is suspected: pudendal block is often advised as a diagnostic tool, though evidence for this approach is lacking.
- Treatment can be initiated in primary care where symptoms are distressing, and includes:
  - Pelvic floor muscle exercises (referral to a women's health specialist physiotherapist is advised).
  - Amitriptyline 10mg nocte (max 50mcg), SSRI (e.g. duloxetine) or anti-epileptic, e.g. gabapentin.
  - Antihistamines may be helpful as an adjunct.
  - Pain commonly starts or becomes worse around menopause. Consider the use of systemic and/or topical oestrogens.
- Specialist treatment often involves pudendal block, sacral neuromodulation, or surgical decompression. CBT and TENS may be helpful.

9.7 Persistent genital arousal disorder

- Persistent genital arousal disorder (PGAD) is a condition of unremitting, unwanted sensations of genital arousal. It is associated with significant and negative psychosocial impact, including suicidal ideation.
- The symptoms can also include distressing genital itch, tingling, buzzing or genital pain without genital arousal, and there may also be urinary urgency and frequency and restless leg symptoms. There has been discussion around changing the name of the condition to genito-pelvic dysthesia (GPD) to reflect that arousal is not always present.
- The symptoms are intrusive and do not go away after orgasm, and can last from hours to days. Orgasmic function/pleasure may or may not be compromised. The condition develops, on average, at around 37 years of age but can present prior to the age of 18. Examination reveals inconsistent evidence of genital arousal (lubrication, swelling of clitoris or labia). The condition has recently been included in the ICD-11.
- There appear to be several diverse biopsychosocial contributors to the condition (e.g. anxiety, depression, trauma, medical comorbidities, pelvic floor muscle dysfunction and medication), but research shows common changes in functional MRI studies in women affected by the condition. The somatosensory cortex shows spontaneous, intense, and more extensive activation of the part of the brain associated with genital stimulation in the absence of any actual physical stimulation occurring. This appears to support a neurological basis for the symptoms and some possible causation or overlap with conditions such as pudendal neuropathy, cauda equina syndrome, spinal cord injury and sacral Tarlov cysts. The condition may also be idiopathic.
- Classification is consistent with that of vulvodynia. There may be overlap between symptoms and aetiologies.
- Treatment of PGAD/PGD requires a full assessment of the potential aetiology of the condition and any overlying biopsychosocial triggers – for example, anxiety or recent cessation of SSRIs. Information should be gathered about the location, severity, timing and triggers of symptoms, and how this is impacting daily living. CBT has been shown to be successful in reducing symptom severity and associated distress.
- PGAD/PGD may be associated with hormonal contraceptive use, due to local depletion of androgens in the strongly androgen-dependent tissues of the vestibule. Menopause may also be a factor due to lower circulating testosterone levels and the presence of GSM. In these situations, local and systemic hormone therapy or changing from combined oral contraception to non-hormonal or intrauterine methods may be of some symptomatic benefit.
- Thyroid levels should also be checked, as hyperthyroidism has been found to be a contributing factor.
- Assessment of the pelvic floor by a specialist (e.g. pelvic floor physiotherapist) is often beneficial in understanding If hypertonicity is contributing to the condition and in improving symptoms.
- Patients should be referred to secondary care for further investigation and management – usually within a chronic pain setting.
- Waiting lists may be long and patients are often very distressed by symptoms. Treatment may therefore be initiated in primary care. The pharmacological options mimic those used in other neurological pain conditions such as vulvodynia, and include anticonvulsants (e.g. gabapentin, pregabalin and topiramate), benzodiazepines and TCAs.
- Useful further reading can be found in the International Society for the Study of Women's Sexual Health (ISSWSH) 2021 review article on the epidemiology, pathophysiology and management of the condition (see *Further reading* below).

9.8 Further reading

BMJ Best Practice (2018) *Faecal incontinence in adults*. BMJ Publishing Group.

Bornstein, J., Goldstein, A.T., Stockdale, C.K. *et al.* (2016) 2015 ISSVD, ISSWSH and IPPS consensus terminology and classification of persistent vulvar pain and vulvodynia. *Obstetrics & Gynecology*, **127(4):** 745–51.

Chalmers, K.J. (2024) Clinical assessment and management of vaginismus. *Aust J Gen Pract*, **53(1–2):** 37–41.

DeLancey, J.O., Masteling, M., Pipitone, F. *et al.* (2004) Pelvic floor injury during vaginal birth is life-altering and preventable: what can we do about it? *Am J Obstet Gynecol*, **230(3):** 279–94.

Dexter, E., Walshaw, J., Wynn H. *et al.* (2024) Faecal incontinence – a comprehensive review. *Front Surg*, **11:** 1340720.

European Association of Urology (2025) *EAU Guidelines on Urological Infections*. Available at: https://d56bochluxqnz.cloudfront.net/documents/full-guideline/EAU-Guidelines-on-Urological-infections-2025.pdf

Giarenis, I. and Robinson, D. (2014) Prevention and management of pelvic organ prolapse. *F1000Prime Rep*, **6:** 77.

Goldstein, A.T., Belkin, Z.R. and Krapf, J.M. *et al.* (2014) Polymorphisms of the androgen receptor gene and hormonal contraceptive induced provoked vestibulodynia. *J Sex Med*, **11(11):** 2764–71.

Goldstein, I., Komisaruk, B.R., Pukall, C.F. *et al.* (2021) International Society for the Study of Women's Sexual Health (ISSWSH) review of epidemiology and pathophysiology, and a consensus nomenclature and process of care for the management of persistent genital arousal disorder/genito-pelvic dysesthesia (PGAD/GPD). *J Sex Med*, **18(4):** 665–97.

Haylen, B.T., Maher, C.F., Barber, M.D. *et al.* (2016) Erratum to: An International Urogynecological Association (IUGA) / International Continence Society (ICS) joint report on the terminology for female pelvic organ prolapse (POP). *Int Urogynecol J*, **27:** 655–84.

Leslie, S.W., Antolak, S., Feloney, M.P. and Soon-Sutton, T.L. (2024) Pudendal neuralgia. *StatPearls*.

Li, J., Yi, X. and Ai, J. (2022) Broaden horizons: the advancement of interstitial cystitis/bladder pain syndrome. *Int J Mol Sci*, **23(23):** 14594.

Nguyen, R.H., Ecklund, A.M., Maclehose, R.F. *et al.* (2012) Co-morbid pain conditions and feelings of invalidation and isolation among women with vulvodynia. *Psychol Health Med*, **17(5):** 589–98.

NICE (updated 2019) *Urinary incontinence and pelvic organ prolapse in women: management* [NG123]. Available at: www.nice.org.uk/guidance/ng123/resources/urinary-incontinence-and-pelvic-organ-prolapse-in-women-management-pdf-66141657205189

Reddy, R.A., Cortessis, V., Dancz, C., Klutke, J. and Stanczyk, F.Z. (2020) Role of sex steroid hormones in pelvic organ prolapse. *Menopause*, **27(8):** 941–51.

Schulten, S.F., Claas-Quax, M.J., Weemhoff, M. *et al.* (2022) Risk factors for primary pelvic organ prolapse and prolapse recurrence: an updated systematic review and meta-analysis. *Am J Obstet Gynecol*, **227(2):** 192–208.

Steenstrup, B., Lopes, F., Cornu, J.N. and Gilliaux, M. (2022) Cognitive-behavioral therapy and urge urinary incontinence in women. A systematic review. *Int Urogynecol J*, **33(5):** 1091–101.

Vergeldt, T.F., Weemhoff, M., IntHout, J. and Kluivers, K.B. (2015) Risk factors for pelvic organ prolapse and its recurrence: a systematic review. *Int Urogynecol J*, **26(11):** 1559–73.

Wu, X., Zheng, X., Yi, X., Lai, P. and Lan, Y. (2021) Electromyographic biofeedback for stress urinary incontinence or pelvic floor dysfunction in women: a systematic review and meta-analysis. *Adv Ther*, **38(8):** 4163–77.

Zolnoun, D., Lamvu, G. and Steege, J. (2008) Patient perceptions of vulvar vibration therapy for refractory vulvar pain. *Sex Relation Ther*, **23(4):** 345-353.

Websites

- https://bsac.org.uk/patient-spotlight-the-symptoms-are-debilitating-ive-spent-the-last-four-years-in-significant-pain-and-in-fear
- https://thepogp.co.uk
- https://vulvalpainsociety.org.uk
- www.baus.org.uk
- www.patientsafetycommissioner.org.uk/resource-for-patients-with-pelvic-mesh
- www.pelvicorganprolapsesupport.org
- www.theurologyfoundation.org/urology-health/uti-information-service-and-helpline
- www.thevaginismusnetwork.com

Chapter 10
Vulval dermatology

10.1 Introduction

- Vulval dermatoses are a group of dermatological conditions that affect the vulva. The vulva is used to describe the external parts of the female genital region and is an area that includes the skin over the mons pubis, labia majora and minora, glans clitoris, clitoral hood, vestibule and the urethral meatus and vaginal introitus (see *Section 1.1.2*).
- Vulval dermatoses can significantly impact a woman's quality of life, causing symptoms such as itching, burning, pain, or changes in the appearance of the vulva. This in turn can impact self-esteem, body image, intimacy and relationships.
- It can be an embarrassing and difficult topic for patients to raise with their doctors, but especially hard for women from certain ethnic groups and transgender patients who may avoid genital exams, so it needs to be raised and explored in a sensitive manner.
- For healthcare professionals, recognising and managing vulval dermatoses is crucial, because early intervention can prevent progression and improve patient outcomes and quality of life.
- This chapter provides a practical guide to understanding, diagnosing and managing vulval dermatoses in primary care. It is divided into vulval dermatoses that are common at different stages of life. Where possible photographs to aid diagnosis have been included, but readers are advised to use high-quality online image libraries for a broader range: www.dermnetnz.org and www.pcds.org.uk are particularly helpful.

10.2 Prepubertal girls

The prepubertal vulval tissue can be prone to dermatological problems for several reasons:

- **Thin, atrophic vulval and vaginal tissue** due to **low oestrogen.**
- **Neutral vaginal pH (6–8)** (unlike the acidic pH in post-pubertal females, which protects against infections).
- **Close proximity of the vulva to the anus**, increasing risk of faecal contamination.
- **Lack of pubic hair and labial fat pads**, reducing physical protection.
- **Poor perineal hygiene**, especially in young children.

Girls usually present with symptoms of redness, inflammation, pain and itch. There are several different causes: inflammatory, infectious or caused by trauma.

10.2.1 Inflammatory and dermatitis-related conditions

Irritant contact dermatitis

- Commonly due to soaps, bubble baths, wet wipes, or exposure to urine/faeces or chlorine from pools.
- Avoid triggers, wash and moisturise with emollients.
- Wipe from front to back, change nappies frequently and use a barrier cream each time.

Atopic dermatitis (eczema)

- Often seen in children with a history of allergies, asthma or eczema.
- Avoid triggers, wash and moisturise with emollients; mild topical steroids (hydrocortisone 1%) may need to be used for short periods.

Allergic contact dermatitis

- Caused by allergens such as fragrances, preservatives or certain fabrics.
- May need allergy testing.
- Avoid allergens. Wear light-coloured cotton underwear that does not have dyes in it, or change brand of nappy.

Psoriasis

- Presents with itchy, well-demarcated, erythematous plaques with silvery scale that can involve the genital area.
- It is a remitting and relapsing skin condition that requires long-term topical management with emollients and vitamin D creams. Mild- to moderate-potency corticosteroids may need to be used for flare-ups.

Lichen sclerosus

- A chronic inflammatory condition that can peak prepubertally; presents with white, thin, wrinkled skin and itching; there is a risk of potential scarring so it must not be missed.
- Potent steroids may be required, and it is best managed under paediatric dermatology.

Lichen planus

- Rare in children but can present with erosions, inflammation and discomfort.

10.2.2 Infectious dermatoses

Candidiasis (thrush)

- More common in nappy-wearing toddlers or after antibiotic use.
- Presents with erythema, satellite pustules and discharge.
- Treat with antifungal creams such as topical clotrimazole or miconazole creams.

Bacterial infections

- Examples include impetigo and folliculitis.
- Main pathogens: *Staphylococcus aureus* or *Streptococcus pyogenes*.
- Symptoms of honey-coloured crusting and weeping discharge.
- Swab skin and treat with topical and/or oral antibiotics, depending on severity.

Viral infections

Molluscum contagiosum

- Dome-shaped papules, white, pink or brown-coloured, shiny, umbilicated (small central pit) papules.
- Usually self-limiting within 12–18 months but may persist for 2–3 years. No treatment necessary.
- Avoid scratching and ensure good hygiene; avoid sharing towels and use barrier cream to protect skin.
- Medical treatments are best avoided or are not licensed for young children in this sensitive area.

Human papillomavirus (HPV, warts)

- Less common in young girls but possible through non-sexual transmission.

Herpes simplex virus (HSV)

- Rare in prepubertal girls unless there is perinatal transmission. Consider if painful ulcers are present.

Parasitic infections (threadworms)

- Can migrate around from the anal to the vulval area causing severe itching, especially at night.
- Consider threadworm tape test and treat the whole family with mebendazole and repeat course after 2 weeks.

10.2.3 Trauma and other causes

Trauma or non-accidental injury (NAI)

- Must be considered in unexplained cases of vulval irritation or bruising.
- Careful documentation and history and discussion with safeguarding lead / paediatrician should be considered.

Labial adhesions

- Presents between ages of 13 and 23 months.
- Often associated with hypoestrogenic states and chronic inflammation.
- Labia minora fused at the bottom with small opening at urethra, or fully fused.
- Usually asymptomatic and no treatment needed; improves with time/adolescence.
- If symptomatic with vulval irritation or urinary symptoms, then oestrogen cream daily for up to 6 weeks can help. Consider surgery for severe cases or if not responsive to oestrogen cream.

10.3 Girls and women of reproductive age

The vulval tissue in women undergoes changes from adolescence to reproductive age due to hormonal variations, primarily in oestrogen.

- The labia minora increase in size and become more prominent to enhance sexual pleasure and protect the vestibule.
- Labial fat pads develop and subcutaneous fat is deposited in the labial folds.
- Pubic hair develops over the mons pubis, which increases physical protection.

These changes enhance the vulva's protective mechanisms and prepare the body for reproduction.

10.3.1 Normal vulval skin variants

Before diagnosing a dermatosis, it is important to be aware of normal vulval anatomy (see *Section 1.1.2*), such as:

- Labial asymmetry
  - Many young women feel distressed about the asymmetry, shape and size of their labia, and this can affect their self-esteem, body image and confidence sexually.
  - Due to the influence of social media and pornography in particular, there has recently been a rise in requests for labiaplasty.
  - It is important to educate women about the normal variation in labial size and asymmetry and make them aware that it can be normal for the inner labia to protrude more than the outer labia in 50% of women.
  - If they are open to looking, then labial libraries are a good way to reassure them about the diversity in normal labia. Two great resources are www.thegreatwallofvulva.com and www.labialibrary.org.au.
  - Despite this, some women may still want to proceed with surgery, and the psychological impact must not be underestimated. However, they should be informed that as labia has erectile tissue with lots of nerve endings, surgery may be associated with loss of sensation and scarring.
- Sebaceous glands (Fordyce spots) – these are small (1–5mm) slightly elevated yellowish or white papules which can be solitary or multiple. Easier to see when the skin is stretched.
- Vestibular papillomatosis (often mistaken for genital warts) – these are benign, skin-coloured, symmetrical bumps which usually appear in a linear array.

10.3.2 Common vulval dermatoses

Inflammatory dermatoses

Lichen sclerosus

This is a chronic scarring dermatosis of unknown aetiology. Prevalence is 3% in women. It is associated with autoimmune conditions, especially in women. Usually peaks in prepuberty and postmenopausal women but can happen at any age.

- **Clinical features**: (*Figure 10.1*) often presents with:
  - white, atrophic plaques, commonly described as 'parchment-like'
  - intense itching, burning pain, soreness or dyspareunia
  - 'figure-of-eight' distribution (vulva and perianal area)
  - scarring, resulting in fusion or narrowing of the vaginal introitus in chronic cases.
- **Diagnosis**: primarily clinical and confirmed by biopsy if the presentation is atypical or non-responsive to treatment.
- **Management**:
  - **First-line**: if you are confident of the diagnosis then a potent topical corticosteroid can be initiated such as clobetasol propionate 0.05% ointment. It should be used once daily for 1 month, then alternate days for 1 month, then twice weekly for 1 month, tapering slowly. Advise a daily dose of ½ fingertip unit; a 30g tube should last at least 3 months. Review progress after 3 months.
  - **If unsure of the diagnosis**: due to the nature of this condition, it is important to diagnose it correctly. The algorithm in *Figure 10.2* states that if you have any doubt about the diagnosis, the use of 1% hydrocortisone ointment, in preference to a more potent corticosteroid, is recommended until a biopsy can be done. This is because use of a potent corticosteroid can reverse the histology and signs, so the specialist may not be able to make the diagnosis. Referral to a gynaecologist/dermatologist is advised. It may be necessary to call them for advice, if there is a long wait for an appointment.
  - **Care of skin**: continue long-term emollients to wash, to reduce irritation and for barrier protection (e.g. Epaderm, Hydromol). Ointments are better than creams.
  - **Follow-up**: review 3 months after treatment has been started. A referral to secondary care dermatology / gynaecology may be needed for a biopsy to confirm the diagnosis if the diagnosis is not clear or if not responding to treatment. Regular reviews are required to monitor for potential progression to squamous cell carcinoma (SCC), which occurs in about 5% of cases. Risk can be mitigated with prompt diagnosis and treatment. Pallor may not resolve completely, and treatment should be titrated to maintain symptom control and resolution of skin changes. Advise an annual review with a GP or secondary care, and patients should self-examine, and return sooner for review if any ulcer/erosion or new lesions appear.

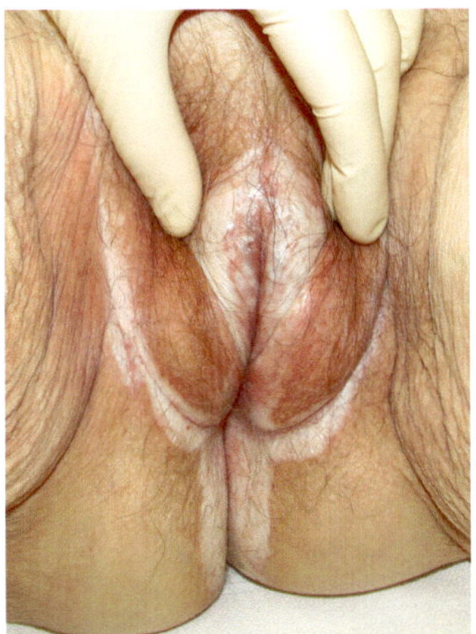

Figure 10.1: Vulval lichen sclerosus. Reproduced from *Dermatology Made Easy* 2e, with permission.

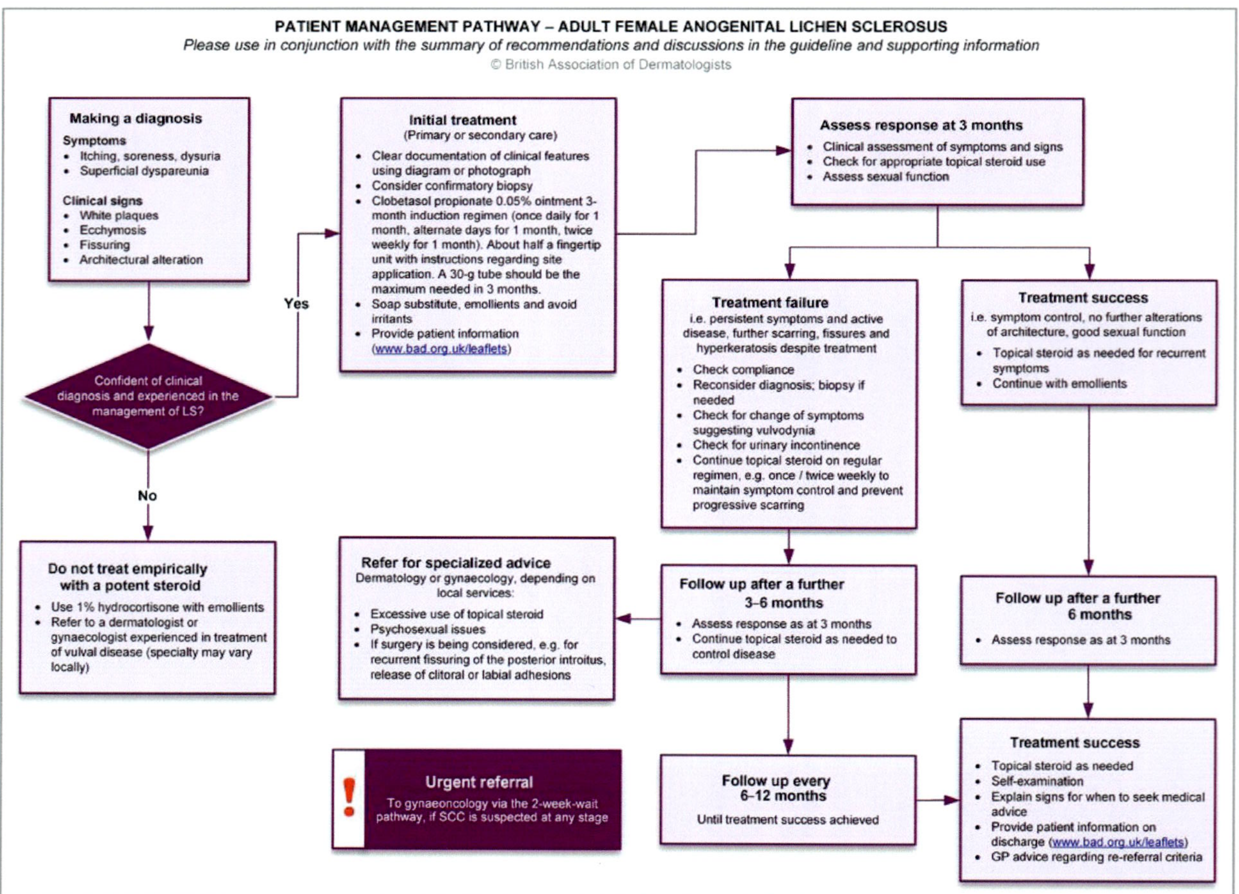

Figure 10.2: Management pathway for anogenital lichen sclerosus. Reproduced from Lewis, F.M., Tatnall, F.M., Velangi, S.S. *et al.* (2018) British Association of Dermatologists guidelines for the management of lichen sclerosus. *Br J Dermatol,* 178: 839, with permission.

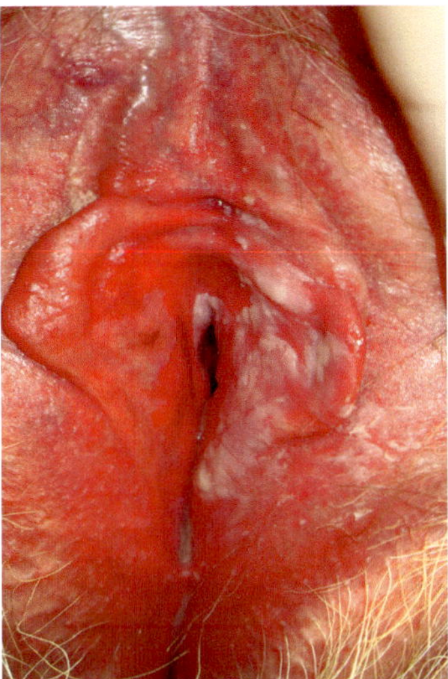

Figure 10.3: Vulval lichen planus. Reproduced from *Dermatology Made Easy* 2e, with permission.

Lichen planus

- **Clinical features** (*Figure 10.3*):
  - This may appear as erosive lesions with a glazed, red surface or as reticular white lines (Wickham's striae).
  - It may involve the vaginal tissue as well.
  - The main symptoms include pain, itching, postcoital bleeding and dyspareunia.
- **Diagnosis**: clinical evaluation supported by biopsy.
- **Management**:
  - **Topical corticosteroids**: moderate–potent preparations, e.g. clobetasol propionate 0.05%.
  - **Calcineurin inhibitors** (e.g. tacrolimus for steroid-resistant cases).
  - **Systemic therapy**: for refractory cases, systemic immunosuppressants (e.g. methotrexate) may be required.
  - A collaboration with gynaecologists or dermatologists is recommended for complex presentations.

Lichen simplex chronicus

- **Clinical features**:
  - Chronic itching leads to lichenification and hyperpigmentation.
  - Patients often present with thickened, leathery skin and itching which is worse at night.
- **Diagnosis**: based on clinical history and examination.
- **Management**:
  - **Topical corticosteroids**: to reduce inflammation, e.g clobetasol propionate 0.05%.
  - **Antihistamines**, e.g. hydroxyzine for night-time itching.
  - **Emollients**: to repair the skin barrier.
  - **Behavioural interventions**: to address underlying itch–scratch cycles.
  - **Education**: avoid irritants such as perfumed soaps or tight clothing.

Eczematous dermatoses

Atopic dermatitis

- Chronic, itchy, dry skin; often with a history of eczema.
- Managed with mild to moderate topical steroids, emollients and antihistamines.

Contact dermatitis (irritant/allergic)

- See *Fig. 10.4*.
- Due to soaps, sanitary products, perfumes or latex condoms.
- Patch testing may help identify allergens.
- Treatment: avoid irritants, use emollients, and apply mild topical steroids.

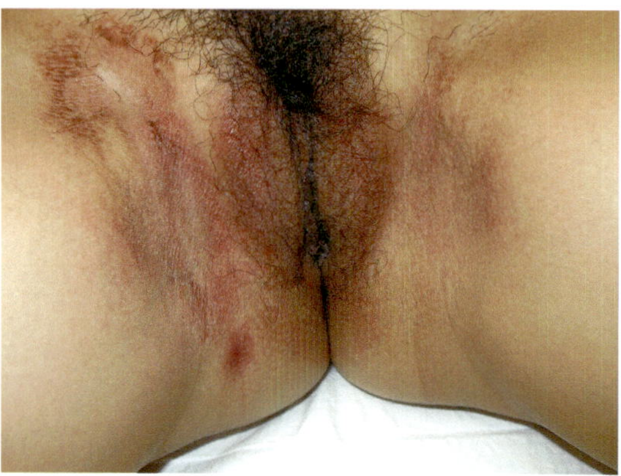

Figure 10.4: Contact irritant dermatitis due to inadequately rinsed underwear. Reproduced from *Dermatology Made Easy* 2e, with permission.

Psoriasis

- See *Fig. 10.5*.
- Well-demarcated pink plaques with minimal scale and mild itch.
- No involvement of the vaginal mucosa (helps differentiate from lichen planus).
- Psoriasis looks different in the genital area. Look for clues elsewhere such as scalp, umbilicus and nails.
- **Management**: mild to moderate topical steroids or calcineurin inhibitors (e.g. tacrolimus) to avoid skin atrophy from long-term use of steroids, vitamin D analogues (e.g. calcipotriol) and emollients.

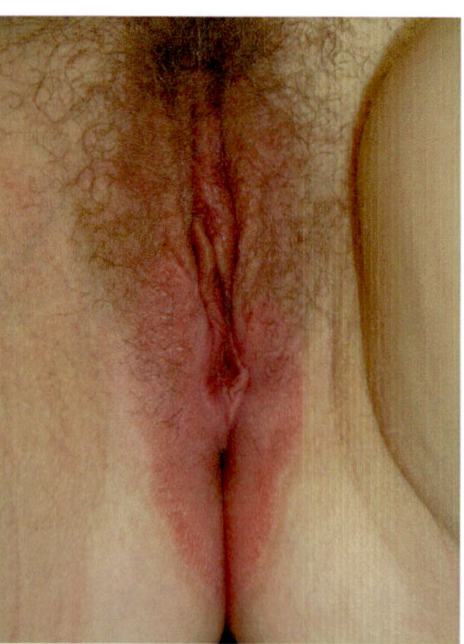

Figure 10.5: Vulval psoriasis. Reproduced from *Dermatology Made Easy* 2e, with permission.

Infectious vulval dermatoses

Candidiasis (thrush)

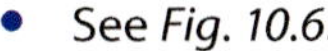

- See *Fig. 10.6*.

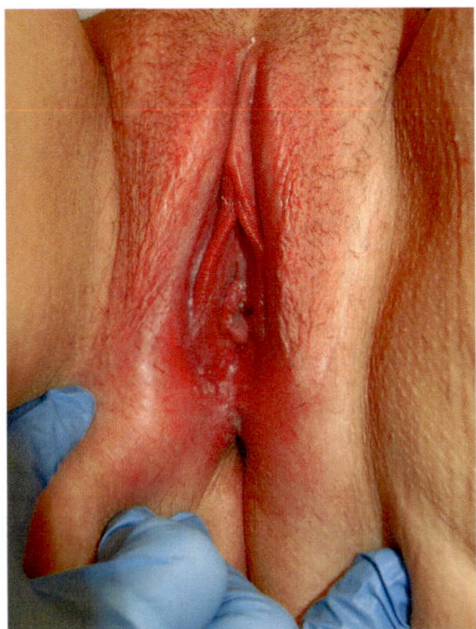

Figure 10.6: Vulval itch due to *Candida albicans*. Reproduced from *Dermatology Made Easy* 2e, with permission.

- Intense itching, erythema, thick white curd-like discharge.
- Treatment: topical (e.g. clotrimazole) or oral (e.g. fluconazole) antifungals.
- Consider recurrent candidiasis if four or more episodes per year and treat with antifungal medication regime as per BNF.
- Many women wrongly assume they have 'recurrent thrush', so patients with recurrent symptoms or failure to improve with treatment must be examined. Candida is less common in postmenopausal women.

Bacterial infections

- **Impetigo**: honey-coloured crusts, treated with topical mupirocin.
- **Erythrasma**: well-demarcated, reddish-brown patches, diagnosed with Wood's lamp (coral pink fluorescence) and treated with topical fusidic acid or oral erythromycin.
- **Syphilis**: since 2001 infection rates have risen rapidly and there has been a marked increase among heterosexuals, especially UK-born heterosexual women.
  - Syphilis is caused by the bacterium *Treponema pallidum*. It is an STI that is curable with antibiotics.
  - It can be divided into early infectious syphilis (<2 years of infection) – primary, secondary and early latent – and late non-infectious syphilis (>2 years since infection).
  - The incubation period for primary syphilis is 9–90 days.
  - Here we will discuss the possible vulval changes. The primary ulcer (chancre) occurs at the site of inoculation so may be seen in the mouth or the genitals. It is classically solitary and painless but can be multiple and painful. It may resolve spontaneously after a few weeks or may go unnoticed. For this reason, it is important not to be falsely reassured if a genital ulcer resolves spontaneously. The syphilis blood test is often negative in the primary chancre stage, so repeat it in those with an ulcer, even if it resolves.
  - For more information about syphilis see *Section 4.13*.

Viral infections

Herpes simplex virus (HSV, genital herpes)

- Painful vesicles and ulcers on vulva.
- HSV-1 and HSV-2 can cause genital lesions. 70% of UK adults carry HSV-1 and 23% HSV-2.
- Infection is lifelong, with periodic episodes of reactivation, as the virus rests on dorsal ganglion.
- Asymptomatic shedding may happen sporadically; not just when there are symptoms.
- Always attempt to confirm the diagnosis. Swab the lesion (pop the blister if necessary) and request HSV PCR using a viral swab. Consider testing for other STIs including chlamydia, gonorrhoea, HIV and syphilis.
- **Treatment**: oral aciclovir (topical does not work) or valaciclovir can be used either prophylactically for frequent episodes or episodically when it appears. Key to treatment is to start as soon as symptoms start.
- Saline bathing as needed may ease symptoms, advise to micturate in the bath and use oral analgesia or lidocaine gel to ease the pain.
- The symptoms and signs of recurrent HSV are not as severe as primary HSV. Recurrences are more likely with HSV-2 and decrease in frequency with time.
- This diagnosis can cause anxiety, particularly about having sex and transmitting the infection to others.
    - Women need reassurance that this infection is like a cold sore on their lip.
    - Most people who are infected with HSV are not aware that they have it; only one-third will experience symptoms and get diagnosed.
    - Some people experience recurrences, but taking antiviral treatments can prevent outbreaks.
    - The website https://herpes.org.uk contains helpful patient information.

Human papillomavirus (HPV, genital warts)

- HPV infection is common and often asymptomatic. It may clear spontaneously. It is a clinical diagnosis.
- Flesh-coloured growths with irregular surface; mainly caused by HPV-6 and -11 which are non-oncogenic; see *Fig. 10.7.*
- One-third regress spontaneously, but if not, then management is cosmetic, and they can be treated with:
    - 5% imiquimod cream (review monthly for up to 4 months)
    - podophyllotoxin cream or solution (review monthly for up to 4 months)
    - catephen ointment for up to 4 months
    - weekly liquid nitrogen.
- There is a lot of stigma attached to this condition, and it can lead to anxiety and depression.
- An STI screen should be done, testing for gonorrhoea, chlamydia, HIV and syphilis.

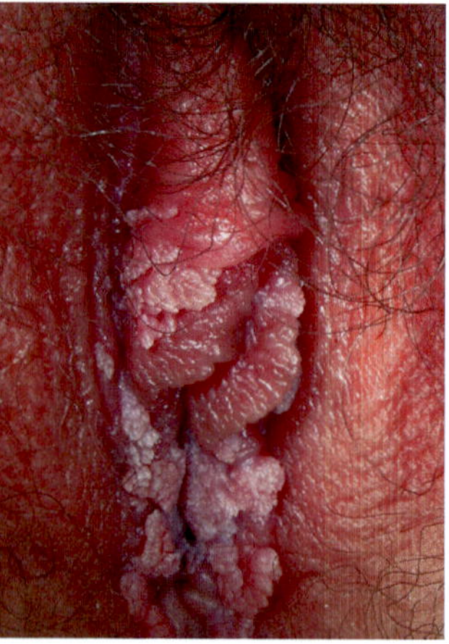

Figure 10.7: Vulval viral warts. Reproduced from *Dermatology Made Easy* 2e, with permission.

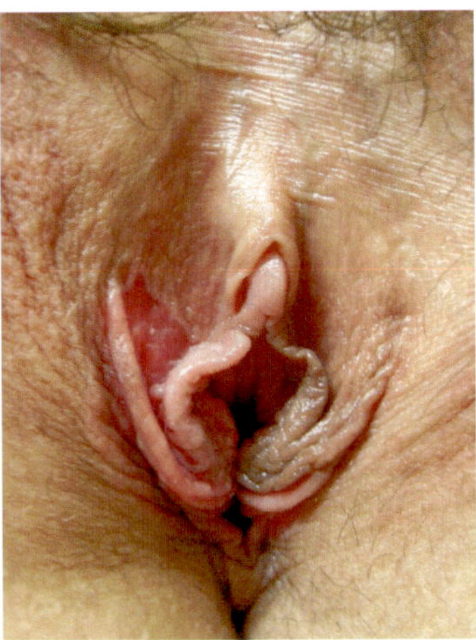

Figure 10.8: Vulval intraepithelial neoplasia (VIN). Reproduced from *Dermatology Made Easy* 2e, with permission.

Neoplastic and premalignant conditions

Vulval intraepithelial neoplasia (VIN)

- See *Fig. 10.8*.
- High-risk HPV-associated precancerous condition.
- Presents with chronic vulval irritation/itch, burning, or asymptomatic white, red or pigmented plaques and psychosexual dysfunction.
- Requires biopsy for diagnosis.
- Treatment: topical imiquimod, laser therapy or surgical excision; HPV vaccine is available for prevention in young girls (licensed from age 9 years).

Vulval squamous cell carcinoma (SCC)

- See *Fig. 10.9*.
- Persistent ulcerated or indurated lesion.
- Lichen sclerosus is a risk factor.
- Requires urgent referral to gynaecology/dermatology for biopsy and treatment.

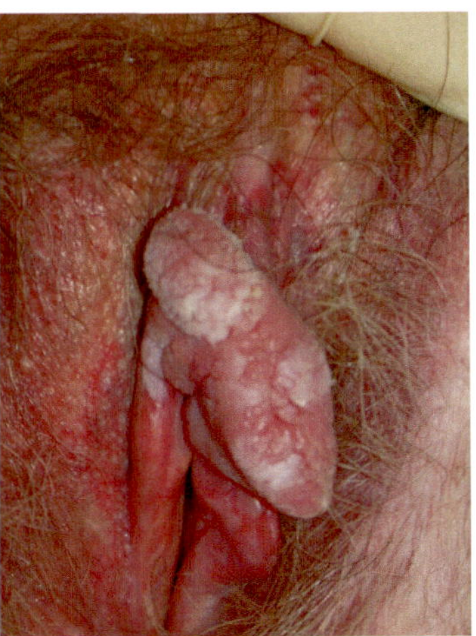

Figure 10.9: Invasive vulval squamous cell carcinoma. Reproduced from *Dermatology Made Easy* 2e, with permission.

10.3.3 Female genital mutilation

- It is estimated that 230 million girls and women worldwide have undergone some form of female genital mutilation (FGM).
- FGM is any procedure that partially or fully removes the external genitalia for non-medical reasons and may involve the clitoral and labial tissues; the vaginal opening may be closed except for a small hole allowing blood and urine to pass through.
- It can lead to long-term problems with infertility, dyspareunia and impaired sexual function, and complications in childbirth, as well as psychological trauma.
- It is mainly practised in parts of North Africa, Southeast Asia or the Middle East to suppress sexuality or as a rite of passage; in some areas it is a prerequisite for marriage. Usually carried out from infancy to age 15 years.
- FGM is a violation of girls' and women's fundamental human rights and is illegal in the UK. If you suspect FGM in any patient below the age of 18 it is mandatory in the UK to report this as a safeguarding issue.
- Gynaecological referral may be necessary.
- See *Section 13.2.1* for more information on FGM.

10.3.4 Vulval pain syndromes

Vulvodynia

- See *Section 9.6* for more information.

Clinical features

- Chronic pain like burning or soreness in the vulva area for 3–6 months.
- There is chronic pain without any obvious visible pathology on examination.
- It may be provoked (triggered by touch) or unprovoked.
- This is due to irritation or hypersensitivity of the nerve fibres in the vulva.
- It can be very distressing for patients and impact them psychologically and sexually.

Management

- Multidisciplinary approach including pelvic floor physiotherapy, psychological support and pain management.
- Topical lidocaine, lubricants, emollients and vaginal oestrogen cream may all help.
- Neuropathic pain medication such as amitriptyline or nortriptyline, simple analgesia and antidepressants may be needed.

Vestibulodynia

- Severe pain on touch or attempting vaginal entry on the vestibule; tenderness to pressure localised only within the vestibule.
- Vestibular erythema is the only physical sign.

Management

- Topical lidocaine, lubricants, emollients and vaginal oestrogen cream may all help.
- Neuropathic pain medication such as amitriptyline or nortriptyline, simple analgesia and antidepressants may be needed.

10.4 Postmenopausal women

Postmenopausal women can experience many of the same conditions as women of reproductive age (as discussed above), but the main issues arise from chronic lack of oestrogen and aging. This may aggravate pre-existing skin conditions or make it hard to know what the cause is.

10.4.1 Common vulval dermatoses seen in postmenopausal women

- Lichen sclerosus – peaks at this time.
- Lichen planus.
- Lichen simplex chronicus.
- Psoriasis.
- Eczema/dermatitis.
- Infectious dermatoses.
- Vulvodynia and vestibulodynia.

These dermatoses have been covered in detail in *Section 10.3*.

Menopausal changes in the vulva together with the vagina, pelvic floor and bladder symptoms are now termed genitourinary syndrome of the menopause, and 50% of women will experience some or all of these symptoms. GSM is covered in more detail in *Section 6.7* and only vulval issues are discussed here.

10.4.2 Vulval changes during menopause

Post menopause there is reduced blood flow to the pelvic floor and the vulval tissue is particularly vulnerable.

- Vulval tissue thins, becomes drier and itchy and loses its elasticity so can tear easily.
- The labia minora and the clitoris shrink in size and the clitoris becomes less sensitive to touch; this leads to reduced arousal.
- The vestibule does not stretch as much, causing superficial dyspareunia.
- All these changes can impact sexual function.
- In addition, the urethral opening can become more prominent and the vulval tissue can also become irritated when it is exposed to urine if there are bladder incontinence issues.

Management

- Washing with emollients such as Epaderm or Hydromol.
- Patting dry rather than rubbing vulval tissue.
- Moisturising with an emollient as above or coconut oil (warn that oil-based creams/ointments may damage latex condoms).
- For external vulval symptoms, apply a fingertip-size amount of estriol 1% cream or Blissel gel daily for 2 weeks then reduce to 2–3 times a week for maintenance of the tissue. This can be added on top of internal vaginal oestrogen if the internal treatment does not help external symptoms. Vaginal oestrogen can be continued long term at a maintenance dose.
- If symptoms persist despite adequate care and topical oestrogen cream, consider referral to dermatology to rule out other causes.
- If sexual problems persist, refer to a psychosexual therapist.

10.5 Practical tips to help manage vulval dermatoses

Building rapport

- Many patients still feel ashamed, embarrassed or vulnerable discussing vulval symptoms.
- Take the time to get a good history and establish a rapport before any examinations.
- Create a safe, non-judgemental space for consultations.
- Use female interpreters if needed.
- To avoid missed or delayed diagnoses always see in person and examine the vulva.
- Ensure that all intimate examinations are trauma-informed (see *Section 4.6* for more details on how to carry out a trauma-informed examination).

History-taking

- Lack of knowledge about vulval anatomy is common amongst women, so take time to ask questions and clarify what they mean.
- Consider asking about hygiene practices – what they use and how often – as they may have been over-vigorous with cleaning the genital area.
- Ask about any triggers, e.g. soap, fragranced products, wet wipes, because even natural or organic products may also be a trigger. There are still persistent scripts that vaginas are 'dirty' or 'smelly' or 'need cleaning' and many sanitary products are bleached or fragranced which adds to the problem and these products can then irritate the skin. Education about this can be helpful in tackling these myths.
- Is it an acute or chronic condition?
- How often does it happen? What treatment has been tried so far?
- Any itching, open sores, pain, burning, discharge, urinary symptoms?
- Any other dermatological conditions in other parts of the body such as the mouth, scalp, nails?
- Always be sure to ask how it impacts them psychologically and sexually.
- Past medical history including asthma, eczema, hay fever, other skin conditions, diabetes, immunosuppressive conditions. Medication used. Family history, especially psoriasis. Occupation.

Thorough examination

- First, gain consent by explaining the examination procedure and why it is necessary, because there may be a reluctance to be examined.
- Always offer a chaperone and document any refusal. Explore refusals in a trauma-informed way, as some women may find these intimate examinations very difficult (see *Section 4.6*).
- Ask if they prefer a female clinician.
- Inform them that they can ask to stop the examination at any time and are always in control.
- Be alert to signs of discomfort or distress during the exam.
- Always examine the vulva in good lighting.
- Use a systematic approach to assess each area of the vulva and the surrounding skin or skin on other parts of the body, e.g. in eczema/psoriasis.
- Ask the patient to highlight the area of concern if unsure.
- A vaginal speculum exam may also be needed.
- It is always helpful to document the examination carefully with the exact location of the problem and correct terminology. A helpful list of dermatology terminology is given below:
    - Macule: a flat non-palpable area of colour change (<1.0cm in diameter).
    - Patch: a larger (>1.0cm) non-palpable area of colour change.
    - Papule: a small, elevated, palpable lesion (<0.5cm in diameter).
    - Nodule: a large papule (>0.5cm in diameter).
    - Plaque: elevated, palpable and flat-topped (>0.5cm).
    - Lichenification: thickened skin with increased prominence of skin markings.
    - Cyst: cavity lined by epithelium containing fluid or semisolid material.
    - Vesicle: a small, fluid-filled blister (<0.5cm in diameter) with clear fluid.
    - Pustule: a vesicle with yellow fluid.
    - Bulla: a large vesicle, containing clear fluid.
    - Scale: a hyperproliferative response of the epidermis; grey, white or silver.
    - Erosion: shallow defect affecting epidermis to basement membrane; dermis is intact.
    - Ulcer: a deeper defect affecting the epidermis and some or all of the dermis.
    - Fissure: a thin, linear erosion of the skin surface.

Testing

- Vulval bacterial or viral skin swabs.
- Blood tests may be needed (pruritus screen, tests for diabetes, hypothyroid, iron deficiency and impaired kidney function).
- Skin scrapings for mycology.

Education

- Provide clear explanations and written materials to empower patients to manage their condition. The British Association of Dermatologists has lots of useful patient leaflets (www.bad.org.uk/patient-information-leaflets).
- Highlight the importance of self-examination and general care of the vulval tissue (see *Section 10.6*).

Holistic care

- Address the psychological impact of chronic vulval conditions, because they can significantly affect self-esteem, body image and sexual intimacy.

Treatments

- Explain how they work and give clear instructions on where to apply, how often and length of use of treatments, and any side-effects that may occur.

10.6 General care of the vulval skin and self-examination

Many women never examine their vulvas and knowledge of vulval anatomy is poor, making it difficult to explain where the problem is. It is vital to educate women on how to self-examine their vulvas and how to care for their vulval skin, and it should be included as part of the management of all vulval conditions.

The British Society for the Study of Vulval Disease has a helpful self-examination leaflet and video on its website that women can be directed towards (https://bssvd.org/practitioner-portal/external-resources).

For general vulval skin care the Primary Care Dermatology Society has a helpful leaflet that can be given to women (www.pcds.org.uk/files/pils/Vulval-care-Dec-23-for-PDF.pdf).

The general advice is to:

- Avoid perfumed, chemical products and irritants such as soap, bubble baths, shampoos, talcum powder, wet wipes and feminine sprays.
- Avoid tight clothes and use cotton underwear.
- Use plain, unperfumed condoms and lubricants (note that oil-based lubricants can damage condoms).
- Use plain white unfragranced toilet paper to wipe.
- Emollients and barrier creams that suit the patient can be used to wash and as a moisturiser. Ointments are better than creams (as they do not have preservatives) on the vulval tissue, e.g. Epaderm, Hydromol, Cetraben. Any cream or ointment may make the bath slippery and may be a fire hazard.

10.7 Red flags and when to refer

- **Persistent lesions:** unresponsive to standard treatments, especially persistent itch.
- **Suspected malignancy:** ulcerated or nodular vulval lump, non-healing sores, vulval bleeding.
- **Extensive scarring or functional impairment:** particularly in lichen sclerosus.

- **Diagnostic uncertainty:** biopsy may be required.
- **Care with darker skin tones:** clinical signs may be harder to recognise, and so doctors should have a lower threshold for referral. The British Association of Dermatologists has a list of resources for this (https://cdn.bad.org.uk/uploads/2022/02/29200007/Educational-Resources-for-Clinicians-on-Skin-of-Colour-in-Dermatology-2020.pdf).
- **Sexual problems:** if any vulval condition impacts sexual function then consider referral to a psychosexual therapist.

Always consider referring to a specialist vulval dermatology clinic if available locally, otherwise refer to a dermatologist or via urgent suspected cancer (USC) pathway if cancer is suspected.

Vulval dermatoses are diverse but manageable with a systematic approach to diagnosis and treatment. As a healthcare professional, early recognition and empathetic care are key to improving outcomes for women with these conditions. Regular updates on vulval dermatology and collaborative care with specialists can further enhance your practice.

10.8 Further reading

British Association of Dermatologists for patient leaflets: www.bad.org.uk/patient-information-leaflets

Oakley, A. (2022) *Dermatology Made Easy*, second edition. Scion Publishing Ltd.

Pictures of normal vulva: www.thegreatwallofvulva.com and www.labialibrary.org.au

Primary Care Dermatology Society: www.pcds.org.uk for leaflets and pictures.

Psoriasis in sensitive area leaflet: www.psoriasis-association.org.uk/media/InformationSheets/SENSITIVE_2016.pdf

Resources for skin of colour: https://cdn.bad.org.uk/uploads/2022/02/29200007/Educational-Resources-for-Clinicians-on-Skin-of-Colour-in-Dermatology-2020.pdf

Self-examination leaflet and video: https://www.bssvd.org/practitioner-portal/external-resources

Vulval care leaflet: www.pcds.org.uk/files/pils/Vulval-care-Dec-23-for-PDF.pdf

Vulval Pain Society: https://vulvalpainsociety.org.uk

Chapter 11
Female cancer and screening

11.1 Introduction

- Cancers that specifically affect the female population include breast, endometrial, cervical, ovarian, vulval and vaginal cancers.
- These cancers significantly impact women's health in the UK, and it is vital that healthcare professionals are aware of the prevalence, risk factors, clinical presentation, diagnosis, management and screening of these cancers.
- It is important to educate patients about these cancers and how they can mitigate the risks, and the signs/symptoms for early detection, as well as actively encouraging women to attend the free screening services available in the UK.
- Gynaecological cancers can affect all women, but also non-binary and trans males, and so it is important to be inclusive and sensitive to the needs of those individuals whose gender identity does not align with the sex they were assigned to at birth, so as not to miss cancers in these groups.
- As diagnosis and treatments continue to improve, there are now a growing number of women who are survivors of gynaecological cancers, and they suffer from the long-term impacts of the treatments and the ongoing anxiety of a cancer coming back. These women will need long-term support for their mental, physical and sexual health, and as clinicians we need to be aware of the issues they may face and how best to support them.
- This chapter will cover the different gynaecological cancers and screening services in the UK and describe the long-term support required for women who have survived cancer.

11.2 Breast cancer and the NHS breast screening programme

This chapter focuses specifically on cancer, but readers should also refer to *Chapter 12* on breast problems for additional information.

11.2.1 Epidemiology

- Breast cancer is the most common cancer in UK women, accounting for approximately 30% of all female cancer cases.
- In the UK, 56 800 women are diagnosed annually. A quarter of these are picked up by screening mammography.
- Incidence rises with age and the highest incidence is in women in their 90s.
- Invasive ductal carcinoma is the most common type of breast cancer, followed by invasive lobular cancer.
- Ductal carcinoma *in situ* (DCIS), where the abnormal cells are present in the lining of the milk ducts but have not spread from this area, and lobular carcinoma *in situ* (LCIS), are less common. LCIS is not strictly a cancer but rather a collection of abnormal cells in the lobules (milk-producing glands) of the breast tissue.
- Other types of cancers include triple-negative breast cancer (this type of breast cancer has no hormonal receptors) and Paget's disease of the breast (which is associated with skin changes in the nipple and is linked to breast cancer).
- Rare types include inflammatory breast cancer, medullary, metaplastic and mucinous breast cancers.

11.2.2 Risk factors

- Age – breast cancer risk rises with age; 25% are diagnosed after the age of 75.
- Family history of breast cancer – risk increases with the number of close relatives with breast cancer and the age at diagnosis (see *Section 12.4*).
- Previous history of breast cancer.

- Genetic mutations in the *BRCA1* and *BRCA2* genes produce a 45–65% risk of developing breast cancer by the age of 70 (see *Section 12.4*). There are also new mutations being discovered that can increase the risk of breast cancer, such as *CHEK2*.
- Obesity – postmenopausal women have a breast cancer risk that is 13% higher per 5 units of BMI increase and 50% higher in those with the highest waist-to-hip ratio as compared to the lowest.
- Smoking – can increase the risk of all cancers.
- Alcohol consumption – the risk increases with increasing units; drinking 2 units per day increases the risk by 9% and drinking 6 units a day by 60%.
- Low activity levels – being sedentary increases the risk. 2.7 hours of moderate exercise per week can reduce the risk of developing breast cancer by 20%.
- Combined oral contraceptive pill – risk increases with years of use and reduces after stopping. The actual risk differs depending on the preparation.
- Hormone replacement therapy – can increase the risk depending on type of HRT used and length of treatment (see *Chapter 7* for more details).
- Early menarche or late menopause.
- Never having had a child, or first child born after the age of 30.
- Not having breastfed – the risk is 16% lower in women who have breastfed.
- Breast density is an independent risk factor, increasing risk up to 2–4-fold.
- Ionising radiation – 1% of breast cancers are thought to be caused by radiotherapy and to a lesser extent by diagnostic radiology.

11.2.3 Clinical presentation

Women with breast cancer may present with the following symptoms that are suggestive of breast cancer.

- Unexplained breast lump – with or without pain *over* the age of 30.
- Unexplained axillary lump over the age of 30.
- Nipple changes that are concerning on one side, including a rash, retraction and discharge over the age of 50.
- Skin changes that are suggestive of breast cancer such as puckering or dimpling.
- Women who present with a breast lump, with or without pain, *below* the age of 30 can still be referred to the breast clinic as a non-urgent referral.
- Women with just breast pain and no lumps are referred if symptoms persist longer than 12 weeks and measures such as well-fitting bras, NSAIDs, and evening primrose oil have not helped. Follow-up appointments should be arranged to monitor the impact of treatment options on the pain and if not settled then to refer to the breast clinic.

11.2.4 Diagnosis

- All women with breast symptoms should be offered a face-to-face exam after seeking consent – a chaperone should always be offered. Compare both breasts, palpate the breasts and nipples and the axillae looking for any skin changes, lumps, pain and discharge from the nipples. This is a good opportunity to educate and encourage women to do self-exams. Helpful leaflets such as one from Breast Cancer Now can be given to patients (https://breastcancernow.org/media-assets/l1nbmxbe/bcc2-know-your-breasts-booklet-web.pdf).
- Women with suspicious features should be referred to the breast clinic via the urgent suspected cancer (USC) pathway. Follow up any referrals for safety-netting to make sure they have been seen within an appropriate timeframe (ideally 2 weeks).
- Women will be offered a mammogram with or without an ultrasound, depending on symptoms. The tests are usually done in a one-stop clinic on the same day. Suspicious lumps may need a biopsy to get a histological diagnosis.
- For any women that are not referred and are being monitored, a follow-up appointment should be arranged to check on symptoms between 2 and 4 weeks, depending on level

of concern. They should be informed of symptoms/changes to look out for in between appointments that should be brought to the attention of a doctor. These would be any suspicious symptoms listed in *Section 11.2.3*.

11.2.5 Treatment

- Treatments offered will depend on several different aspects of the cancer, such as the type, grade, size, stage, whether it has oestrogen and progesterone receptors, and if HER2 protein (human epidermal growth receptor 2) is present or not.
- Cancer grading – each cancer will fall into one of three grades (1–3) depending on how different the cells look to normal tissue and how fast they are growing. Women with a grade 3 cancer are more likely to be offered chemotherapy because they are fast growing.
- The size of a cancer or how many cancerous lesions there are may affect the extent of surgery or whether chemotherapy or radiotherapy is given prior to surgery to shrink the lesion.
- Cancer staging – this signifies how far the cancer has spread; there are four stages each with substages, with stage 1 the least invasive and stage 4 showing widespread involvement (see *Box 11.1*).
- Hormones can help cancers grow, and some cancer cells have receptors for oestrogen and progesterone: 80% of breast cancers are oestrogen receptor-positive cancers (ER-positive) and others are progesterone receptor-positive cancers (PR-positive). Hormone therapy, which either reduces the woman's circulating hormones or blocks the receptors, may be offered to patients with hormone receptor-positive cancers. Hormone receptor-negative cancers won't respond to hormone therapy.
- Some breast cancers express androgen receptors (i.e. are AR-positive) too but this is not something that is routinely tested. However, there are several trials going on looking at anti-androgen medication in women who have cancers that are AR-positive, and it is a growing area of interest.
- HER2 is a protein that promotes the growth of some breast cancers. Some cancers produce a higher amount of this protein and are termed HER2-positive. These patients should be offered targeted biological therapy alongside or after chemotherapy.
- The surgery offered to women with breast cancer is either breast-conserving surgery such as wide local excision or lumpectomy, or a mastectomy where all the breast tissue and nipple is removed. Chemotherapy, hormone therapy or targeted therapy is sometimes offered before surgery. Some women will also have to have their lymph nodes removed (this can lead to lymphoedema at a later stage). Some women may opt to have a breast reconstruction at the same time as surgery for removal of the breast, but this can also take place at a later stage.
- Radiotherapy is usually given after recovery from surgery and chemotherapy to reduce the risk of breast cancer recurrence. It is usually given daily over 1–3 weeks.
- Chemotherapy can be given before surgery to shrink the cancer or after surgery to reduce the risk of the cancer returning or spreading. It is also used to treat metastatic cancer.
- Hormone therapy reduces the risk of cancer coming back, and if the cancer is ER- or PR-positive then drugs such as tamoxifen, letrozole, exemestane or anastrozole, goserelin injections or leuprorelin injections are used. They are usually started after other treatments and women may be advised to take them for 5–10 years. These drugs can have menopausal side-effects, which can affect compliance, so women should be directed to their oncologist as the drugs may need to be changed/reviewed over time due to these side-effects.
- Targeted biological therapies block the cancer from growing and spreading and are used in HER2-positive cancers. Different types are used but the most common is Herceptin.
- Bisphosphonates may be used to reduce the risk of cancer spreading to the bones. They are also used to treat osteoporosis and when the cancer has already metastasised to the bones. Zoledronic acid is usually given via IV infusion every 6 months for 3 years.

BOX 11.1: Breast cancer staging

Stage 1A – cancer is ≤2cm and has not spread outside the breast.

Stage 1B – cancer is ≤2cm. Tiny numbers of cancer cells have spread to lymph nodes in the armpit (micrometastases).

Stage 2A – cancer is ≤2cm and has spread to 1–3 lymph nodes, or 2–5cm and has not spread to the lymph nodes.

Stage 2B – cancer is 2–5cm and spread to 1–3 lymph nodes, or cancer is 5cm and has not spread to the lymph nodes.

Stage 3A – cancer is ≤5cm and has spread to 4–9 lymph nodes, or >5cm and has spread to 3 lymph nodes.

Stage 3B – cancer has spread to the skin of the breast or chest muscle and may have spread to 1–9 lymph nodes.

Stage 3C – any size of cancer that has spread to the skin of the breast or chest muscle and spread to ≥10 lymph nodes. The cancer has spread to lymph nodes below the breastbone and above or below the collarbone. It has spread to ≥4 lymph nodes in the armpit.

Stage 4 – cancer has spread to other parts of the body, such as the bones, liver or lungs.

11.2.6 UK screening recommendations (NHS breast screening programme)

Mammography

- Women aged 50–70 are invited for mammography screening every 3 years.
- Women will be invited for their first mammogram any time between the ages of 50 and 53.
- Women at higher risk (e.g. *BRCA* mutation carriers) may be offered earlier and more frequent screening.
- Screening can be extended past age 70 if a woman wishes it to.
- Results are sent to patients after 2 weeks.
- Some women do not attend when invited for screening, and their reasons and concerns should be explored.
- If any suspicious features are seen on the mammogram, women will be automatically referred to the local breast clinic for further examinations/tests.
- Trans men and non-binary people may not be invited for screening if they are not registered as female at the surgery. If they have breasts, they can contact their GP or the NHS breast screening programme to be screened.

Self-examination and clinical breast examination

- Not routinely recommended but it may help with awareness. Women should be shown how to examine their breasts (see *Sections 12.1.2* and *12.2.3*) and advised what symptoms to look for that need to be reported to their doctor.

Genetic testing

- Consider for women with a strong family history or known *BRCA* or *CHEK2* mutations – 10% of breast cancer cases are caused by genetic mutations inherited from a parent. Referral to a genetic specialist may be warranted.

11.2.7 The role of the clinician

- Encourage participation in the NHS breast screening programme.
- Recognise red flags such as palpable lumps, nipple changes or unexplained pain.
- Coordinate referrals for diagnostic imaging and specialist evaluation.

11.3 Endometrial cancer

11.3.1 Epidemiology

- Endometrial cancer is the fourth most common cancer in women in the UK and 9700 women are diagnosed with it every year.
- The incidence has risen by 12% over the last 10 years.
- Although it can develop at any age, incidence rates are highest in females aged 75–79. 80–90% of endometrial cancers are oestrogen-dependent.

11.3.2 Risk factors

These are mainly related to chronic exposure to oestrogen.

- Age: mainly a problem in postmenopausal women, but 10% of cases occur in premenopausal women.
- Obesity due to oestrogen being produced by adipose tissue.
- Early menarche and late menopause.
- Low parity.
- Unopposed oestrogen exposure.
- PCOS.
- Diabetes.
- Tamoxifen – this can block the impact of oestrogen on the breast, but it is pro-oestrogenic on the uterus and bones. 1 in 500 women on tamoxifen may be affected.
- Lynch syndrome is an inherited condition that increases risk of developing several types of cancer, especially colorectal, endometrial and ovarian.
  - Lifetime risks for endometrial cancer can vary between 40 and 60%.
  - If women have completed their family they may be advised to have risk-reducing surgery, a total hysterectomy with bilateral salpingo-oophorectomy (BSO).
  - They should be advised of the symptoms of cancer so they can seek medical advice promptly.

11.3.3 Clinical presentation

- The most common presentation is irregular bleeding in postmenopausal women.
- Unscheduled bleeding on HRT.
- Intermenstrual bleeding at any age.
- Unusually heavy bleeding.
- Blood-stained vaginal discharge.
- Haematuria with anaemia or haematuria with vaginal discharge, or thrombocytosis in women with postmenopausal bleeding.

11.3.4 Diagnosis

- A pelvic and abdominal examination, together with a speculum inspection with swabs to rule out other causes for symptoms. Blood and urine tests may also be needed to rule out other causes, especially if presenting with irregular bleeding.
- A pelvic ultrasound scan will report whether there is thickening of the endometrium and suspicion of endometrial cancer. If there is any thickening concurrent with other risk factors, a USC referral to gynaecology will be needed. Referral will be required for linings:
  - ≥4mm on continuous combined HRT
  - ≥7mm on sequential HRT.

  If not on HRT and the lining is >4mm then an urgent investigation is required.

- A hysteroscopy with endometrial biopsy will be needed to make the diagnosis. This can be done either locally with pipelle sampling, or under general anaesthetic if the patient is not able to tolerate it, if inadequate sampling or in women with a history of cervical stenosis.

11.3.5 Treatment

- The most common treatment for endometrial cancer is a total hysterectomy and BSO. If women have not gone through the menopause, this clearly impacts their fertility and causes a surgical menopause (see *Section 6.10*).
- Some women may need radiotherapy either externally to the pelvis/vagina or internally (brachytherapy) to the vagina.
- Chemotherapy is not usually effective, but there are some newer immune therapy treatments being considered.

11.3.6 UK screening recommendations

- Routine screening for endometrial cancer is **not** recommended for asymptomatic women.
- High-risk individuals (e.g. Lynch syndrome carriers) may require transvaginal ultrasound and endometrial biopsy.

11.3.7 The role of the clinician

- Investigate abnormal uterine bleeding, particularly postmenopausal bleeding.
- Identify at-risk women and provide lifestyle advice for women who are at increased risk of endometrial cancer due to obesity.
- Facilitate early specialist referral for suspicious cases.

11.4 Cervical cancer and the NHS cervical cancer screening programme

11.4.1 Epidemiology

- Cervical cancer can occur at any age, but the highest incidence is between the ages of 30 and 35 years. It is very rare below the age of 25.
- Approximately 3200 women are diagnosed with cervical cancer in the UK each year.
- The type of cervical cancer depends upon the type of cell the cancer started in.
  - The two main types of cervical cancer are squamous cell carcinoma (SCC) and adenocarcinoma.
  - 80–90% are SCCs. Squamous cells are flat, skin-like cells covering the ectocervix, which is the outer surface of the cervix.
  - 10–20% are adenocarcinomas and these start in the glandular cells of the endocervix.
  - SCC and adenocarcinoma are treated in the same way.
  - There are some rarer types of cervical cancer such as small cell cancer of the cervix, which tends to grow quickly and is treated differently.

11.4.2 Risk factors

- Age – it is more common in younger women and 50% occur below the age of 45.
- Persistent infection with high-risk HPV.
  - HPV is a very common group of viruses affecting around 80% of people at some point in their lives. It is transmitted by skin-to-skin sexual contact.
  - HPV usually causes no symptoms and is cleared by the body within 2 years; however, some types of HPV can cause genital warts or cancer.

    - There are over 100 different types of HPV, most of which are harmless; however, HPV-16 and -18 are common high-risk HPV subtypes and contribute to 70% of cervical cancers worldwide.
    - Other cancers linked to high-risk HPV include cervical, anal, penile, vulval and vaginal and some types of head and neck cancer.
- The introduction of the HPV vaccine and HPV testing in smear tests should gradually reduce the incidence of cervical cancer.
- Smoking can impact the immune system, making it less likely to clear HPV infections.
- Immunosuppression with drugs can impact the immune system, making it less likely to clear the HPV virus.
- Early sexual activity.
- Multiple sexual partners.
- Infection with other sexually transmitted disease, e.g. chlamydia.
- Low socioeconomic status.
- Combined oral contraceptive use – this may increase risk by reducing the capacity to clear HPV infections.

11.4.3 Clinical presentation

- In the early stages, most women have no symptoms and so most cervical cancers are found on routine cervical screening.
- In those women under 25 years who have not been invited for routine screening, persistent symptoms such as those listed below should be investigated or referred to gynaecology, even though cervical cancer is rare in this age group.
- If women do have symptoms, then cervical cancer can present as irregular vaginal bleeding. Bleeding could be postcoital, intermenstrual or postmenopausal.
- If smear tests are normal, the cervix looks normal and swabs are clear, but if abnormal bleeding persists for more than 6–8 weeks, then refer to gynaecology for colposcopy.
- Malodorous vaginal discharge may not be thought of as a symptom of cervical cancer, so it can lead to a delay in presentation and diagnosis. Consider cervical cancer in those whose symptoms persist, or do not respond to treatment for co-existing genital infections.
- Dyspareunia.
- Low back pain.
- In advanced cancer, women may present with recurrent urine infections, bone pain, leg swelling, constipation, loss of appetite, fatigue and weight loss.

11.4.4 Diagnosis

- Vaginal speculum examination should always be undertaken in any woman presenting with abnormal vaginal bleeding; the cervix should be visualised. If the cervix looks abnormal, refer for colposcopy urgently.
- It is important to be aware that early cancerous changes may not be visible on examination and the cervix may appear normal, so refer to gynaecology if symptoms persist for more than 6–8 weeks.
- Most women are picked up by cervical screening. Screening can allow detection and early treatment of abnormal cell changes that could lead to cervical cancer, therefore helping to prevent cancer rather than diagnose it.
- Cervical screening tests for high-risk strains of HPV. If these are found, cytology is performed to check for any abnormal changes to the cells. Anyone who has high-risk HPV with abnormal cells on cytology will be referred for colposcopy to make the diagnosis.
- If a smear test cannot be carried out due to pain, or the cervix cannot be visualised, the patient should be referred to the colposcopy clinic.

11.4.5 Treatment

- Colposcopy looks closely at the cells on the cervix and a biopsy will be taken. This identifies abnormal cells, for example pre-cancerous changes called cervical intraepithelial neoplasia (CIN) or cancerous cells.
- The grade of CIN is determined by the depth of invasion of abnormal cells which, if left untreated, can progress to cervical cancer.
  - CIN 1 (mild): one-third depth of invasion of the surface cervix layer.
  - CIN 2 (moderate): two-thirds depth of invasion.
  - CIN 3 (severe): full thickness invasion of the surface layer of the cervix. This is more likely to develop into cancer if not treated.
- Depending upon the grade of CIN, management could be conservative, or treatment to remove the abnormal cells. A conservative approach involves monitoring of the cells over time, through colposcopy, cervical screening or biopsies, to see if the cells revert to normal.
- If the changes persist, or in moderate–severe CIN, then treatment options are typically used to remove abnormal cells using electrical diathermy to the surface of the cervix (this is known as a large loop excision of the transformation zone (LLETZ). In some cases, surgery may be needed, with a deeper excision in the shape of a cone (cone biopsy).
- There is no prescribable treatment to cure HPV infection.

11.4.6 UK screening recommendations (NHS cervical screening programme)

- Cervical screening test (CST): women aged 25–64 are invited for screening.
- Since 1st July 2025 there has been a change in the way women are invited for cervical cancer screening in the UK.
  - Previously women aged 25–49 were screened every 3 years, and those aged 50–64 were screened every 5 years in England.
  - Now, younger women (aged 25–49) who test negative for HPV, will be invited at 5-year intervals, rather than 3 years, offering a more personalised approach dependent upon individual results.
  - Those that test positive for HPV will be invited more frequently.
  - The interval for those aged 50–64 remains every 5 years.
  - The NHS is now using digital invitations and reminders to invite eligible women, through the NHS app. Women will subsequently receive text messages and reminder letters if they do not book an appointment.
  - The update aligns England with Scotland and Wales, where the cervical screening process has always been different, and women between the ages of 25 and 64 are invited for cervical screening every 5 years. Some high-risk women may be offered smears up to the age of 70.
- The NHS Cervical Screening Programme involves primary human papilloma screening, to identify people with high-risk HPV strains.
  - Liquid-based cytology is performed only if high-risk HPV is found.
  - Cytology reports the level of dyskaryosis or abnormal changes in the cells. They can be borderline, mild, moderate or severe, or reported as inadequate if not enough cells were sampled.
  - Colposcopy is used to diagnose CIN and to differentiate high-grade lesions from low-grade abnormalities in people with abnormal cytology.
- Those who test negative for high-risk HPV on their cervical screening test will be invited for a routine recall.
- Those who test positive for high-risk HPV but have normal cytology will be invited for a repeat cervical screening test in 1 year. At this stage:
  - If they test negative for high-risk HPV, they will revert to routine recall for future cervical screening.
  - If they test positive for high-risk HPV, they will be referred for colposcopy.

- If results show that high-risk HPV is positive and cytology is abnormal at any time, they will need to be referred to colposcopy.
- Women who have had a sub-total hysterectomy and whose cervix remains will need to continue having cervical screening. Some women may need vault smears after a hysterectomy if there has been a history of CIN, and secondary care should advise about follow-up vault smears.
- For those women who have GSM, cervical smears can be very painful.
    - It can be a good opportunity to discuss the symptoms of GSM and treatment options.
    - Using vaginal oestrogen locally for at least 3–4 weeks can improve the vaginal tissue and make the smear more comfortable. It should be stopped 48 hours before a smear test.
- Cervical screening uptake can be suboptimal and barriers to attending for screening can be:
    - age – either young women or those over 50 years
    - ethnic minorities
    - low socioeconomic status
    - previous sexual trauma or sexual problems such as vaginismus
    - lack of knowledge or awareness about smear tests
    - concern and embarrassment about the procedure
    - fear of cancer and pain associated with speculum procedure.
- Actively inviting women for screening and exploring the reasons they do not attend as well as explaining the procedure can help.
    - Informing women of options such as smaller speculums, female staff or female chaperones, double appointments and being able to stop at any time.
    - HPV self-sampling kits, which are sent to the homes of individuals, has been piloted; evidence shows this could boost uptake for screening and there is a possibility they may be introduced in early 2026.
- Women who have sex with women are at risk of cervical cancer, and the prevalence of HPV is 3–30%. In lesbian women who have never had heterosexual intercourse the prevalence is 19% because HPV can be transmitted through lesbian sexual contact. They should be actively encouraged to attend for screening. Trans men may not get invited for screening if they are registered as male in their surgery. If they still have a cervix they are at risk of cervical cancer and should be invited for a smear test.
- HPV vaccination is now offered to all adolescents regardless of gender aged 12–13 as part of the NHS immunisation programme. This will hopefully reduce the incidence of cervical cancer in women in the future. These vaccines protect against the types of HPV which are likely to cause cervical cancer, but not all types, so it is still necessary to take part in cervical screening.
- Pregnant women should defer their routine cervical screening test until 12 weeks post-delivery to give the cervix a chance to return to normal and avoid false positive tests.

11.4.7 The role of the clinician

- Promote HPV vaccination among eligible patients.
- Ensure regular screening compliance and follow up on abnormal results.
- Counsel patients on HPV transmission, smoking cessation and safe sexual practices.
- Encourage practice nurses to report any suspicious findings on vaginal exams / smears promptly to the GP.

11.5 Ovarian cancer

11.5.1 Epidemiology

- In the UK ovarian cancer is the sixth most common cancer in women. 7500 women are diagnosed every year.

- Ovarian cancer is not one disease – it is a group of cancers that start in different types of cells within the ovary, fallopian tube or peritoneum.

There are many different types of primary ovarian cancer: 85–90% are epithelial ovarian cancers. These start in the layer of cells covering the ovary or lining the fallopian tube / peritoneum. Subtypes include:

- High-grade serous carcinoma (HGSC) – most common and aggressive form.
- Low-grade serous carcinoma (LGSC) – slower growing, less common.
- Endometrioid carcinoma – sometimes linked to endometriosis.
- Clear cell carcinoma – may also be associated with endometriosis.
- Mucinous carcinoma – produces mucus, rarer.
- Transitional cell (Brenner) tumour – rare variant.

2–3% of primary ovarian cancers are germ cell tumours, which originate from the cells that form eggs. Subtypes include:

- Dysgerminoma – most common germ cell type, often in younger women.
- Yolk sac tumour (endodermal sinus tumour) – aggressive but often curable if caught early.
- Immature teratoma – contains embryonic tissue.
- Embryonal carcinoma – rare, aggressive.
- Choriocarcinoma – extremely rare in ovaries.

1–2% of primary ovarian cancers are sex cord–stromal cell tumours which develop from the ovarian connective tissue that produces hormones. Subtypes include:

- Granulosa cell tumour – can produce oestrogen; sometimes slow-growing.
- Thecoma – often produces oestrogen.
- Sertoli–Leydig cell tumour – may produce testosterone, leading to virilisation.

Other rare types include:

- Small cell carcinoma of the ovary – very aggressive, rare and affects young women.
- Primary peritoneal carcinoma – behaves like epithelial ovarian cancer but starts in the peritoneum. Treated the same way as ovarian cancer.
- Metastatic tumours to the ovary – e.g. Krukenberg tumour (often from stomach, breast or colon).
- Fallopian tube cancer is a type of ovarian cancer called a high-grade serous cancer. It is treated the same as ovarian cancer.

11.5.2 Risk factors

- Age – 50% occur over the age of 65, mainly in postmenopausal women, but it can occur at any age.
- Family history of ovarian cancer.
- Two inherited genetic conditions that are linked to ovarian cancer are *BRCA* gene mutations and Lynch syndrome.
- Nulliparity.
- Endometriosis.
- Being overweight, smoking, HRT (carries a 1% risk of ovarian cancer), asbestos and radiation exposure and diabetes.

11.5.3 Clinical presentation

- Ovarian cancer is often diagnosed late due to the symptoms being quite vague and similar to other conditions. It can be easy to miss the diagnosis.
- It is often mistaken for irritable bowel syndrome.
- In women, especially those over 50 years, presenting with one or more of the following symptoms on a persistent (for at least 1 month) or frequent (12 times per month) basis should be investigated further:

- Persistent abdominal distension or bloating.
- Pelvic or abdominal pain.
- Increased urinary urgency/frequency.
- Change in bowel habit: constipation or diarrhoea.
- Symptoms that suggest new-onset irritable bowel syndrome in women >50 years.
- Feeling full (early satiety) and/or loss of appetite.
- Unexplained weight loss.
- Unexplained fatigue.
- Less common: irregular vaginal bleeding, back pain.

11.5.4 Diagnosis

- Abdominal and pelvic examination – a mass may be detected or ascites found.
- Blood test – CA125 is often used as a marker for ovarian cancer. It can be raised in 50% of women with an early-stage ovarian cancer. However, CA125 is not specific for ovarian cancer, and it is important to be aware it can be raised in other conditions, such as benign ovarian tumours, endometriosis, pelvic inflammatory disease, fibroids, pregnancy and liver disease. It can also be raised in endometrial and cervical cancer.
- If CA125 is raised >35IU/ml, an ultrasound scan of the abdomen/pelvis should be requested.
- If ovarian cancer is suspected, refer via the USC pathway to gynaecology and secondary care will investigate further with CT scans to check for metastases and for staging.
- Biopsies for histological confirmation and type of cancer and genetic tests may also be needed, depending on biopsy results and family history.

11.5.5 Treatment

- Usually, a combination of chemotherapy and surgery is used to treat ovarian cancer.
- Surgery involves primary debulking surgery, which can include removal of ovaries and fallopian tubes, womb and cervix and parts of the vagina. Sometimes omentum and parts of the bowel may need to be removed, depending on how far it has spread, which may result in the need for a stoma.
- Chemotherapy is either given before or after surgery or used on its own for non-surgical cases due to extensive disease.

11.5.6 UK screening recommendations

- Routine screening for ovarian cancer is **not** recommended for asymptomatic women in the general population, because CA125 lacks the sensitivity and specificity to be used as a screening test for ovarian cancer.
- High-risk women (e.g. *BRCA* mutation carriers, family history of two or more cases of ovarian or breast cancer diagnosed at early age in first-degree relatives) may be offered transvaginal ultrasound and CA125 testing under specialist guidance.

11.5.7 The role of the clinician

- Recognise non-specific symptoms such as bloating, pelvic pain, early satiety and urinary frequency.
- Consider ovarian cancer in differential diagnoses and facilitate prompt specialist referral.
- Support risk-reducing strategies, including contraceptive pill use and risk-reducing surgery in high-risk women.

11.6 Vulval cancer

11.6.1 Epidemiology

- Vulval cancer is rare, accounting for only approximately 5% of gynaecological cancers.
- In the UK, about 1300 women are diagnosed annually.

- It predominantly affects postmenopausal women, with a higher incidence in those over 65 years.
- The incidence rates are increasing in younger populations (i.e. those aged 50–59) due to the rise in HPV-related VIN (vulval intraepithelial neoplasia) in these groups. However, over time with the introduction of the HPV vaccine the risk of HPV-related VIN should reduce in the vaccinated population.
- Approximately 90% of vulval cancers are SCCs due to high-risk HPV and inflammatory dermatoses such as lichen sclerosus and lichen planus. The other 10% are due to primary vulval melanomas, basal cell carcinomas, Bartholin's gland carcinoma, adenocarcinoma and rarely sarcomas.

11.6.2 Risk factors

- Age – higher risk in those over 65 years, but increasing incidence in the age group 50–59 years.
- HPV infection – particularly HPV types 16 and 18. They can cause VIN, a potentially precancerous condition, which if left untreated can result in vulval cancer.
- Chronic vulvar conditions, such as lichen sclerosus and lichen planus.
- Smoking increases susceptibility to HPV infections.
- Immunosuppression including HIV infection.
- History of CIN or cervical cancer.

11.6.3 Clinical presentation

- Persistent vulvar itching or pain/soreness.
- Lump or ulceration on the vulva.
- Thickened, raised, red, lighter or darker patches on the skin of the vulva.
- Bleeding or blood-stained discharge not related to menstrual cycles or any postmenopausal bleeding.
- Mole on the vulva that changes in size/shape/colour, or bleeds.
- A visible lesion with associated symptoms of pain and/or bleeding is highly suspicious.
- Groin lymph node enlargement may be present in advanced lesions.

11.6.4 Diagnosis

- To diagnose vulval cancer, all women will need a clinical examination with inspection and palpation of the vulva. Suspicious cases will need referral to gynaecology or dermatology, depending on the findings.
- A vulval skin biopsy at the edge of the lesion is essential for histopathological confirmation. Clinical drawings and photographs will also be undertaken in secondary care.
- Further imaging such as MRI or CT scans may be needed to assess the extent of disease spread.

11.6.5 Treatment

- Surgery is the main treatment option, ranging from local excision to radical vulvectomy.
- Radiotherapy may be used pre- or post-surgery, with or without chemotherapy, or as primary treatment in non-surgical candidates.
- Chemotherapy is often combined with radiotherapy for advanced cases. Sometimes chemotherapy is given to shrink the cancer prior to surgery.
- Treatment decisions should be made within a multidisciplinary team, considering tumour stage and patient health and preferences.

11.6.6 UK screening recommendations

- There are currently no screening tests to prevent vulval cancer.
- HPV vaccines prior to HPV exposure are likely to reduce the incidence of vulval SCC in the future, as more young girls are vaccinated. Studies are ongoing to see if HPV vaccination following the

diagnosis of VIN can reduce the risk of recurrence or development of vulval SCC, but there is currently not sufficient evidence to support HPV vaccination for secondary prevention.
- Any woman with high-risk HPV should be referred for colposcopy.
- Monitoring and good control of lichen sclerosus or lichen planus with high-dose topical steroids may reduce the incidence of vulval SCC.
- Women who are not responding to steroid treatment within 1–2 weeks should be referred urgently to secondary care via the USC pathway.
- Women with known VIN will need monitoring with vulvoscopy.

11.6.7 The role of the clinician

- Always offer face-to-face examination for any woman with suspicious vulval symptoms.
- Practice nurses should report any suspicious lesions/symptoms to a clinician for further examination.
- Consider annual reviews of those patients with lichen sclerosus.
- Encourage girls to have their HPV vaccine and women over 25 years to attend cervical screening.
- Possible long-term issues following vulval cancer treatment include lymphoedema, psychosexual issues, body image issues and altered bowel and bladder function post radiotherapy.

11.7 Vaginal cancer

11.7.1 Epidemiology

- Primary vaginal cancer is rare: it is the least common gynaecological cancer, with approximately 250 cases diagnosed annually in the UK.
- It most commonly affects women over 60.
- The majority (90%) of vaginal cancers are SCCs and 10% are adenocarcinomas.
- Other very rare causes may be melanomas, lymphomas or sarcomas.

11.7.2 Risk factors

- Age – 40% are aged >75.
- HPV infection – 75% of vaginal cancers are linked to HPV.
- Previous gynaecological malignancies – history of cervical or vulvar cancer. Be vigilant in women with CIN or VIN.
- *In utero* exposure to diethylstilboestrol (DES) – associated with clear cell adenocarcinoma.
- Smoking.
- Immunosuppression, e.g. lupus or HIV/AIDS.

11.7.3 Clinical presentation

- 1 in 5 may have no symptoms and may be detected on routine examination.
- Abnormal vaginal bleeding – postcoital, intermenstrual or postmenopausal.
- Vaginal discharge – persistent and possibly malodorous.
- Persistent pelvic or vaginal pain and pain during intercourse.
- Palpable mass felt by patient or detected during pelvic examination.

11.7.4 Diagnosis

- Offer all women with suspicious symptoms a pelvic examination with a speculum, including inspection of the vaginal walls.
- A colposcopy exam will be carried out in secondary care to look at lesions in detail on the cervix and vaginal wall.

- A biopsy will need to be taken for histological confirmation.
- Further imaging may be needed such as an MRI or CT/PET scan to determine the extent of any disease that may have spread.

11.7.5 Treatment

- Radiotherapy – mainstay treatment, especially for localised disease. It can either be external or internal (brachytherapy) where a small device may be placed internally for a few hours at a time.
- Surgery – depending on extent of disease the surgery may be partial or radical. Usually reserved for small, accessible tumours or recurrent disease. In some cases they may also be offered vaginal reconstruction.
- Chemotherapy – often combined with radiotherapy for advanced stages.
- Management should be individualised within a multidisciplinary framework.

11.7.6 The role of the clinician

- Early recognition: identify and evaluate symptoms promptly.
- Timely referral: adhere to NICE guidelines for suspected cancer referrals.
- Patient education: promote awareness of symptoms and risk factors.
- Preventive measures: encourage HPV vaccination and safe sexual practices using condoms.
- Managing long-term complications: mainly psychosexual issues with psychosexual therapy referral.

11.8 Support after cancer

- Caring for patients who have survived breast and gynaecological cancers presents a unique set of challenges that extend well beyond the completion of active treatment.
- Survivors often face long-term physical effects such as fatigue, brain fog, lymphoedema, menopausal symptoms and sexual dysfunction, alongside emotional challenges including anxiety, depression and fear of recurrence.
- Maintaining a good quality of life involves a holistic, patient-centred approach that addresses three areas: physical, psychosocial and psychosexual needs. Healthcare professionals play a vital role in this phase of care. They should:
  - provide regular follow-up to monitor for recurrence and late effects.
  - offer support for managing chronic symptoms including bone and heart health.
  - ensure timely referrals to specialists such as pelvic floor physiotherapists, counsellors, or sexual health experts.
- Sexual problems after gynaecological cancers such as vaginal dryness, vaginal stenosis, vaginismus, dyspareunia, reduced arousal and desire, altered orgasm and reduced pleasure are common and can impact relationships.
- Women also experience psychological challenges around their sexuality in relation to altered body image, loss of femininity and fertility. They may feel less safe in their bodies following the trauma of a cancer diagnosis and this can often cause dissociation and again contribute to sexual problems.
- These issues are difficult to raise but important for some women and many think that there are no treatment options.
- Healthcare professionals should explore this area sensitively with patients because it is not always discussed in secondary care; inform them of treatment options such as lubricants, vaginal moisturisers, vaginal oestrogen for some women following discussion of risks/benefits with their oncologist, dilator therapy, pelvic floor physiotherapy and trauma-specific and/or psychosexual therapy.
- GPs should also actively listen to patients' concerns, promote healthy lifestyle changes, and coordinate care with oncology teams to ensure continuity and reassurance.

- Empowering patients with information, emotional support, and access to resources is key to helping them rebuild their lives and maintain wellbeing after cancer.
- Women should be directed to organisations such as Macmillan and Maggie's, which offer information and support as well as menopause after cancer workshops for women with cancer.

11.9 Conclusion

Healthcare professionals play a crucial role in cancer prevention, screening and early detection. By staying informed on screening guidelines and risk factors, we can guide patients to make informed health decisions and improve overall cancer outcomes in women and support them with holistic care to have a good quality of life after a cancer diagnosis.

11.10 Further reading

Breast exam leaflet: https://breastcancernow.org/media-assets/l1nbmxbe/bcc2-know-your-breasts-booklet-web.pdf

British Gynaecological Cancer Society (BGCS) Guidelines for Ovarian and Endometrial Cancer: www.bgcs.org.uk

https://eveappeal.org.uk for patients with information about all the gynaecological cancers.

Macmillan Cancer Support (2019) *Cancer and your sex life*. Available at: https://cdn.macmillan.org.uk/dfsmedia/1a6f23537f7f4519bb0cf14c45b2a629/2948-10061/mac17968-e01-sex-life-pdf

Morrison, J., Baldwin, P., Hanna, L. *et al.* (2024) British Gynaecological Cancer Society (BGCS) vulval cancer guidelines: an update on recommendations for practice 2023. *European Journal of Obstetrics and Gynecology and Reproductive Biology*, **292:** 210–38. Available at: www.ejog.org/article/S0301-2115(23)00813-8/fulltext#f0010

NHS Breast Screening Programme: www.nhs.uk/conditions/breast-cancer-screening

NHS Cervical Screening Programme: www.nhs.uk/conditions/cervical-screening

NICE (updated 2023) *Familial breast cancer* [CG164]. Available at: www.nice.org.uk/guidance/cg164

RCOG (2014) *Guidelines for the diagnosis and management of vulval carcinoma*. Available at: https://www.rcog.org.uk/media/dqwnw2a1/vulvalcancerguideline.pdf

UK National Screening Committee: www.gov.uk/government/groups/uk-national-screening-committee-uk-nsc

www.macmillan.org.uk for cancer information and support.

www.maggies.org for ongoing support during and after a cancer diagnosis; offer menopause after cancer workshops in all the centres.

Chapter 12
The breast

12.1 The breast

Breasts are composed of skin, fatty tissue, glandular (milk-producing) tissue, connective tissue, blood vessels, lymphatic system and nerves (see *Fig. 12.1*). Most of the breast consists of glandular tissue and fatty tissue. The ratio of glandular to fatty tissue varies among women.

The pectoralis major muscle forms the base of the breast. The breast is anchored to the pectoralis major fascia by flexible Cooper ligaments which allow the breast to move.

The breast is composed of two regions: the circular body, the largest part of the breast, and the axillary tail, the smaller part, which runs along the inferior lateral edge of the pectoralis major, towards the axillary fossa.

Breast development begins in puberty. Cyclical hormonal changes promote development and proliferation of the fatty tissue and glandular tissue.

- Adipose (fatty) tissue fills the space between the connective tissue and glandular tissue, and determines breast size.
- Connective (fibrous) tissue provides structural support and helps hold the breast tissue together.
- Glandular tissue (also known as the mammary gland) makes up the functional aspect of the breast.
  - It includes lobes and lobules (alveoli; milk-producing units) and lactiferous ducts (milk ducts, which carry milk to the nipple).
  - This ductal system is largely dormant until pregnancy. Hormones of pregnancy trigger crucial changes in the breasts:
    - Oestrogen promotes the development of lactiferous milk ducts (which are ultimately responsible for storage and delivery of milk).
    - Progesterone stimulates alveolar-lobular formation (which are ultimately responsible for production of milk).
- The nipple is surrounded by a darkened area of skin called the areola. The areola contains small, sebaceous (oil-producing) glands known as Montgomery glands which are naturally enlarged in pregnancy and lactation.

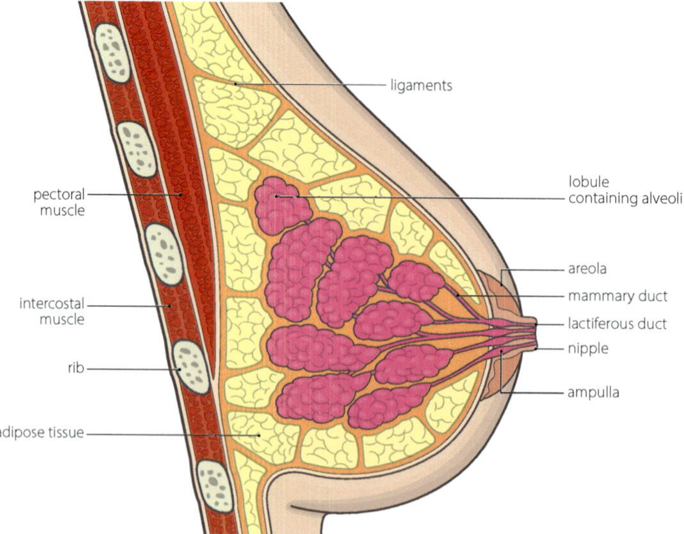

Figure 12.1: The breast. Reproduced from *Anatomy and Physiology: an introduction for nursing and healthcare* (2020) with permission from Lantern Publishing Ltd.

12.1.1 Breast size and density

Breast size and symmetry

It is common for a woman's breasts to be a different size and shape from each other, and to change at different times in the month, during pregnancy and after menopause.

Breast asymmetry refers to a noticeable difference in the appearance of one breast, in comparison to the other. Asymmetry may occur due to overdevelopment or underdevelopment of one breast. Changes can often be seen with puberty and menopause, or if there is a change in body weight; however, new-onset asymmetry may be suggestive of an underlying breast mass and should be referred.

Breast density

The breasts are made up of dense breast tissue (glandular tissue and connective tissue) and fatty breast tissue. Dense breasts have a higher proportion of glandular and connective tissue compared to fatty tissue.

Breast density cannot be assessed on examination. Dense breast tissue refers to the way the breast tissue appears on a mammogram. About 10% of women have very dense breasts and up to 50% have some mixed dense and fatty tissue.

On a mammogram fatty breast tissue is transparent, and it is easy to look for anything concerning, but very dense breast tissue is seen as white or opaque, making interpreting the mammogram more difficult, and making a tumour harder to detect. There is a link between higher breast density and an increased risk of breast cancer.

In 2019, the UK National Screening Committee (UK NSC) looked at the evidence for whether offering extra ultrasound screenings after a standard mammogram test could help women with dense breasts. The review concluded that the routine use of ultrasound could not be recommended, and there was not enough evidence to support a change in the screening programme.

12.1.2 Breast awareness

Encourage patients to be breast aware by regularly feeling their breasts, looking for changes and checking anything new or unusual with their doctor.

Breast symptoms to be aware of include a lump in the breast or armpit, nipple discharge, new indentations or dimpling, and thickened or reddened skin.

Patient information websites include:

- Breast Cancer Now (https://breastcancernow.org/about-breast-cancer/awareness/signs-and-symptoms-of-breast-cancer)
- CoppaFeel! (https://coppafeel.org/breast-cancer-info-and-advice/how-do-i-check).

12.2 Breast symptoms

It is understandable that any breast symptom can cause significant anxiety. Most primary care consultations that relate to breast symptoms represent benign breast disease. Benign breast disease can present with symptoms such as pain, nipple discharge, nodularity and swelling.

It is important to take a thorough history and examine the breast. The questions can be guided by the patient's symptoms.

Please use local guidelines when considering management of individual patients.

12.2.1 History-taking

- Is there a breast lump: when was it first noticed, and has it changed in size or in any other way?
- Has the nipple changed: is there a discharge, is it blood-stained, is there nipple inversion or retraction?
- Are there skin changes: a change in colour or appearance, a rash or 'peau d'orange' where the skin appears thickened and pitted and resembles orange peel, tethering or a pinched appearance? Where did the rash start (nipple or areola)?
- Menstrual history: age of menarche, last menstrual period, changes noted through the menstrual cycle, menopause history (natural, surgical, early or late).
- Family history: include breast and ovarian cancer, sarcoma under 45 years, complicated cancers at young age, glioma or childhood adrenal carcinomas. Is there a need a referral to secondary care or genetics? See *Section 12.4.3* and also check:
  - NICE guideline NG242: *Ovarian cancer: identifying and managing familial and genetic risk.*
  - NICE guideline CG164: *Familial breast cancer: classification, care and managing breast cancer and related risks in people with a family history of breast cancer.*
- History of breast pain.
- History of trauma to the breast.
- Lifestyle: include BMI, smoking, alcohol and exercise.
- History of hormone use: HRT and hormonal contraceptives.
- Breastfeeding, family size and age when had children.
- If implants are in place, ask about unexplained breast enlargement, asymmetry, fluid build-up and type of implant used.
- Previous breast disease or investigations.
- Risk factors: obesity, Ashkenazi Jewish ancestry, chest wall radiation, smoking, excess alcohol.
- Most recent mammogram.
- Past medical history.
- Medication and supplements.

12.2.2 Risk factors for breast cancer

- Previous breast cancer.
- Family history of breast cancer.
- Advancing age.
- Early menarche or late menopause.
- Never having had a child, or first child born after the age of 30.
- Not having breastfed.
- Breast density is an independent risk factor, increasing risk up to 2–4-fold.
- Lifestyle:
  - Physical activity may reduce the risk.
  - Being overweight or having a high alcohol intake can increase the risk.

12.2.3 Breast examination

As with any examination, explain to the patient what you intend to do and why. Obtain consent for the examination and offer a chaperone; document this and the discussion (see *Section 4.6.3*).

- Breast inspection, sitting and with the hands pushed into the hips, and then repeat with the hands above the head.
  - Look for lumps, swelling, bloody discharge, lumps in the axilla, dimpling, skin rash or thickening and nipple inversion/retraction.
- Palpation of the breast
  - This should be thorough and take about 3 minutes each side. There is no best method, but one technique is to examine sitting up and then ask the patient to lie supine, with their

hands above their head and repeat, including turning them on their side to examine all of the breast tissue.
    - Using the flat of the hand, in a circular motion or up and down motion, feel the whole breast including the axilla and up to the clavicle. Include the nipple and ask the patient to squeeze to check for discharge.
    - If a lump is found, note size, consistency and whether it is attached to skin or underlying tissue.
- If the patient feels a lump but you cannot feel it, it is sensible to reassess after 6 weeks and if you still cannot palpate the lump, but the patient is sure they can feel it, refer to breast clinic.
- Document all history and examination findings and document if you have given safety-netting advice, for example, "patient asked to return at 6 weeks if symptoms have not resolved".

12.3 Benign breast conditions

While most palpable breast lumps are not cancerous, distinguishing between benign and potentially malignant features is essential. The decision on how urgently to refer should be guided by a thorough history, physical examination, and an assessment of individual breast cancer risk factors.

Benign breast conditions are often due to age-related or hormonal changes.

When considering the following diagnoses, all unexplained lumps should be referred for assessment in a specialist breast clinic, with those in patients aged ≥30 being sent via the urgent suspected cancer (USC) pathway.

12.3.1 Benign breast swelling and tenderness

Causes include:

- Puberty
    - Breast enlargement, sometimes initially unilateral, is the first obvious sign of puberty in girls.
- Pregnancy
    - Normal changes to breasts during pregnancy and breastfeeding include tenderness, increase in size, areolar and nipple changes, and leaking of colostrum or milk.
    - Problems in breastfeeding can include sore or cracked nipples, thrush or engorgement.
- Cyclical mastalgia
    - Breasts change throughout the menstrual cycle.

12.3.2 Breast cysts

- Most common causes of a breast lump, most often affecting women over 35 years.
- Can be unilateral or bilateral; painful or painless; soft or hard; can be multiple in number and range in size.
- Can develop naturally as the breast changes with age, due to normal changes in hormone levels.
- Less common after menopause, unless HRT is taken.

12.3.3 Fibroadenoma

- Can occur at any age, most common in younger women in their 20s and 30s, often start to develop in puberty.
- Usually feels like a smooth lump in the breast that moves easily under the skin.
- Complex fibroadenomas are associated with a slight increased risk of breast cancer.

12.3.4 Fat necrosis

- Usually caused by trauma or surgery to the fatty tissue of the breast, and it can present as a lump or a bruise on the breast with a lump underlying this.
- The lump is usually painless and the skin around it may look red, bruised or dimpled.
- Once the diagnosis is confirmed, it usually requires no treatment and self-resolves over time.

12.3.5 Benign phyllodes

- Phyllodes tumours are smooth, firm lumps in the breast and are usually benign, but they can be malignant.
- They are most common in women age 40–50 who have not yet been through the menopause.
- They can be difficult to diagnose, as they can look like a fibroadenoma.
- They are treated by surgical removal.

12.3.6 Intraductal papilloma

- A wart-like lump develops in one or more of the milk ducts in the breast, usually close to the nipple, but it can be found anywhere in the breast.
- There may be a lump and/or nipple discharge, which could be clear or blood-stained.
- More common in women over 40 years.
- Often discovered on routine mammogram.
- If there are multiple intraductal papillomas, there may be a slightly higher risk of developing breast cancer.
- These are treated by removal of the lesion.

12.3.7 Atypical hyperplasia

This is a benign hyperplasia (increase in the number of cells) which can occur in the ducts or lobes. Atypical cells are ones which develop an unusual pattern or shape. The cells may not necessarily change further to become cancer cells; they may die off or revert to normal.

- Can sometimes develop as the breast changes with age.
- More common in women over 35 years.
- Diagnosis is usually by chance after a routine mammogram, or from examination of tissue from a biopsy or after breast surgery.
- Can increase the risk of developing breast cancer in the future.

12.3.8 Sclerosing adenosis

A benign condition where there is extra growth of tissue within the breast lobules, that may occur as part of the aging process.

- Mostly asymptomatic but can cause a lump or pain.
- Often only diagnosed during routine mammogram or following tests for a different breast problem.
- Can look like breast cancer on a mammogram.
- Once diagnosed, it does not need follow-up, and it does not have malignant potential.

12.3.9 Duct ectasia

- Ductal ectasia is when the milk ducts behind the nipple shorten and widen with age.
- Clinically this can mimic invasive carcinoma.
- Can cause nipple discharge, non-cyclical breast pain, a lump behind the nipple, with tenderness and nipple inversion.

12.3.10 Periductal mastitis

- The tissue around the ducts becomes inflamed.
- Most common in younger women and smokers.
- Can cause a tender, hot or reddened breast, nipple discharge (which can be blood-stained or pus), nipple inversion, or a lump behind the nipple.

12.3.11 Granulomatous mastitis

- Granulomatous mastitis is a rare inflammatory condition of tender lumps in one or both breasts that can discharge pus.
- The cause is unclear, but it is more common in women with diabetes, who use oral contraceptives, have autoimmune disease, are of South Asian, Chinese or Black heritage (so there may be a genetic component).
- Symptoms can include a tender lump or lumps in the breast, pain, redness and swelling, nipple inversion, skin pitting, inflammation or ulceration, axillary swelling or lumps and abscesses on the breast.
- Treatment involves the use of oral steroids or NSAIDs. It usually resolves spontaneously over a period of 1–2 years.

12.3.12 Infection – mastitis

- Mastitis is inflammation of the breast, and it can be infective or inflammatory. The management of mastitis is divided into that for lactating and non-lactating women.
- Lactating women
    - Most common organism is *Staphylococcus aureus.*
    - Risk of abscess formation and sepsis.
    - Managed with analgesia, warm compress, continue milk flow (breastfeeding or expression), and prescribe antibiotics.
        - Flucloxacillin can be considered first-line.
        - If penicillin allergy, then erythromycin (preferred if pregnant) or clarithromycin 250–500mg every 6 hours or 500mg every 12 hours for 10–14 days.
        - Encourage breastfeeding and advise regular paracetamol.
        - If it does not settle, refer to breast clinic for ultrasound scan and guided aspiration.
- Non-lactating women
    - This non-lactational infection often occurs around the nipple: periductal mastitis. This is usually associated with a tender lump in the nipple area, erythema and nipple discharge. It can be chronic and is associated with smoking. Offer smoking cessation advice.
    - The most common organisms are *Staphylococcus aureus,* enterococci and anaerobic bacteria.
    - Prescribe co-amoxiclav 500/125mg every 8 hours for 10–14 days.
    - If penicillin-allergic consider erythromycin, clarithromycin or metronidazole. Refer to NICE CKS: *Mastitis and breast abscess*.
    - If it does not settle in 2 weeks, refer to breast clinic.
- If there is any evidence of an underlying mass, a failure to respond to treatment or if breast cancer is suspected as part of the mastitis diagnosis, then refer under the USC pathway.

12.3.13 Skin lesions on the breast

- Although skin lesions on the breast can cause some concern, benign lesions such as sebaceous cysts, benign moles and skin tags do not require referral to breast clinic, but consider red flags for skin lesions which require urgent referral to Dermatology.

- At any age refer urgently to the breast clinic skin changes that suggest cancer, such as tethering, fixation, ulceration, peau d'orange, inflammation that does not settle after one course of antibiotics, and non-responsive eczema.

12.3.14 Breast nodularity

- Breast nodularity is common (particularly in the upper, outer quadrants). It is often bilateral and can occur cyclically. The breast can feel lumpy and there should not be a discrete mass.
- It is not necessary to refer breast nodularity to the breast clinic if:
  - it is diffuse (not a discrete lump)
  - it is symmetrical
  - it is associated with tenderness
  - it fluctuates with the menstrual cycle
  - there are no skin, nipple or axillary changes
  - the history and breast exam are otherwise normal.
- You can reassess soon after a next period and, at reassessment, if there is asymmetrical, persistent nodularity, a new discrete lump, or persistent focal change, or there are any features suggestive of breast cancer, refer to the breast clinic.

12.4 Breast cancer

Breast cancer (see also *Section 11.2*) is the most common cancer in females in the UK. Treatment has improved and patients are surviving longer. This has resulted in women living for many years after their cancer diagnosis, managing the treatment and the risk of recurrence.

- 1 in 7 women in the UK will develop breast cancer at some point in their lifetime.
- 9 out of 10 women who develop breast cancer do not have a family history of breast cancer.
- Around 55 000 cases of breast cancer are diagnosed in women and 400 in men in the UK each year.
- A further 7000 people are diagnosed with ductal carcinoma *in situ* (DCIS), which is an early form of breast cancer, in the UK every year.
- In the UK, breast cancer is less common in women from South Asian, Black, Chinese, mixed and other communities, than in white women, but women from these groups face lower survival rates, later diagnosis and different levels of care.
- A clinical examination, imaging and biopsy will detect over 99% of breast cancers. In patients under 40 years, imaging is usually an ultrasound scan rather than a mammogram.
- Risk factors for breast cancer are discussed in *Section 12.2.2*.

12.4.1 Signs and symptoms suggestive of breast cancer

- An unexplained discrete breast or axillary lump, ulceration, skin dimpling, puckering or tethering, and breast distortion.
- Bloody or serous unilateral nipple discharge (particularly single duct nipple discharge).
- Persistent nipple eczema, nipple ulceration, new nipple retraction or distortion.
- Breast infection or inflammation that fails to respond to antibiotics. Consider an inflammatory breast cancer, which is rare, but evolves quickly.
- New asymmetric nodularity (lumpy or knobbly texture of breast tissue, often felt as small bumps or lumps) persisting after menstruation or for 2–3 weeks.
- Non-lactational mastitis in women over 50 years, or mastitis which fails to respond to antibiotics.
- Ask about previous breast cancer.
- Ask about significant family history of breast or ovarian cancer.

12.4.2 Referral

Follow local referral guidelines. NICE CKS: *Referral for breast cancer* states:

- **Refer people using a suspected cancer pathway referral** for breast cancer if they are:
  - Aged ≥30 and have an unexplained breast lump with or without pain, or
  - Aged ≥50 with any of the following symptoms in one nipple only:
    - Discharge.
    - Retraction.
    - Other changes of concern.
- **Consider a suspected cancer pathway referral** for breast cancer in people:
  - With skin changes that suggest breast cancer, or
  - Aged ≥30 with an unexplained lump in the axilla.
- **Consider non-urgent referral** in people aged <30 with an unexplained breast lump with or without pain.
- Refer to https://cks.nice.org.uk/topics/breast-cancer-recognition-referral/management/referral-for-breast-cancer.

12.4.3 Family history of breast cancer

If a woman with no personal history of breast cancer presents with breast symptoms or has concerns about her relatives with breast cancer, take a family history from both sides of the family to assess her risk.

Refer to a secondary care or a specialist genetic clinic, following NICE guidelines CG164: *Familial breast cancer: classification, care and managing breast cancer and related risks in people with a family history of breast cancer.* This guidance summarises which women can be cared for in primary care, which women require referral to secondary care, and which to specialist genetic clinics, depending upon their family history.

At her referral appointment, her risk of breast cancer can be assessed, and she will be given an individualised image surveillance strategy. For some women this will involve more frequent breast monitoring, for others this will include chemoprevention (with tamoxifen or an aromatase inhibitor) or a risk-reducing mastectomy.

In summary, NICE guidance CG164 states:

"People without a personal history of breast cancer can be cared for in primary care if the family history shows only 1 first-degree or second-degree relative diagnosed with breast cancer at older than age 40 years (in most cases, this will equate to less than a 3% 10-year risk of breast cancer at age 40 years), provided that none of the following are present in the family history:

- *bilateral breast cancer*
- *male breast cancer*
- *ovarian cancer*
- *Jewish ancestry*
- *sarcoma in a relative younger than age 45 years*
- *glioma or childhood adrenal cortical carcinomas*
- *complicated patterns of adrenal cancer at a young age*
- *paternal history of breast cancer (2 or more relatives on the father's side of the family)."*

Women who do not meet the criteria for referral can be cared for in primary care and should be given information about risk of family history, as stated in the NICE CG164 guidelines.

Seek advice from secondary care if the criteria above are present in the family history, in addition to breast cancers in relatives, but the patient does not fulfil the referral criteria below, there is uncertainty about whether to refer or not, or the woman is not reassured by the information provided.

12.4.4 Referral from primary care for family history of breast cancer

NICE guidance CG164 advises which women should be referred to secondary care and which women should be referred to a specialist genetic clinic. It is important to refer to the full NICE guidelines as they cannot be covered in detail here. We are able to cover some of the criteria for referral to secondary care, where NICE states:

"People without a personal history of breast cancer who meet the following criteria should be offered referral to secondary care:
- *One first degree female relative diagnosed with breast cancer aged younger than 40, or*
- *One first degree male relative diagnosed with breast cancer at any age, or*
- *One first degree relative with bilateral breast cancer where the first cancer was diagnosed at younger than aged 50 years, or*
- *Two first degree relatives, or one first degree and one second degree relative, diagnosed with breast cancer at any age, or*
- *One first degree or second degree relative diagnosed with breast cancer at any age and one first degree or second degree relative diagnosed with ovarian cancer at any age (one of these should be a first degree relative), or*
- *Three first-degree or second-degree relatives diagnosed with breast cancer at any age"*

Discuss with secondary care if you are not certain about a referral, for example in cases where family history is unusual.

If a high-risk gene mutation such as *BRCA1* or *BRAC2* has been identified in a family member, then the first-degree relatives of that person (for example brothers and sisters) have a 50/50 risk of having the faulty *BRCA* gene and need to be referred to a specialist genetic service to have genetic testing to determine if they have gene mutation; see *Section 12.4.6*.

Provide women with written information and support. This should cover breast cancer risk, breast awareness, the NHS breast screening programme, lifestyle advice regarding breast cancer risk (alcohol, weight, exercise and smoking) and advice on hormonal contraception and HRT, where relevant. Advise them to contact you if their family history changes.

12.4.5 Risk of breast cancer

A family history of breast cancer is a risk factor for developing the disease. The risk increases with the number of relatives affected and the age at diagnosis of the relative (the younger the age of diagnosis, the greater the risk). Risk is also affected by other factors, including weight, drinking alcohol, level of physical activity, age at menopause, parity, hormonal contraception, hormone replacement therapy (HRT) and history of breastfeeding.

- General population risk, or baseline risk:
  - Any woman in the UK has a 1 in 7 chance of developing breast cancer over the course of her lifetime.
  - This equates to around a 14% risk (140 in every 1000 women), but breast specialists consider up to 17% lifetime risk is within normal limits.
  - In the general population, most breast cancers develop after the age of 50.
- Moderate risk:
  - Women who have a moderate risk of breast cancer have a higher risk of getting breast cancer than women at baseline risk who have no family history of the disease.
    - There may be several relatives with breast cancer.
    - Breast cancer could affect people in several generations in the family.
  - A woman may be told she has a moderate risk if one close relative developed breast cancer under the age of 40.
  - Women with moderate risk have a lifetime risk of developing breast cancer of between 17% and 30%.

  - There is a 3–8% chance of developing breast cancer between the ages of 40 and 50.
  - There is a slightly higher chance of developing breast cancer at a younger age than the general population.
- High risk:
  - Women in this risk group are more likely than those at moderate risk to develop breast cancer, but this doesn't mean they will develop breast cancer.
    - Usually, they will have several close relatives (maternal or paternal) diagnosed with breast cancer, ovarian cancer or both, over several generations (such as grandmother, mother, daughter). They will usually have been diagnosed at a younger age, often under 50 years.
  - Women with a high risk have a 30% or greater chance of developing breast cancer in their lifetime.
  - These women have an 8% or greater chance of developing breast cancer between the ages of 40 and 50 and have a much higher chance of developing breast cancer at a younger age than the general population.
  - All women who have a gene mutations *BRCA1, BRCA 2* or *TP53* genes are at high risk.

Women without breast cancer, but at moderate or high risk may be offered regular surveillance scans. The type of surveillance depends upon the age and level of risk. They may also be offered drug treatment (chemoprophylaxis) or risk-reducing surgery.

This information may be helpful for women:
- www.nice.org.uk/guidance/cg164/resources/familial-breast-cancer-breast-cancer-in-the-family-pdf-246406340293
- https://breastcancernow.org/about-breast-cancer/awareness/breast-cancer-in-families

12.4.6 Inherited genetic mutations increasing risk of breast cancer

Most breast cancers happen by chance. Researchers estimate that only around 5–10% of breast cancers are caused by an inherited genetic mutation on their chromosomes. The *BRCA* gene is one example, and everyone has *BRCA1* and *BRCA2* genes. BRCA stands for BReast CAncer gene. These genes stop cells from growing and dividing out of control. A mutation in these genes means that cells can grow out of control. Around 1 in every 450 people have a faulty *BRCA1* or *BRCA2* gene; this rate is significantly higher in some groups (e.g. Ashkenazi Jewish ancestry).

Patient resources:
- The Royal Marsden's A beginner's guide to *BRCA1* and *BRCA2* (https://patientinfolibrary.royalmarsden.nhs.uk/brca1brac2).
- Breast Cancer Now's information on family history of breast cancer (https://breastcancernow.org/about-breast-cancer/awareness/breast-cancer-in-families).
- Maggie's is a charity providing cancer support.
- Future Dreams is a charity providing practical and emotional support for those diagnosed with breast cancer.

12.5 Breast pain

The recommendations from the RM Partners NW & SW London Cancer Alliance (https://rmpartners.nhs.uk/wp-content/uploads/2022/09/RM-Partners-Breast-Referral-Guidance-for-Primary-Care-June-2022.pdf) are that most women will present with breast pain at some stage in life. Breast pain as a sole symptom is normal and does not require referral, investigation or in most instances treatment, unless a breast lump has been identified. Pain will usually settle spontaneously with time and may be recurrent and episodic.

There is no association between breast pain and breast cancer, when no lump is identified, according to the *British Journal of General Practice* (https://bjgp.org/content/72/717/e234). In most cases reassurance is required. Women can be given the following information:

- RM Partners video: *Understanding breast pain* (https://rmpartners.nhs.uk/new-video-to-help-understand-breast-pain).
- Breast Cancer Now article: *Breast pain* (https://breastcancernow.org/about-breast-cancer/breast-lumps-and-benign-not-cancer-breast-conditions/breast-pain).
- CoppaFeel! article: *Breast pain* (https://coppafeel.org/breast-cancer-info-and-advice/understanding-breast-changes/breast-pain).

12.5.1 What to include in the history and examination

- Timing of pain related to the menstrual cycle – ask about recurring pattern.
- Nature of the pain, duration, position and radiation; exacerbating or relieving factors.
- Presence or absence of other breast symptoms such as lump, breast changes, nipple discharge, or axillary symptoms.
- A family history of breast disease can cause stress, and this may lead to the patient to experience breast pain.
- History of hormonal medications and other medications.
- Consider puberty or pregnancy as a cause.
- Ask about symptoms of premenstrual syndrome.
- Assess risk factors for breast cancer.
- Date of last mammogram.
- Perform a breast examination, as described in *Section 12.2.3*.

12.5.2 Types of breast pain

- True breast pain:
  - Cyclical breast pain.
  - Hormonal or medication-related, such as HRT or hormonal contraception.
  - Non-cyclical and non-hormonal breast pain.
- Extra-mammary breast pain, such as referred musculoskeletal.

Cyclical breast pain

- This is common, affecting up to two-thirds of women, with 10% having moderate to severe pain. It resolves spontaneously in 20–30% of women but tends to recur in 60%.
- The pain and tenderness are linked to the menstrual cycle; it is thought to involve hormonal changes affecting the breast tissue.
- Usually starts during the luteal phase, increasing until menstruation begins, and improves after menses.
- Dull, heavy or aching in nature.
- Usually bilateral.
- May be poorly localised, cause a burning pain into the nipple and extend to the axilla.
- May worsen in perimenopause, when HRT or hormonal contraception is used.

Management of cyclical breast pain

- Reassurance to reduce anxiety, that most women can expect to experience an episode of breast pain in their lifetime.
- Wearing a well-fitting supportive bra, and a soft one at night.
- Consider a breast pain diary.
- Change in medication: SSRIs and the oral contraceptive pill can both cause breast pain, so considering alternative options may help. Use of HRT can cause breast pain in some women. Adjustment of HRT, reducing to a lower dose of oestrogen can be helpful, then weaning up slowly, if necessary.
- Analgesia:
  - Consider paracetamol at maximum daily dose, daily, for 2 weeks, stop if no improvement, but continue for a further 2 weeks if improvement.

    - A topical NSAID preparation for 2–3 months. There is evidence that topical diclofenac is effective in relieving breast pain, and this should be considered first.
    - OTC treatment (not prescribed). Natural remedies containing gamma-linolenic acid, such as star oil or evening primrose oil (EPO), can be tried.
        - There is no objective evidence that they are better than placebo, but they work for some women.
        - A standardised capsule of EPO (500mg) contains approximately 40mg of gamma-linolenic acid. A gamma-linolenic acid dose of 120–160mg twice a day may be beneficial for some women.
        - Check there are no contraindications before advising about this; for example, pregnant women should not take EPO.
    - If breast pain is severe enough to affect quality of life and sleep, and does not respond to first-line treatment, refer to local guidelines and consider referral to the breast clinic.

Non-cyclical breast pain

- Not related to the menstrual cycle.
- Constant or intermittent.
- Unilateral and variable positions.
- Causes include mastitis, pregnancy, trauma, previous surgery, fibrocystic disease, malignancy and stretching of Cooper's ligaments.

Extra-mammary breast pain (chest wall pain)

- This is more common than true mastalgia and is the commonest type of breast pain referred to breast clinic.
- Unilateral, can be brought on by activity such as breathing, coughing, heavy lifting.
- Can be reproduced by palpation on a specific area of the chest wall. It is helpful, on examination, to demonstrate this to the patient to reduce anxiety.
- Causes include musculoskeletal conditions such as costochondritis, soft tissue injury, rib or vertebral fracture; fibromyalgia, herpes zoster; referred pain from cardiac or gastrointestinal conditions (such as ischaemic heart disease, peptic ulcer, gallstones or gastro-oesophageal reflux).

Management of non-cyclical and extra-mammary breast pain

- Consider causes of pain referred to the breast, such as costochondritis, infection, axilla, periductal mastitis.
- Can consider paracetamol at maximum daily dose, daily, for 2 weeks, stop if no improvement but continue for a further 2 weeks if improvement. An alternative is an NSAID, such as ibuprofen, topically for 2–3 months.

Referral to secondary care for breast pain

- Co-existing symptoms such as breast lump, bloody nipple discharge, ulceration, skin distortion, recently-acquired nipple retraction/distortion, new asymmetric nodularity persisting after menstruation for 2–3 weeks, previous breast cancer.
- Family history of breast cancer. The psychology of breast pain associated with significant family history of breast cancer leading to anxiety as a reason for breast pain has been explored. Eliciting an accurate family history is important. Those with a moderate or high risk of breast cancer need referral to secondary care family history services, if this has not already been done. They do not require a clinical breast team review prior to this, if the presenting complaint is breast pain, with a normal examination.
- Persistent cyclical breast pain requiring referral is defined by the NICE CKS as being pain for over 3 months. This is because 20–30% will resolve over this time. After 3 months, if true mastalgia is present, treatments such as tamoxifen or danazol can be considered in a secondary care setting, and a referral can be considered.

12.6 Nipple discharge

Nipple discharge is very common. Fluid can be obtained from the nipples of between 50 and 70% of normal women. The discharge of fluid from a normal breast is called physiological discharge. It is not a cause for concern and is usually yellow, milky or green. It does not happen spontaneously and often can be seen coming from more than one duct.

12.6.1 Taking a history

- Take a breast history, as described in *Section 12.2.1.*
- Ask about the discharge. Is it unilateral or bilateral; affecting a single duct or multiple ducts; is it spontaneous or does it only occur if the breast is expressed?
- What is the discharge like? Patients might use words like milky, clear, sticky, coloured, blood-stained (with fresh blood or old blood).
- Ask about red flag symptoms, such as breast implant-associated anaplastic large cell lymphoma, previous breast cancer and significant family history of breast or ovarian cancer.

Signs and symptoms suggestive of breast cancer

- Single duct unilateral blood-stained or watery discharge.
- Unexplained discrete breast or axillary lump, ulceration, skin dimpling, breast distortion.
- Persistent nipple eczema, ulceration, new breast contour change.
- Breast infection or inflammation that fails to respond to antibiotics.
- New asymmetric nodularity persisting after menstruation or for 2–3 weeks.

12.6.2 Differential diagnosis

- Physiological nipple discharge (for example occurs with **pregnancy, lactation, hormonal fluctuation, nipple stimulation and some medications**).
- Galactorrhoea:
  - Refers to the discharge of a milky fluid from the breasts, unrelated to pregnancy or breastfeeding.
  - It is usually bilateral, and the milky discharge arises from multiple ducts. The amount of discharge can vary and may be secreted either spontaneously or expressed.
  - It most commonly results from **hyperprolactinaemia**, due to medications, pituitary pathology or endocrine disorders such as primary hypothyroidism.
- A pathological cause, such as breast cancer.
- Ductal carcinoma *in situ* (DCIS): can cause a clear, sticky discharge.
- Duct ectasia: yellow/green/brown discharge from more than one duct. This is a benign condition due to inflammation of the walls of the ducts. It usually affects postnatal women. The discharge is usually bilateral. In most cases, no treatment is needed, but if the discharge is a problem for the patient, then the ducts behind the nipple can be removed.
- Periductal mastitis is a benign condition, more common in younger women and smokers. Symptoms include breast pain, tenderness, redness, nipple discharge, and sometimes a mass or abscess.
- Fresh blood coming from the nipple can be associated with intraductal papilloma.

12.6.3 Management of nipple discharge

Decide if the discharge has a physiological cause **or if you suspect underlying pathology**.

Suspected pathological cause – refer:

- Single duct, unilateral, blood-stained or watery discharge or other associated symptoms or signs suggestive of malignancy.

Classic physiological features and a normal breast exam with no features suggestive of malignancy – reassure: no referral is needed. Features of physiological discharge include:

- Bilateral discharge; the patient may not be aware it is bilateral, so she can be asked to check by applying firm pressure.
- Multi-duct discharge, she can be asked to check by applying pressure to see if it is coming from more than one duct.
- Bilateral or multi-duct discharge that occurs only with pressure.
- Discharge on areola caused by excoriation and eczema.
- Safety-net and advise to avoid nipple stimulation. Review medications, consider testing prolactin and thyroid function if the discharge is milky and persistent.

Galactorrhoea

- If you suspect galactorrhoea take a history and perform an examination to consider a cause:
  - Causes include: physiological, drugs, thyroid disorder, pituitary tumour.
  - Galactorrhoea is most commonly caused by **hyperprolactinaemia**, but may also occur with **normal prolactin levels**.
  - Prolactin stimulates milk production, so high levels often lead to **bilateral milky discharge**.
  - Symptoms of hyperprolactinaemia include oligo-/amenorrhoea, galactorrhoea (when not pregnant or breastfeeding), vaginal dryness, acne, hirsutism, headaches and visual impairment.
- Check prolactin and thyroid function.
- Exclude pregnancy and lactation (not recommended to routinely measure prolactin).
  - Review physiological causes: the levels of prolactin in normal individuals tend to rise in response to physiological stimuli, including sleep, exercise, pregnancy, breastfeeding and surgical stress.
    - In the absence of breastfeeding, prolactin levels return to normal within 3 weeks of giving birth.
  - Review medications: medications which cause hyperprolactinaemia include high-dose oestrogens (COCP), some antipsychotic drugs, antidepressants including SSRIs, antihypertensives including verapamil, and opiates.
  - Consider pathological causes of hyperprolactinaemia, which include pituitary adenomas (prolactinomas), diseases of the hypothalamus, renal failure, hypothyroidism and ectopic tumours.
  - Prolactin levels >1000mIU/L usually warrant further investigation by the endocrinologist. Refer according to local guidelines for prolactin levels.

12.7 Nipple changes

Nipples vary in shape, size and colour. They can point up or down, be dark or pale and can look different on each breast. Their appearance can be influenced by genetics, age and hormonal changes (for example with pregnancy or use of CHC).

12.7.1 Taking a history

- Take a breast history, as described in *Section 12.2.1*.
- Ask about signs and symptoms suggestive of breast cancer, e.g.:
  - Bloody or serous unilateral nipple discharge.
  - Unexplained discrete breast or axillary lump, ulceration, breast distortion.
  - Peau d'orange, skin dimpling, skin tethering, contour change.
  - Persistent nipple eczema, ulceration, new breast contour change.
  - Breast infection or inflammation that fails to respond to antibiotics.
  - New asymmetric nodularity persisting after menstruation or for 2–3 weeks.
- Ask about red flag symptoms and history of breast implant-associated anaplastic large cell lymphoma, previous breast cancer and significant family history of breast or ovarian cancer.

12.7.2 Nipple inversion

- Nipple inversion is common and is usually nothing to worry about and doesn't need specific treatment.
- The ducts are elastic and due to this, can cause nipples to turn in. The nipple usually looks folded in, with a horizontal crease. It may remain turned in most of the time.
- It is possible to breastfeed with nipple inversion.
- Other reasons include a congenital cause, a carcinoma or mammary duct ectasia with periductal fibrosis.

12.7.3 Nipple retraction

- Different from nipple inversion; this is a persistent, asymmetric and non-slit-like, eccentric and rarely isolated finding. Usually there is a different clinical reason such as a carcinoma.

12.7.4 Nipple eczema

- Eczema starts in the areola first and rarely involves the nipple.
  - This should be treated with emollients and topical steroids. Consider an occlusive dressing to improve contact time.
  - Review at 4–8 weeks and refer to secondary care if not improving or uncertain about diagnosis.

12.7.5 Paget's disease of the breast

- Paget's disease is a cancer within the epidermis.
- It is a scaly, raw, vesicular or ulcerated lesion that begins on the nipple, and it spreads to the areola.
- This is different from eczema which starts on the areola and rarely involves the nipple.
- Pain, burning or pruritus may be present before the rash/lesion.
  - 50% have an underlying lump.
  - 90% have an associated invasive cancer.
  - Requires an urgent referral.

12.7.6 Referral

RM Partners NW & SW London Cancer Alliance advises as follows.

- Refer:
  - New unilateral nipple inversion.
  - Unilateral 'eczema'. Paget's disease changes start on the nipple; they are eccentric and spread from the nipple to the areola.
- Do not refer:
  - Bilateral nipple inversion.
  - Long-standing nipple inversion.
  - Bilateral nipple or areola eczema – if a patient has a history of eczema and the changes are bilateral then a course of emollients plus topical steroid cream can be prescribed, and symptoms reviewed after 2–4 weeks and if symptoms are not settling, refer.

12.8 Breastfeeding

12.8.1 Lactation physiology

- In the second half of pregnancy prolactin triggers the production of colostrum, but levels of oestrogen and progesterone are high enough to prevent significant lactation. Once the placenta has been delivered there is a sudden drop in these hormones, which leaves the high levels of prolactin to trigger lactation. From this point, prolactin and oxytocin are both responsible for maintaining production and release of breast milk.

- Nipple stimulation (by breastfeeding or expression) causes a surge in oxytocin and a milk ejection reflex (known as the let-down reflex). This is followed by milk moving from the alveoli into the lactiferous milk ducts. As the alveoli are emptied, prolactin activates prolactin receptors in the alveoli, to trigger further milk production so that milk synthesis can meet the requirements of the infant.

12.8.2 Breast milk composition

- Human milk consists of many components including water, fatty acids, triglycerides, lactose, proteins, vitamins, calcium, phosphate, B and T lymphocytes, neutrophils, macrophages, stem cells, enzymes, hormones, growth factors and oligosaccharides.
- The composition of a woman's milk changes both over the course of a day, throughout the time she is breastfeeding and as the infant grows older. The milk towards the end of a feed can contain two or three times the concentration of fat than the first milk of a feed. Because of this, it is important to avoid switching the infant to the second breast before they have 'drained' the first breast, as much as possible.

12.8.3 Breastfeeding problems

Every woman with breastfeeding problems should see a health professional with appropriate training and expertise, to observe breastfeeding and milk expression and offer advice.

Offer support from local or national breastfeeding support groups, e.g.:

- The National Breastfeeding Helpline offers support 24 hours a day, every day. Telephone 0300 100 0212 and www.nationalbreastfeedinghelpline.org.uk
- The Breastfeeding Network: www.breastfeedingnetwork.org.uk
- The Association of Breastfeeding Mothers: https://abm.me.uk
- La Leche League GB: https://laleche.org.uk

Ask about excessive crying and how the parents are coping. Give patient information:

- www.cry-sis.org.uk
- https://iconcope.org

For information about how to assess a woman with breastfeeding problems and manage problems such as engorgement, compressed ducts, a galactocele, ductal infection, mastitis or breast abscess, nipple damage, nipple infection, skin conditions and problems with milk supply refer to:

- www.nhs.uk/baby/breastfeeding-and-bottle-feeding/breastfeeding-problems/common-problems
- https://cks.nice.org.uk/topics/breastfeeding-problems/diagnosis/assessment
- The GP Infant Feeding Network (UK): https://gpifn.org.uk

If problems do not improve with treatment, seek advice from a breast specialist.

- The Drugs and Lactation Database (www.ncbi.nlm.nih.gov/books/NBK501922) contains information on drugs and chemicals to which nursing mothers may be exposed. It includes information on the levels of such substances in breast milk and infant blood, and the possible adverse effects in the breastfeeding infant.

12.9 Breast imaging

12.9.1 Mammogram

This is an X-ray of the breasts, where the breast is placed on an X-ray machine and pressed down firmly on the surface by a plate. At least two pictures of each breast are taken, one from top to bottom and one from side to side to include the armpit.

Breast screening uses mammography radiography to detect changes in the breast before the symptoms or signs of breast cancer have developed. Mammography sensitivity is 78–92% and specificity is 75–94%. Mammography is limited in patients with dense breasts, where sensitivity is reduced to 48%.

Having a mammogram may be uncomfortable, but it only takes a few seconds, and the compression does not harm the breast or any breast implants. The amount of radiation is also minimal.

Mammograms are not usually performed in women under the age of 40, unless there is a very strong family history of cancer, as discussed in *Section 12.4.4.*

The NHS Breast Screening Programme automatically invites all women registered with a GP in the UK every 3 years, between the age of 50 and their 71st birthday. Women should receive an invitation within 3 years of their 50th birthday.

Women older than 70 years will not be sent invitations for routine screening, but they can continue to receive breast screening by self-referral to a local breast screening service.

Women at increased risk of breast cancer (such as those who have a strong family history of breast cancer) may be eligible for breast screening before the age of 50.

Support should be given to women to help them make an informed decision about participation in the breast screening programme. This should include information on the benefits of screening (including early detection of breast cancer) and the harms of breast screening (including exposure to radiation, possibility of over-diagnosis, a false positive result, false reassurance if cancer is missed, discomfort and anxiety).

There is a small risk of radiation-induced cancer for a woman who has full-field digital mammographic screening (2 views) of between 1 in 49 000 and 1 in 98 000 per visit. It is estimated that 400–800 cancers are detected for every cancer induced.

12.9.2 Ultrasound

A breast ultrasound scan uses high-frequency sound waves to produce a picture of the inside of the breast. It may show changes which are not palpable on examination. Breast ultrasound is not a replacement for a mammogram.

12.9.3 Magnetic resonance imaging

MRI scans use magnetism and radio waves to produce an image of the breast and do not expose the breast to radiation. MRI may be used in women with dense breasts to get a better picture, or in women who have a high-risk family history of cancer or who have a genetic abnormality, such as a *BRCA* gene mutation.

12.9.4 Clinician resources

- Breast webinar 2022: https://vimeo.com/royalcornwallnhs/review/694813802/b7ead7e027
- RM Partners NW & SW London Cancer Alliance: https://rmpartners.nhs.uk/wp-content/uploads/2022/09/RM-Partners-Breast-Referral-Guidance-for-Primary-Care-June-2022.pdf

12.10 Further reading

BMJ Best Practice (updated 2024) *Mastitis and breast abscess – symptoms, diagnosis and treatment.* Available at: https://bestpractice.bmj.com/topics/en-gb/1084

Breast Cancer Now website: https://breastcancernow.org

Breastcancer.org (undated). *Dense breasts*. Available at: www.breastcancer.org/risk/risk-factors/dense-breasts

Cancer Research UK (2023) *Risk factors for breast cancer.* Available at: www.cancerresearchuk.org/about-cancer/breast-cancer/risks-causes/risk-factors

Dave, R.V., Bromley, H., Taxiarchi, V.P. *et al.* (2021). No association between breast pain and breast cancer: a prospective cohort study of 10 830 symptomatic women presenting to a breast cancer diagnostic clinic. *BJGP*, **72(717):** e234–43.

Health in Menopause (undated). *Common benign breast conditions*. Available at: https://healthinmenopause.co.uk/breast-conditions-non-cancerous

Hubbard, T.J., Sharma, A. and Ferguson, D.J. (2020) Breast pain: assessment, management, and referral criteria. *BJGP*, **70(697):** 419–20.

King, P. (2022) Breast webinar. Available at: https://vimeo.com/royalcornwallnhs/review/694813802/b7ead7e027

Macdonald, C. (2019) *Anatomy and physiology*. The GP Infant Feeding Network (UK). Available at: https://gpifn.org.uk/anatomy-and-physiology

Macmillan Cancer Support (undated) *The breasts*. Available at: www.macmillan.org.uk/cancer-information-and-support/breast-cancer/the-breasts

National Cancer Institute (updated 2024) *Dense breasts: answers to commonly asked questions.* Available at: www.cancer.gov/types/breast/breast-changes/dense-breasts

NHS Cornwall and Isles of Scilly (2024) *Breast lumps and suspected breast cancer (female).* Available at: https://rms.cornwall.nhs.uk/primary_care_clinical_referral_criteria/primary_care_clinical_referral_criteria/breast_guidelines/breast_lumps_female

NHS Inform (undated) *Nipple inversion (inside out nipple).* Available at: www.nhsinform.scot/illnesses-and-conditions/breast-symptoms/nipple-inversion-inside-out-nipple

NHS Royal United Hospitals Bath NHS Foundation Trust (2025) *Hyperprolactinaemia – a guide for GPs*. Available at: www.ruh.nhs.uk/pathology/documents/clinical_guidelines/PATH_026_Hyperprolactinaemia_A_Guide_for_GPs.pdf

NHS South Tees Hospitals NHS Foundation Trust (undated) *Prolactin*. Available at: www.southtees.nhs.uk/services/pathology/tests/prolactin

NICE (revised 2025) CKS: *Breast cancer – recognition and referral.* Available at: https://cks.nice.org.uk/topics/breast-cancer-recognition-referral

NICE (updated 2023) *Familial breast cancer: classification, care and managing breast cancer and related risks in people with a family history of breast cancer* [CG164]. Available at: www.nice.org.uk/guidance/cg164/ifp/chapter/How-breast-cancer-risk-is-described

NICE (updated 2023) Recommendations of CG164. Available at: www.nice.org.uk/guidance/cg164/chapter/Recommendations#clinical-significance-of-a-family-history-of-breast-cancer

Panay, N. *NAPS guidelines on premenstrual syndrome.* National Association for Premenstrual Syndrome. Available at: www.pms.org.uk/app/uploads/2018/06/guidelinesfinal60210.pdf

Patient.info (updated 2022) *Benign breast disease.* Available at: https://patient.info/doctor/Benign-Breast-Disease

Public Health England (2017) *Radiation risk with digital mammography in breast screening.* Available at: www.gov.uk/government/publications/breast-screening-radiation-risk-with-digital-mammography/radiation-risk-with-digital-mammography-in-breast-screening

RM Partners West London Cancer Alliance (2022) *Breast referral guidance for primary care.* Available at: https://rmpartners.nhs.uk/wp-content/uploads/2022/09/RM-Partners-Breast-Referral-Guidance-for-Primary-Care-June-2022.pdf

Visintin, C. (2025) *UK NSC is reviewing the latest evidence for additional screening based on breast density.* UK National Screening Committee. Available at: https://nationalscreening.blog.gov.uk/2025/05/28/uk-nsc-is-reviewing-the-latest-evidence-for-additional-screening-based-on-breast-density

Chapter 13
Legal and safeguarding

13.1 Consent

13.1.1 What is consent?

- Consent is an ethical and legal term referring to the permission given by a patient before they receive any type of medical treatment. This process is often referred to as 'informed consent' and is a cornerstone of good medical practice.
- Consent is also referred to in the context of sexual activity.

13.1.2 What is required for consent to be given?

- In order to give consent, a person needs to understand exactly what they are consenting to. The exchange of information between medical professionals and patients is therefore essential to good decision-making.
- Serious harm may result when patients are not listened to or if they do not receive the information they need, ***in a way they can understand***. Some patients will need considerable effort made to ensure they can comprehend issues well enough to make informed decisions about their care.
- The GMC has issued guidance on decision-making and consent for UK doctors. It sets out seven principles of decision-making and consent which form the basis of good, ethical and safe medical care. It underlines the basic principle that all patients have the right to be involved in decisions about their care and be supported to make informed decisions if they are able, with decision-making seen as an ongoing process focused on meaningful dialogue and the exchange of relevant information specific to the individual patient.
- Medical professionals must start from the presumption that all adult patients have capacity to make decisions about their treatment and care. A patient can only be judged to lack capacity to make a specific decision at a specific time and only after assessment in line with legal requirements (see the Mental Capacity Act 2005).
- The consent process is proportionate to the decision and circumstance, allowing verbal or non-verbal consent for less complex issues, or in life-threatening emergencies where swift action is required to save life.
- Good-quality, timely documentation is vital.
- NICE has issued specific guidance to support the process of 'shared decision-making' which highlights the need to place the patient's values at the centre of decision-making and to respect their right to autonomy (www.nice.org.uk/about/what-we-do/our-programmes/nice-guidance/nice-guidelines/shared-decision-making).

13.1.3 Young people and consent

- There are specific issues to consider around consent and young people. The legal age for consent is 16, but the law allows younger patients to take decisions around their treatment where they are deemed to have capacity to understand the impacts and consequences of such decisions.
- One well-known example of this is the concept of 'Gillick competence'. If a young person is deemed to have 'Gillick competence' they have:
  - sufficient maturity and mental capacity to consider the issue in question – including the advantages and disadvantages and long-term impacts, and the risks, implications and consequences of their choices
  - adequate understanding of the information they have been given, i.e. that they can understand, retain, use and weigh all the relevant information
  - an understanding of the alternative options, including doing nothing
  - an ability to explain their reasoning around the decision.

- Young people often find it more difficult to access services or defend their rights. Although the GMC guidance on decision-making in young people advises us to take into account the wishes of those caring for them, it is clear that we should make the wellbeing of the child or young person our first concern. We need to remain alert for any safeguarding concerns.
- Supporting young people in decision-making may require us to balance a number of legal and ethical issues such as confidentiality, autonomy, consent and duty of care. If you do not believe a young person is 'Gillick competent' then you should seek consent from their parents before proceeding. Documentation is particularly important in these situations. When decision-making or consent feels challenging in this group, seek the advice of your local named safeguarding lead or your medical defence union.

13.1.4 Learning disability, consent and women's health

- Individuals with learning disabilities and difficulties have diverse needs which may be specific to each decision being made regarding their care.
- Principles of informed consent and shared decision-making, as outlined above and in the GMC, Mental Capacity Act and NICE guidance, underline our duty to do all we can to ensure we support an individual to be involved in as many decisions as possible about their care.
- This may require us to provide support, alternative resources and additional time to explain the information needed to make a decision, and the alternative options available – including doing nothing.
- **Communication difficulties may mean a patient is unable to express an issue and it is easier for us to miss things.** Not providing adequate support or time creates discrimination and contributes to the poorer health outcomes of this group compared to the rest of the population.

Contraception

- A systematic review of contraceptive knowledge and use among women with intellectual, physical or sensory disabilities found that these women use a narrower mix of contraceptive options and have less knowledge about their choices than women without disabilities.
- Evidence suggests women with learning difficulties are not given sufficient information and are not fully involved in decisions about contraception.
- Public Health England reports that the most widely used forms of contraception in this group are the implant (46%), the combined pill (24%) and the progestogen-only pill (7%). In the wider population the combined pill makes up 47% of use.
- Contraception was prescribed at an earlier age (38% prior to 16 years) for those with severe and profound learning disabilities. Management of menstruation is cited as the most common reason for starting contraception.
- A person with a learning disability or cognitive impairment may be competent to make an informed choice regarding method of contraception and may be able to use any method reliably. An assessment of competence should be made. The following resources may help support choice-making:
    - The Family Planning Association has a useful guide on contraception for people with learning disabilities (www.fpa.org.uk/product/contraception-a-guide-for-people-with-learning-disabilities).
    - The Picture of Health website has a selection of easy-read guides and resources, including information on contraception and abortion, how to put on a condom, and STIs (www.apictureofhealth.southwest.nhs.uk/sexual-health).
    - Mencap has information on relationships and sex and learning disability (www.mencap.org.uk/advice-and-support/relationships-and-sex).

  - The Choice Support website has a useful leaflet on love, sex and relationships (www.choicesupport.org.uk/uploads/documents/Love-Sex-and-Relationships-BOC-Easy-Read-Policy-and-Guidelines-Feb-2017.pdf).
- Many sexual and reproductive health services will have a specific clinical service to support the needs of people with learning disabilities – consider referring into this service if you have one locally.
- If sterilisation or abortion are being considered as possible options for a person who is considered to lack capacity, and the person has no one else to support or represent them, an Independent Mental Capacity Advocate must be appointed.

13.2 Understanding our safeguarding responsibilities

- Safeguarding is concerned with protecting people's health, wellbeing and human rights.
- Healthcare professionals must follow the principles in *Working Together to Safeguard Children* (2018) and the Care Act (2014) to safeguard children and vulnerable adults (e.g. the disabled, elderly and those with mental health conditions).
- We need to consider the possibility of sexual violence and exploitation, neglect, abuse, coercion, control, financial, technological, emotional and online abuse in our more vulnerable patients.
- Where concerns arise, they must be reported to the appropriate safeguarding team (child, adult or the police if there is immediate risk of harm).
- Multi-agency working is vital in safeguarding to build an adequate picture of a situation and to share any concerns. This may involve seeking more information from other professionals involved in the care of your patient, e.g. health visitors, nurses, social workers, carers and teachers.
- Documentation is important. Record concerns clearly, factually and promptly in the patient's records. Review and follow up where necessary.
- The RCGP, RCN and PCPCH worked collaboratively to create safeguarding standards for general practice and a toolkit and eLearning modules to support training (www.rcgp.org.uk/learning-resources/safeguarding-standards).

13.2.1 Specific safeguarding concerns: female genital mutilation

- FGM, also known as 'cutting', refers to procedures which result in partial or total removal of the external female genitalia, or other injuries to the female genital organs for non-medical reasons.
- It is estimated that worldwide, over 125 million girls and women have undergone FGM. It is thought that 137 000 women and girls in England and Wales have undergone FGM, including 10 000 girls under the age of 15.
- FGM is practised for a number of complex reasons, usually due to a wrongly-held cultural belief that it is beneficial for the girl.
- FGM is considered a human rights violation and a form of child abuse that breaches the United Nations Convention on the Rights of the Child. It is seen as a severe form of violence against women and girls.

Types of FGM

- Type 1: partial or total removal of the clitoris and/or the prepuce (clitoridectomy).
- Type 2: partial or total removal of the clitoris and the labia minora, with or without excision of the labia majora (excision).
- Type 3: narrowing of the vaginal orifice with creation of a covering seal by cutting and appositioning the labia minora and/or the labia majora, with or without excision of the clitoris (infibulation).
- Type 4: all other harmful procedures to the female genitals for non-medical purposes, e.g. pricking, piercing, incising, scraping and cauterisation.

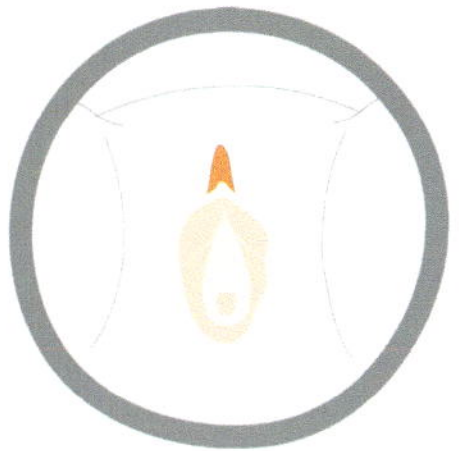
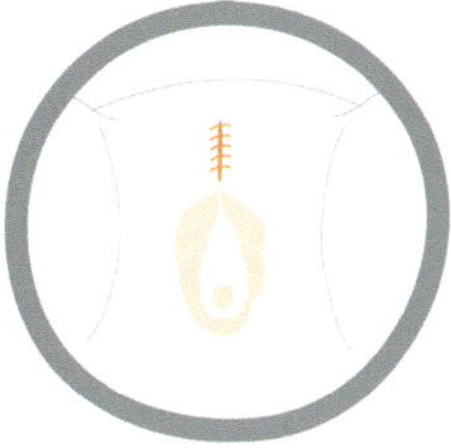

Type 1: Clitoridectomy

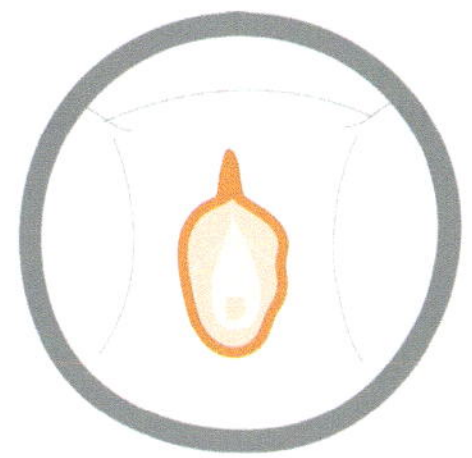
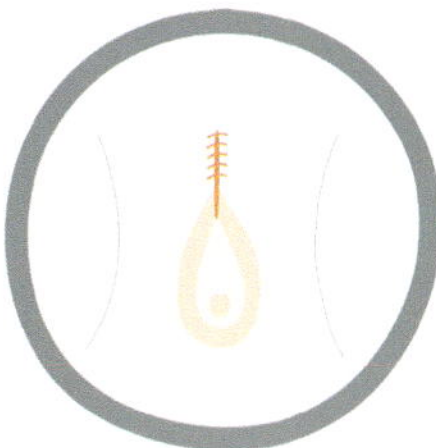

Type 2: Excision

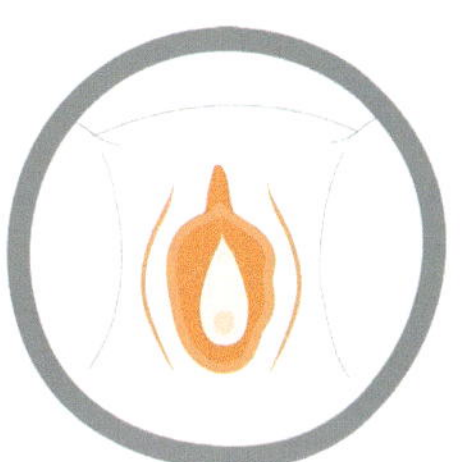
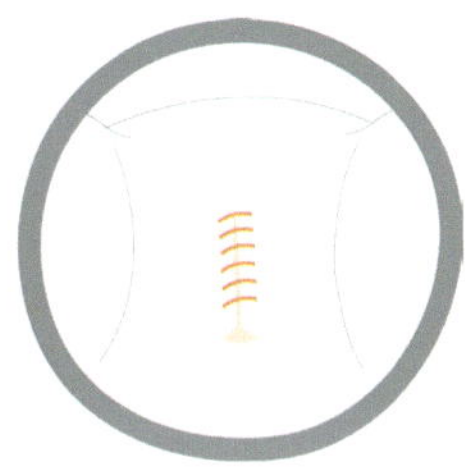

Type 3: Infibulation

Figure 13.1: Types of FGM. Image reproduced from Savera UK, www.saverauk.co.uk.

Legal obligations regarding FGM

- All health professionals must be aware of the Female Genital Mutilation Act 2003 in England, Wales and Northern Ireland and the Prohibition of Female Genital Mutilation (Scotland) Act 2005. The Acts state that:
  - FGM is illegal unless:
    - a surgical operation on a woman or girl irrespective of age is necessary for physical or mental health.
    - she is in any stage of labour, or has just given birth, for purposes connected with the labour or birth.
  - It is illegal to arrange or assist in arranging for a UK national or UK resident to be taken overseas for the purposes of FGM.
  - It is an offence for those with parental responsibility to fail to protect a girl from the risk of FGM.
  - **If FGM is confirmed on a girl aged under 18, reporting to the police within 1 month is mandatory.**
- All female genital cosmetic surgery (e.g. labiaplasty) is prohibited unless it is deemed necessary for the patient's physical or mental health. This requires anyone performing such surgery to ensure they comply with the law.

13.3 Sexual assault

- Sexual assault is common, with 1 in 4 women having been raped or sexually assaulted as an adult.
- The term covers offences ranging from indecent exposure to rape.
- The WHO defines sexual violence as:
  "any sexual act, attempt to obtain a sexual act, or other act directed against a person's sexuality using coercion, by any person regardless of their relationship to the victim, in any setting. It includes rape, defined as the physically forced or otherwise coerced penetration of the vulva or anus with a penis, other body part or object."

- Disclosure of assault remains low, and the Crime Survey in England and Wales (2018) suggests only 17% of women who have been assaulted will report it to the police.
- Sexual assault can present to healthcare professionals in a number of ways. Some women may never disclose to us, and we need to be alert to when we may need to ask sensitively about it.
- Disclosure of an assault must be met with a supportive and non-judgemental approach. **Being believed is crucial to an individual's recovery**.

13.3.1 Responding to a disclosure of a recent sexual assault

- **Women who present after sexual assault should be fast-tracked to appropriate healthcare professionals with minimal delays. Document the initial history (time and nature of the incident, the record of what happened where and with whom).**
- **Treat any injuries with basic first aid but avoid cleaning injuries where possible, to protect DNA evidence. Document the injuries, using a body diagram if possible.**
- **The immediate needs of the woman regarding safety are paramount: consider notifying the police if she consents. If consent is not given, you should only report if you believe there is serious risk to other individuals (including domestic violence or the safety of children).**
- Many areas have Sexual Assault Referral Centres (SARCs). Access to these can be variable, so it is important to familiarise yourself with local policies and services.
- SARCs and emergency departments will have early evidence kits containing swabs, a urine collection pot, mouth swabs and mouth rinse. **It is important that the woman is advised not to eat, drink or pass urine prior to early evidence being collected, should she wish to capture vital evidence.**
- Vaginal rape carries a 5% risk of pregnancy. Consideration should be given to pregnancy protection, i.e. emergency contraception, including a copper IUD.
- Women should be offered post-exposure prophylaxis for HIV, hepatitis B screening and vaccination, and follow-up screening for STIs.

13.3.2 Supporting women after sexual assault

- Sexual assault can have lasting consequences for women, including the impact of post-traumatic stress disorder, drug and substance misuse, self-harm and suicide. In one study, 20% of sexual assault survivors reported mental health problems.
- As clinicians, we need to ensure we provide trauma-informed, sensitive care to all our patients (see *Section 4.6* for more details).

13.3.3 Helpful resources

- Women can be signposted to the following organisations:
  - Rape Crisis England and Wales: www.rapecrisis.org.uk
  - Refuge: www.refuge.org.uk
  - SafeLives: www.safelives.org.uk
  - The Survivors Trust: http://thesurvivorstrust.org
  - Women's Aid: www.womensaid.org.uk
  - List of SARCs in the UK: http://thesurvivorstrust.org/sarc

13.4 Domestic violence

- The WHO considers violence against women an urgent public health priority.
- The Domestic Abuse Act 2021 states that domestic abuse consists of any of the following :
  - Physical abuse.
  - Sexual abuse.

- Violent or threatening behaviour.
- Coercive or controlling behaviour.
- Economic abuse.
- Psychological, emotional and other abuse.

- 1 in 4 women experience domestic abuse during their lifetime. A domestic abuse call is made to the police every 30 seconds, despite it being estimated that less than 24% of domestic abuse crime is reported.
- The risk posed to women is serious. The Femicide Census (www.femicidecensus.org) showed an average of one woman dying at the hands of a man in the UK every 2.7 days in 2021. Risk of serious assault or death is highest for a woman after she leaves an abusive relationship: 38% of women killed by their ex-partner between 2009 and 2018 were killed within the first month of separation and 89% in the first year.
- Healthcare professionals are often in a unique position to identify abuse and support victims in their next steps towards getting to safety. The average woman waits 3 years before getting help and will see their GP 4.3 times during this period.
- Routine screening improves levels of victim identification in primary healthcare settings. The Pathfinder Toolkit created by SafeLives recommends that GPs make targeted inquiries, with a low threshold for asking questions (https://safelives.org.uk/resources-library/health-pathfinder-toolkit-and-practice-briefings/).

13.4.1 Who is most at risk?

- Domestic abuse often starts or escalates in pregnancy. 1 in 3 pregnant women experience domestic violence.
- Risk is also increased in:
  - those of non-heterosexual orientation and trans-gender identity
  - those with long-term illness, disability or mental health issues
  - those who are socioeconomically disadvantaged
  - women aged 16–24.
- 41% of UK girls aged 14–17 in an intimate relationship experienced some form of violence from their partner.
- Women are now able to check with the police under the Domestic Violence Disclosure Scheme ('Clare's Law') if they have concerns that a new, former or existing partner has a history of abuse.

13.4.2 What can we do if a woman discloses that she is experiencing abuse?

- Health professionals may be the first people to whom a woman ever discloses her abuse. It is vital that we respond appropriately, asking the woman what she would like to happen and informing them of sources of support (see *Section 13.4.4*).
- We also need to make a rapid assessment of the level of risk to the woman and any other individuals involved or living in the household, and consider the need for a safeguarding referral.
- The risk of immediate harm is increased when there is:
  - escalating violence
  - substance misuse
  - mental health problems in perpetrator or victim
  - a history of stalking
  - credible threats to kill
  - assault or threatening with a weapon
  - controlling or excessively jealous behaviour
  - assault during pregnancy
  - strangulation
  - 'honour'-based violence.

- There is more information on how to assess risk and what action to take contained in the RCGP Safeguarding Toolkit (https://elearning.rcgp.org.uk/mod/book/view.php?id=15290&chapterid=901).
- Take care when documenting in the notes to follow local safeguarding protocol, e.g. whether to add information to an alleged perpetrator's notes, and alerts to any children who may be in the home. All relevant safeguarding information must be hidden from patient online access. There is a need for detailed and accurate documentation but also several potential pitfalls which require careful thought – the RCGP has excellent guidance on this (https://elearning.rcgp.org.uk/pluginfile.php/205139/mod_book/chapter/901/RCGP%20guidance%20on%20recording%20of%20domestic%20violence_updated%20Jan%202021.pdf).
- Bear in mind that it takes, on average, seven attempts before a woman is able to leave an abusive partner for good – leaving is a process rather than a single act. It is therefore important to build up a trusting and supportive relationship with a woman disclosing abuse, whilst also continuing to make an ongoing assessment regarding the risk they may face, and the risk to any children, young people or vulnerable adults.
- Although adults with capacity are allowed to make unwise decisions, we need to also be alert to how coercion and control may affect a woman's decision-making in domestic violence situations.
- Making the decision to involve the safeguarding team can feel complicated. You may wish to seek advice from your defence union before breaking a patient's confidentiality if they do not consent to the referral being made, and you feel uncertain of the balance of your ethical and safeguarding responsibilities.

13.4.3 Multi-agency risk assessment conferences (MARACs)

- When someone reports experiencing domestic abuse, it is essential to quickly assess the danger they are in. Many agencies use the SafeLives DASH checklist (Domestic Abuse, Stalking, 'Honour'-based violence) to quickly identify who needs the most urgent help, i.e. referral to safeguarding, assignment of an independent domestic violence advisor (IDVA) and referral to MARAC if necessary.
- A MARAC is an information-sharing meeting attended by police, healthcare, child protection, housing practitioners, IDVAs, and other specialists from the statutory and voluntary sectors.
- The primary focus of a MARAC is to share information and create a risk management plan to protect the individuals concerned. The person alleged of the domestic abuse should not be informed of the meeting or the referral to MARAC.

13.4.4 Helpful resources

- The 24-hour freephone National Domestic Abuse Helpline, run by Refuge: call 0808 2000 247 for free confidential advice.
- Refuge: find out more about the services available (https://refuge.org.uk) for women and children.
- Women's Aid: find local support near you (www.womensaid.org.uk/womens-aid-directory).
- Galop: for LGBT+ (https://galop.org.uk).
- Karma Nirvana – support for 'honour'-based abuse: 0800 5999 247 (karmanirvana.org.uk).
- National Stalking Helpline: 0808 802 0300 (www.suzylamplugh.org).
- Revenge Porn Helpline: 0345 6000 459 (revengepornhelpline.org.uk).
- Rights of Women: 020 7251 6575 (rightsofwomen.org.uk).
- Advocate: weareadvocate.org.uk.
- Bright Sky is a mobile app and website (https://uk.bright-sky.org/en) for anyone experiencing domestic abuse.

- Safe Spaces are safe, confidential rooms where victims can take time to reflect, access information on specialist support services or call friends or family. A list of Safe Spaces can be found here: https://uksaysnomore.org/safespaces.

13.5 Non-fatal strangulation

Strangulation is the obstruction of blood vessels and/or the airway by external pressure to the neck. It results in decreased oxygen supply to the brain.

- Section 70 of the Domestic Abuse Act 2021 introduced non-fatal strangulation (NFS) and non-fatal suffocation. Strangulation does not require a particular level of pressure, force or evidence of injury. Applying any form of pressure to the neck (whether gently or with some force) is a serious offence.
- Strangulation is common in interpersonal violence. In domestic abuse, up to 44% of victims report having been strangled. 1 in 11 rape victims report having been strangled during the attack, rising to 1 in 5 when the alleged rapist was a partner or ex-partner.
- NFS is dangerous from both an immediate health perspective and as a red flag for future lethality. Homicide reviews show victims of NFS are 7 times more likely to be killed at a later date. Safeguarding intervention is therefore crucial at presentation. As well as assessing and referring the patient, it is important to consider the safety and welfare of any children under 18 years who are linked to the patient or perpetrator. A MARAC referral is required regardless of DASH (domestic abuse, stalking, harassment and 'honour'-based violence) score.
- If a victim doesn't have children, has capacity (consider confusion and fear) and has declined police or social care involvement, it is important to take time to support and encourage police reporting, with explanation of the future risks.
- Patients presenting with NFS may describe confusion, sore neck, breathing and swallowing difficulties, voice changes, headache or vomiting. Loss of consciousness or continence is common.
- Do not be reassured by the lack of physical signs – 50% will have no visible external injury. Victims are at risk of acute neck and brain injuries. Gold standard imaging is a CT angiogram of the head and neck, with 1 in 47 scans of strangulation patients showing evidence of cerebrovascular injury.
- NFS is extremely traumatic. Many patients report feeling that they were about to die. Offer referral for psychological support and practise trauma-informed care.
- It is important to document carefully, using body maps where possible.
- There is an excellent patient leaflet available at www.ifas.org.uk.

13.6 Further reading

GMC (undated) *0–18 years: about the guidance*. Available at: www.gmc-uk.org/professional-standards/the-professional-standards/0-18-years/about--the-guidance

GMC (undated) *Learning disabilities*. Available at: https://www.gmc-uk.org/professional-standards/ethical-hub/learning-disabilities#Learning-disabilities

GMC (updated 2024) *Decision making and consent*. Available at: www.gmc-uk.org/professional-standards/the-professional-standards/decision-making-and-consent

Horner-Johnson, W., Moe, E.L., Stoner, R.C. *et al.* (2019) Contraceptive knowledge and use among women with intellectual, physical, or sensory disabilities: A systematic review. *Disabil Health J*, **12(2):** 139–54.

Mental Capacity Act 2005. Available at: www.legislation.gov.uk/ukpga/2005/9/contents

Maternal Mental Health Alliance (undated) *Maternal mental health and domestic abuse*. Available at: https://maternalmentalhealthalliance.org/campaign/inequalities/domestic-abuse

NICE (revised 2023) CKS: *Domestic abuse – what are the risk factors?* Available at: https://cks.nice.org.uk/topics/domestic-abuse/background-information/risk-factors

NICE (undated) *About shared decision making*. Available at: www.nice.org.uk/about/what-we-do/our-programmes/nice-guidance/nice-guidelines/shared-decision-making

NSPCC (updated 2022) *Gillick competency and Fraser guidelines*. Available at: https://learning.nspcc.org.uk/child-protection-system/gillick-competence-fraser-guidelines#article-top

ONS (2022) *Domestic abuse in England and Wales overview: November 2022*. Available at: www.ons.gov.uk/peoplepopulationandcommunity/crimeandjustice/bulletins/domesticabuseinenglandandwalesoverview/november2022

RCOG (2015) Green-top Guideline no. 53: *Female genital mutilation and its management*. Available at: www.rcog.org.uk/media/au0jn5of/gtg-53-fgm.pdf

Refuge (undated) *Domestic abuse – facts and statistics*. Available at: https://refuge.org.uk/what-is-domestic-abuse/the-facts

SafeLives (undated) *Health Pathfinder*. Available at: https://safelives.org.uk/research-policy/health/pathfinder

WHO (2024) *Violence against women*. Available at: www.who.int/mediacentre/factsheets/fs239/en/

Index